Making Sense of Research Second Edition

Martha Brown Menard, PhD, CMT

Foreword by Aviad Haramati, PhD

Making Sense of Research, Second Edition
Martha Brown Menard, PhD, CMT
© Copyright 2009

To order copies, please contact:
Curties-Overzet Publications Inc.
330 Dupont Street, Suite 400
Toronto, Ontario
Canada M5R 1V9
Toll Free Phone: 1-888-649-5411
Fax: 416-923-8116
Website: www.curties-overzet.com
E-mail: info@curties-overzet.com

ISBN 978-0-9685256-6-1

Acknowledgements

No one writes a book alone. Many people have contributed to the writing of both editions. Thanks again to publisher and colleague Debra Curties, who initially approached me about turning a continuing education workshop into book form. Debra has always been a terrific editor to work with; I appreciate her attention to detail and patience with the process, and me.

To my teachers over the years who have made science exciting: Paul Lyle (chemistry); Carolyn Bruner (biology); Ron MacVittie (math); John Walsh, who taught me anatomy and physiology; Sue Colletta and Ray Bratton (chemistry); and especially Barry Hinton (gross anatomy) and Bruce Gansneder (research methods). Thanks to Don Ball for demystifying statistics and suggesting that I consider a degree in educational research. A special thanks to Peyton Taylor, MD, and Doug DeGood, PhD, who facilitated my dissertation research at UVA, and to Justine Owens, PhD, and Catherine Kane, PhD, RN, FAAN, who have been mentors to me.

To my all my clients, who over the years have been my greatest teachers, and who were forbearing when I needed to take time away from my practice to write. To all my dear friends, who were so supportive of me during this process, especially Charlotte and David Hisey, Cathy Ayers, Brooke, John, and Evan Boyer, Roger Tolle, and Michael Crear. Hakima Amri, PhD, has been both a scientific colleague and a friend, and I deeply appreciate her support.

To the all the people who read and contributed suggestions to the manuscript, thanks for your tremendous help in improving and polishing the text: Cathy Ayers, Peter Becker, Allan Best, PhD, Stephen Cormier, Trish Dryden, Richard Hammerschlag, PhD, Glenn Hymel, EdD, Jean Ives, Janet Kahn, PhD, Brian Menard, Robert Rodbourne, Beth Rosenthal, MPH, PhD, Jan Schwartz, and Roger Tolle. Thanks again to Bev Ransom for her wonderful artistic talents. A special thanks to Allan Best, PhD, and Adi Haramati, PhD, for writing the respective forewords to the first and second editions. The contributions of Paul Finch, PhD, to the chapters on statistics and case reports were significant and deserve particular mention. The many thoughtful suggestions of Marja Verhoef, PhD, also deserve a special thank you.

Thanks again to the authors and publishers who graciously gave permission to reprint their articles as study examples, and to the New Yorker Cartoon Bank. The quotes at the beginning of each chapter are from the British biologist and physiologist Sir Peter Medawar's book *Advice to a Young Scientist*, still one of my favorite books about the practice of science.

Last but far from least, to my husband, Nate, words cannot express my love and gratitude for your infinite caring and support, sense of humor, and manly domestic skills. Namaste.

Table of Contents

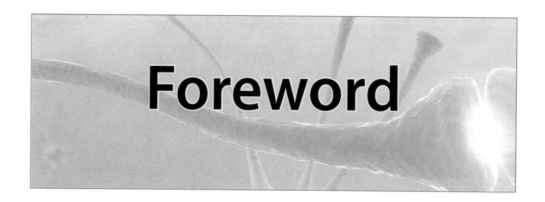

Foreword

As I write these words in early July 2009, I am reflecting on two important, but very different, conferences I recently had the privilege of attending. The first was the North American Research Conference on Complementary and Integrative Medicine, held in Minneapolis, Minnesota, in mid-May. This forum, sponsored by the Consortium of Academic Health Centers for Integrative Medicine, an organization of 43 centers in the US and Canada dedicated to advancing integrative medicine, is held every three years at a site in North America. Approximately 800 participants from 20 countries attended this meeting, which had a rich program of symposia, workshops, featured discussions and over 300 research presentations addressing the state-of-the-science in the field.

What was intriguing, however, was the emphasis that the organizers placed on research literacy and the need to extend a culture of research to complementary and alternative medicine (CAM) training and CAM practice. Indeed, three sessions addressed topics such as: *What are Research Literacy Competencies for the CAM Practitioner?*, *How can CAM Research better Reflect CAM Practice?*, and *Changing the Culture of CAM Institutions towards an Evidence-based Approach*. The sessions were attended by both conventional and CAM researchers, and by educators and practitioners, which underscored a shared desire to work across disciplines in order to advance these laudable goals.

The second meeting was in mid-June in Bethesda, Maryland, convened by the National Center for Complementary and Alternative Medicine (NCCAM) at the National Institutes of Health (NIH). Present at this meeting were about 30 principal and co-investigators of CAM R25 (Education) grants supported by NCCAM. The goal of the CAM R25 grant program is to support educational initiatives in CAM institutions that would create a culture for research literacy and evidence-based practice. For each of these projects, a collaborative partnership is required between the CAM institution and a conventional academic health center. I was invited to address this group on strategies for disseminating, to a broad audience, the progress they made and the lessons they had learned in the process. During the session I was again struck by the consensus expressed by the attendees regarding the imperative for establishing a culture of research in the CAM institutions: from students to faculty to community-based practitioners.

So, why the focus and interest on research literacy? To be frank, the delivery of health care, like any other service, must be based on the best available information about what works, what does not and, most importantly, what is potentially harmful. Indeed, both conventional and complementary health care practitioners are recognizing that treatment options for their patients must be informed by evidence. Decisions about treatment efficacy and effectiveness, and appropriate approaches for a particular instance or individual, all require information that comes from rigorous research. While this notion seems self-evident, it is also true that most health care practitioners are not researchers. Thus, there is a need for all practitioners to be able to read and evaluate the research literature, and to competently assess the quality of the evidence.

Another important rationale is that research literacy can contribute to better understanding and dialogue among health professionals. Increasingly, individual practitioners such as physicians, nurses, massage therapists, chiropractors, acupuncturists and others find themselves working collaboratively in teams, whether in the care of patients with debilitating pain, or in addressing the needs of individuals with chronic illnesses such as cancer or diabetes. The ability to communicate an objective understanding of the relevant research findings represents an essential skill and a common language across all disciplines that will help determine the most appropriate treatment options for the patient.

While the desire for understanding research may be present and growing, many are often stymied by not knowing where or how to begin. With this book, Dr. Menard has provided a wonderful tool to help educators, researchers and practitioners in all health professions to begin the journey towards research literacy.

From the first chapter that introduces the reader to the scientific method, Dr. Menard shares her wisdom and expertise about what constitutes evidence and how evidence-based practice originated, and gives a very useful step-by-step guide to how to read a scientific journal article. Her approach is to demystify science and evidence, without losing any of the rigor.

Those new to scientific discovery are brought up to date with clear descriptions of the types of research studies that are conducted, from case series and cohort studies to randomized, placebo-controlled clinical trials. The section on how to search for relevant research articles is particularly well described, as are the chapters on how to read qualitative and quantitative papers. Dr. Menard very clearly outlines the types of research articles that exist, and focuses appropriately on the importance of meta-analyses and systematic reviews and the emergence of the Cochrane Collaboration as a repository of the highest quality information. For many, these publications will become a key source of information.

Another helpful addition to the book is the chapter entitled "Making Sense of Statistics." Here, Dr. Menard conveys the logic behind statistical significance testing and describes how to tell when tests are being employed appropriately. The statistical concepts are explained in clear and simple terms that even those with limited mathematical backgrounds can easily understand.

I was also impressed that the final chapter takes the reader through the process of writing a case report. Even for practitioners not likely to engage in laboratory bench work or become actively involved in conducting clinical trials, the ability to report on cases they see in their practices is an essential and vitally important skill. In this way, much more can be contributed to the evidence base for the betterment of patients and practitioners alike.

So, in considering Dr. Menard's valuable contribution to fostering research literacy, I found this book to be a clearly written, carefully crafted, practical guide to understanding research that is suitable for any student embarking on a career in the health professions, be it a conventional discipline or one within the broad area of CAM. It will also be very useful for the practitioner who desires to inform his or her clinical practice with an evidence-based perspective. My sincere hope is that individuals and institutions will seize upon the lessons that Dr. Menard offers, and use this accessible and insightful book as a stepping off point towards developing skill and familiarity with what has often seemed an intimidating subject. As integrative medicine increasingly brings us together, I look forward to the next series of conferences in the coming years where it will be patently evident that research literacy is now part of the culture of health care across the many disciplines. Enjoy the journey.

Aviad Haramati, PhD

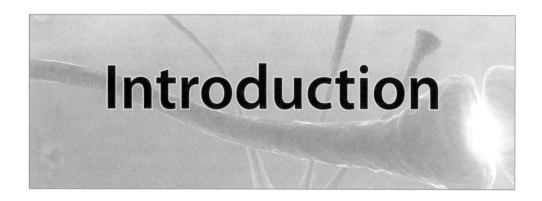

Introduction

The beginner must read, but intently and choosily and not too much.

P.B. Medawar

I believe that reading health care research offers every complementary practitioner a valuable tool for improving the quality of care you are able to offer your clients, and for ensuring that you and your loved ones receive the best possible health care. Understanding research is vital to the continued development of complementary therapies. Yet it remains a critical gap in the professional education of many practitioners.

Much has changed in the landscape of health care research since the first edition of this text was published. When I wrote the preceding paragraph in 2002, research literacy was almost nonexistent in the curricula of many complementary practitioner training programs. Research literacy has gained a much larger foothold in many CAM professional programs. To see the critical evaluation of research as a mandated competency for new practitioners is a most welcome development in several disciplines. Research literacy remains vital to the continued advancement of complementary and integrative health care, and the reasons that it matters are true as much today as they were then.

Why I Wrote this Book

After I graduated from massage school in 1982, research was the farthest thing from my mind. I was more concerned with getting my practice off the ground and working as a teaching assistant. Although the training I received was excellent, I realized after a few months of private practice and keeping up with students' questions that there was much more to learn, and decided to go back to school.

Despite a wonderfully eclectic academic program that allowed me to combine courses in gross anatomy, physiology, and biochemistry with others in psychology and athletic training, after a few more years of practice I found myself still dissatisfied with my level of knowledge. I began to read medical, nursing, and psychology journal articles about massage therapy, searching to find the relatively few that appeared in the health care literature at that time.

At first, I was pleased to find any research and interpreted any study with positive findings as proof that massage really worked. However, as I carefully read more studies with both negative and positive results, I realized that the reality was more complicated. It also seemed to me that many studies were designed by people who knew very little about the clinical practice of massage therapy. The more I read, the more I thought I could develop a study that would reflect a more accurate assessment of what massage could do in a given situation. In 1992, I entered the graduate clinical psychology program at the University of Virginia knowing that I wanted to design a study evaluating some aspect of massage therapy for my master's thesis.

Through discussions with professors and fellow students, I learned more about how to read journal articles critically. I realized that some of the studies I had been reading had other issues besides the massage protocols. Understanding the reasoning behind design features such as blinding and random assignment, and understanding how these features supported or undermined the evidence presented in other research studies helped me in developing my own. In many ways, this book is the one I wish had been available to me when I was a student.

I went on to complete my Ph.D. in education, specifically in research methodology, the theory and practice of how to design and conduct research. The study I designed for my thesis on the effect of massage on postoperative outcomes was among the first projects to be funded by the new NIH Office of Alternative Medicine. It became my doctoral dissertation. With experience gained from conducting my own study, I began speaking to other massage practitioners in the United States and Canada about my own work and about research in general.

Many of the practitioners I spoke with were excited about research and its potential to help massage therapy become more accepted within the larger health care field. But without any background or training, most seemed to feel that research was something mysterious, difficult, and almost impossible for the average complementary practitioner to understand. Motivated by these conversations, I began teaching workshops on how to read a clinical research article. This book developed from the material presented at these workshops, and has been expanded and updated to provide a thorough introduction to the topic. Through it, I hope to convey a necessary and important skill to a wider audience than I could ever expect to reach in person.

Why Does Research Literacy Matter?

Why do I think research literacy is important? First, research is a fundamental aspect of each of the conventional health care disciplines: medicine, nursing, psychology, physical therapy, speech therapy, occupational therapy, and so on. Research supports the theoretical foundation of any discipline and helps to distinguish useful treatments and practices from those that offer no benefit or prove harmful to patients. In addition, complementary therapies such as chiropractic and acupuncture have developed a sizable body of research to support their use. Research on the effectiveness of these therapies has helped facilitate their acceptance by conventional health care and the general public, and is a cornerstone of the shift towards evidence-based practice.

Key to this acceptance is the effort to reduce the language barrier between conventional health care and complementary approaches to health. As complementary practitioners we still are in the minority within the larger health care field, and it is particularly important that we be able to explain our work in terms that others can grasp. Understanding research greatly improves our ability to communicate effectively with other health care professionals through a shared frame of reference and a common language. With the growing trend towards integrative health care, the ability to have meaningful dialog across disciplines will continue to assume greater importance.

Next, being able to locate and critically evaluate research in one's field is essential to providing the best possible care for clients. Evidence-informed practice is rapidly becoming the new standard across health care generally, and complementary and integrative therapies will be held to it. Reading research is one way to stay current on the latest developments, and it can be part of what keeps the work intellectually stimulating. Because news about recent research is often reported in the popular media, clients or other health care providers may approach practitioners with questions about what implications a new study might have. It is incumbent upon practitioners to be able to discuss questions that arise from research in their field. Understanding how to evaluate research findings helps one to do this knowledgeably, with ease and confidence.

Finally, research is increasingly important for all of us as consumers in the health care system. As patients, we are beginning to assume a more active role in the health care partnership; more of us are seeking out research studies for the most current information about our own care. Popular media often do not report study findings in enough detail to determine how much confidence to place in the results or whether they apply to particular groups such as women or minorities. The media are also more likely to emphasize the most newsworthy angle instead of the usually more cautious interpretation found in peer-reviewed journals. Understanding research may be important to all of us at some point in helping us ask doctors the right questions to make sure that we and those close to us get the best possible care.

Currently, more and more people are using complementary therapies, and the number of medical schools offering integrative medicine programs has increased several times over. Evidence-based health care is definitely here to stay, and policy decisions regarding what treatments will be reimbursed are increasingly based on research. And more than ever, consumers in today's health care system need to be research literate in order to get the best possible health care, and make informed decisions with their providers.

Goals of This Book

The primary goal of this book is to increase your ability to locate and evaluate relevant research articles to enhance your work and your health. Its intent is to make health care research more accessible to all who are interested, especially those without a background or formal training in science. As complementary therapies become more integrated into conventional health care, and as every health care discipline moves towards evidence-based practice, it is increasingly necessary that we as practitioners become research literate. While the book was originally intended to fill a critical gap in the education of complementary therapists, this edition has been revised and expanded so that any health care practitioner or interested layperson will find the concepts and skills presented here useful. To that end, I have tried as much as possible to write in plain English, keeping technical terms to a minimum and providing clear explanations where needed. A glossary is also provided for easy reference.

As you become more proficient in the critical evaluation of research, you will likely find yourself becoming a bit more skeptical about accepting what you read at face value. You will also notice yourself honing your critical thinking skills. For those who may be interested in actively participating in research in some capacity, this book introduces basic concepts as a foundation for further education. One of the best ways to learn how to conduct research is to read the findings of other investigators and study their successes and mistakes. Reading research gives you a feel for how scientists think. In addition, critically reviewing and integrating existing research on a topic is a necessary first step in designing any study.

As I said at the beginning of this introduction, I believe research literacy is an essential skill that can improve the quality of care practitioners are able to offer their clients. A major result of becoming research literate is the enhancement of one's knowledge and professional abilities, for example, in developing treatment plans and in communicating more effectively with other health care providers. Becoming research literate creates a basis for improved clinical decision-making, successful outcomes for your clients, and increased professional recognition. Simply put, making sense of research can help you become a better practitioner.

How to Use This Book

The book is structured so that the reader begins with a broad perspective on understanding research and then progresses to more specific aspects in subsequent chapters. General concepts, including the underlying assumptions of scientific research, are introduced first. A primary focus of the book remains the evaluation of quantitative health care research because quantitative studies are still the majority published; however, more information and discussion of qualitative approaches to health care research has been added. Next, different types of research studies are identified and their strengths and weaknesses described. The various sections of a journal article and how to read them critically are then outlined in detail.

Following this discussion, studies are provided as examples of how to evaluate both quantitative and qualitative journal articles, using a question and answer format. This edition has expanded, adding new chapters on understanding basic statistics, designing and preparing case reports for publication, more information on ethics in health care research, more study examples, and updated information on how to locate health care research online. To assist students and faculty, I have again listed learning objectives at the beginning of each chapter and provided questions or activities to reinforce knowledge and enhance skills at the end of most chapters. To assist schools wishing to integrate research literacy into the curriculum, I am developing an online version of my course on research literacy, which this text can accompany, and interested readers may contact me for more information.

My hope for every health care practitioner who uses this book remains that the knowledge and skills gained as a result will create a solid foundation for greater confidence and understanding. As you begin the important task of integrating research into an evidence-based practice, I hope that you will use research to inform your clinical decision-making skills and choices among available treatment options. I continue to wish each reader the very best. May this book help you continue a lifelong commitment to learning, caring, and excellence in your chosen field.

Martha Brown Menard, PhD, CMT

Let the beauty we love be what we do.
There are hundreds of ways to kneel and kiss the ground.

Rumi

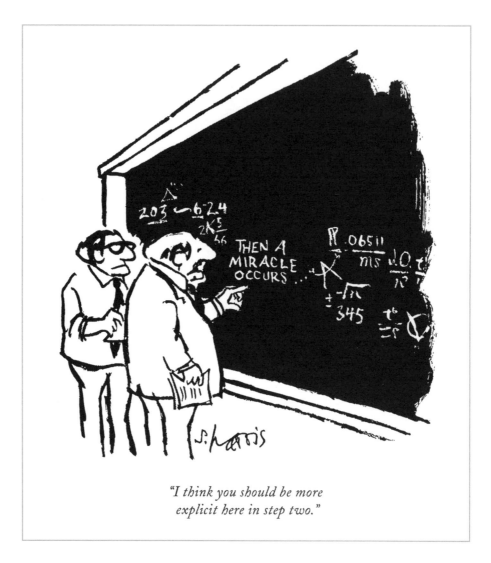

"I think you should be more
explicit here in step two."

Chapter 1:

A Brief Introduction to the Scientific Method

"The scientific method,"
as it is sometimes called, is a potentiation of common sense.

P. B. Medawar

Learning Objectives

After completing this chapter,
the reader should be able to:

- *Name the bases upon which knowledge claims can be made.*

- *Understand the concepts of falsification and reproducibility.*

- *Explain the two basic principles and three core values that underlie ethical clinical research.*

- *Describe three differences between quantitative and qualitative methods.*

- *Define evidence-based medicine and evidence-based practice.*

- *Describe the hierarchical model of levels of evidence and the evidence circle.*

- *Discuss the relationship between research literacy and evidence-based practice.*

Chapter 1: A Brief Introduction to the Scientific Method

Before one begins reading health care journal articles and evaluating their merits, it is helpful to understand some general principles about the processes involved in scientific research. This chapter introduces fundamental concepts and provides an overview of the underlying and often unspoken assumptions about how scientific research is conducted. Two basic concepts, falsification and reproducibility, that are necessary to critically evaluate research studies are also introduced in this chapter. The ethical principles and values that support scientific research are explained, and evidence-based medicine is defined. The idea of "weighing" the evidence presented in journal articles is discussed, and two models for examining the relative strength of evidence are presented. Finally, the importance of research literacy to implementing an evidenced-based practice is considered.

Science as a Way of Thinking

When people hear the word "science" various types of images come to mind. Associations with science can be positive or negative, depending on how it is portrayed in the popular media or based on personal experiences with education. A different way to think about science may be to simply consider it as a way of looking at the world with a spirit of open-minded curiosity and inquiry.

Science is not, however, the only way of seeking or gaining knowledge about the world. Claims about knowledge may be made on grounds such as tradition, intuition, or authority. For example, we may have learned that a familiar procedure should be performed in a certain manner because it has always been done that way. In some situations, such as choosing a family's holiday activities, this kind of knowledge claim is acceptable. In another setting, we might sense that a person we are being introduced to is untrustworthy because we "just know it," and this intuition may prove to be correct. Or, we may have been taught that massage is contraindicated for people with cancer because that is what our massage teacher was taught and passed on to us, based on a text written at the turn of the 20th century. In this latter example, our teacher's assertion is not a valid knowledge claim based on more recent and accurate information.

There are two other methods upon which scientific knowledge claims are more likely to be based: rationalism and empiricism, which have their foundations respectively in critical thinking and sensory experience.

Rationalism is a way of acquiring knowledge through the use of reason or logic. A classic example of a logical deduction is the following argument:

> *All men are mortal. (premise)*
>
> *Socrates is a man. (premise)*
>
> *Therefore Socrates is mortal. (conclusion)*

There is one problem with this approach: the conclusion is valid only when the premises are accurate. In the example above, the reader has no way to independently verify that Socrates is really a man and not the name of a fishing boat or a software program. Without some way to assess the accuracy of a premise, both it and any resulting conclusion are based on assumption alone. To have more confidence in the results of this process, each premise or step must be tested.

Empiricism is a way of acquiring knowledge through observation and experience. An empiricist accepts a statement as true only if he or she can demonstrate it through physical assessment. Something cannot exist, nor can a statement be true, unless it can be verified through the senses. This method of gaining knowledge requires observation and analysis, and provides a way to test the premises and conclusions of rationalism. Science creates the basis for knowledge claims by marrying the rational and empirical approaches. It seeks to validate the assumptions of rationalism through careful observation, measurement, and evaluation of sensory information. This way of thinking defines science and scientific research.

Above all, scientific research is about asking questions. "What," "how," and "why" are questions scientists often ask about the natural world. They look to get their answers through the development and testing of hypotheses. A **hypothesis** is a highly specific statement that can be demonstrated to be true or false through methodical gathering and analysis of empirical information or data. Qualitative research methods are often employed in the development of scientific hypotheses, while quantitative methods are more frequently used to test hypotheses. The different methods used to conduct scientific investigation through testing hypotheses will be discussed in more detail later in this and in subsequent chapters.

An essential feature of almost every research question is that it seeks to describe or explain relationships among variables. For example, pollsters may want to know whether men and women plan to vote differently on an issue, teachers may want to know if different teaching methods can improve reading comprehension, complementary practitioners may want to uncover the process through which clients make treatment decisions, and physicians may want to understand the patient's experience of living with a chronic illness.

Another aspect of science is that it is systematic. Once a research question or hypothesis is identified, information or data related to it is gathered in a methodical way. The researcher attempts to ensure that no relevant information is overlooked or left out, whether from personal preference or forgetfulness. Particularly at the beginning stages of a scientific inquiry, no one knows what observation or piece of data may prove to be important. If the information collected can be expressed in numerical form, a systematic approach often includes the use of statistical calculations to determine whether there are any changes among the variables or outcomes being studied and, if so, whether it is possible that these results could have occurred due to chance alone. If the information is collected in the form of words, detailed descriptions are made and then analyzed for similar themes, patterns, and meaning.

Science also ideally has an antiauthoritarian element. As suggested earlier, part of the essence of science is not taking someone else's word for it. Rather than relying on history, opinion, the experience of others, revelation, or individual desire that a hypothesis be true or false, science accepts the assertion that something is true based on evidence. Peer-reviewed journals, where scientific articles are published after being vetted by colleagues and experts in the researcher's field, allow for sharing study results and their implications with a wider audience. Readers are free to make up their own minds about the worth and credibility of the author's methods, results, and conclusions.

As the noted biologist Peter Medawar wrote, another way to define the scientific method is to view it as a high-powered version or "potentiation" of everyday common sense. This common-sense standard is one that we will apply thoughtfully when weighing evidence presented in health care research articles.

Falsification and Accumulation of Knowledge

Falsification is an idea first put forth by the philosopher Karl Popper.[1] It can be summarized as follows: because it is always possible that new information could be discovered at any time, even about a research question that seems to have been thoroughly investigated, we can never say that "such and such is certainly true." We can only say that a hypothesis is provisionally true to date because no evidence to disconfirm it has come to light. Popper's view is that rather than working toward verification, that is, demonstrating a thing to be true, science works best when attempting to prove it false. When a hypothesis fails to be demonstrated as false enough times, it becomes part of the body of accepted knowledge. However, the idea of falsification implies that this status is always provisional and that there are degrees of certainty. Lee Cronbach[2] may have put it best when he described the pursuit of scientific knowledge as "reducing uncertainty."

In this way, although errors and mistakes may be accepted for a time, science is essentially self-correcting because it is understood that knowledge is provisional. As new information becomes available, accepted knowledge eventually changes to accommodate and include it. Sometimes this assimilation takes place over a long time, particularly if the new information stands in contradiction to previously held beliefs, but if the evidence is strong enough it will eventually become integrated into the body of accepted knowledge.*

Given this perspective, one study alone rarely provides enough information or evidence to conclusively answer a question. It is much more common for a body of evidence to accumulate over time. One study builds upon another. This is what Einstein meant when he said, "If I have seen farther than other men, it is because I have stood on the shoulders of giants." As more studies are conducted and more information becomes available, a more complete and detailed picture is formed. We will return to this idea when we discuss the evidence circle.

Reproducibility of Results

Reproducibility refers to the capacity of a study to be repeated, preferably by a different investigator, and still produce the same or similar results. Another type of replication can be found in studies that build upon previous work or knowledge. Reproducibility adds a great deal of weight to the body of scientific evidence on a particular question; it is the highest standard in terms of validating a hypothesis. Experimental results that cannot be replicated by others using the same methods and materials are viewed quite skeptically by the scientific community. Repeated failure to reproduce results under reasonably similar conditions is usually considered

* *The amount of time necessary is sometimes a generation or more, as younger scientists who may be more open to new ideas come up through the ranks. There is a well-known saying that ironically acknowledges the social and cultural nature of scientific revolutions: "Science progresses one death at a time."*

evidence of disconfirmation. A standard practice in reporting research findings is to give sufficient detail for a fellow scientist to reproduce the study.

Science as a Social Activity

Science takes place via human interaction, through informal communication among colleagues with similar interests, more formal presentations and discussions at conferences, and publication of completed research findings in peer-reviewed journals. Knowledge-building is a social process as much as it is a scientific one.

Because human beings are fallible, the social norms of science help to minimize the presence and/or influence of personal bias in the processes through which speculation becomes knowledge. These norms include an expectation of integrity in the design, conduct, interpretation, and publication of research studies. One example is the practice among peer-reviewed journals of requiring disclosure of all sources of financial support for a study, so that readers can judge the extent to which the study could be biased because of who funded the research. As an example, a study concluding that smoking poses no substantial health risks in spite of numerous contradictory studies would be viewed even more suspiciously if it were funded by the Tobacco Institute. By the same token, research on herbs and dietary supplements has sometimes been viewed more critically when funded by companies that manufacture these products.

The philosopher of science Thomas Kuhn articulated the idea that scientific world views or paradigms define the kinds of research questions that may legitimately be asked.[3] What is thought to be "legitimate" can vary according to the social norms and assumptions of a culture and what is considered within that culture to be useful or important knowledge. Other writers since Kuhn have detailed ways in which the practice of science has sometimes been distorted by dominant cultural biases, such as the idea that women[4] or people of color[5] were somehow biologically inferior to white males.

Ethics in Health Care Research

It is also important to define how research may legitimately be conducted, a subject that has been influenced by social norms and cultural bias as well. Present-day scientists involved in health care research have a code of ethical principles that must be applied to research involving both human and animal subjects.

With respect to human subjects, two of the most basic principles of ethical clinical research are:

1. to fully inform prospective participants about what the study procedures will entail, so that they can make an informed decision about whether or not to take part in the study

2. to do everything possible to minimize potential harm to study participants; this is derived from the Hippocratic Oath – to do no harm

Experimental studies are especially susceptible to ethical concerns because they involve direct intervention by the researcher in the lives or health of the participants. For this reason, the researcher is expected to make every effort to protect the human rights and well-being of the study's participants.

Current standards for research ethics have been formalized since World War II. In the US, the Nuremberg Code (1947) and the Declaration of Helsinki (1964, revised in 1975) became the foundation for the formation of the National Commission for Protection of Human Subjects and Behavioral Research. This commission produced a document known as the Belmont Report, which is available from the United States Printing Office for a fee. It can also be viewed online at no charge at: ohsr.od.nih.gov/guidelines/belmont.html.

The Belmont Report proposes that three core values should underlie all research endeavors: respect for persons, beneficence, and justice. The practical implications of each value are as follows:

Respect for persons refers to treating people as autonomous beings, with the right to make decisions based on their own interests or preferences. This value requires that people participate in research studies voluntarily, with adequate information regarding study procedures, and has resulted in the legal protections found in informed consent documents. People whose circumstances involve less autonomy, such as prisoners, children, or mentally challenged individuals, must receive special protections because they cannot give fully informed consent. For example, children participating in research must have a parent or guardian give consent in the child's best interests.

Beneficence refers to the value of doing no harm. This concept obligates researchers to give thought to maximizing the potential benefits and minimizing the potential risks that might occur from participating in a research investigation.

Researchers are required to communicate an accurate assessment of the potential risks and benefits of participation, so that prospective subjects can decide for themselves whether the putative benefits outweigh the possible risks. Beneficence underlies much public debate about exploring new areas of research, especially as new technologies expand the types of interventions that are possible. An example is the historical controversy over stem cell research, where the moral value of relieving suffering through developing effective treatments for debilitating chronic diseases contended with the potential moral cost of using embryos to provide the necessary stem cells (which can now be cultured).

Justice refers to the value of fairness in the distribution of the benefits and burdens associated with participation in research. In the 19th and 20th centuries, a disproportionate share of research participants came from poor, disenfranchised, and/or captive populations. The exploitation of Nazi prisoners in medical experiments is a particularly flagrant example of such injustice. While we might like to think that the abuse of research participants could never happen here or now, the need for justice remains current.

A disturbing example is found in recent US history. The Tuskegee Syphilis Study was initiated by the Public Health Service in 1932. Its subjects were rural black men diagnosed with syphilis, for which no effective treatments existed at the time; the study set out to observe the untreated natural course of the disease. The men were told that they were participating in a study of "bad blood." When penicillin became available in 1943 the men were not offered this new treatment and the study was allowed to continue. Only when public health workers leaked the truth to the media and the National Association for the Advancement of Colored People filed suit was the study stopped – in 1972. During the 40 years that the study was conducted, 28 men died directly as a result of the disease, 100 died from complications, and 40 wives and 19 children were infected. In 1997, former president Bill Clinton acknowledged publicly that the study had been morally reprehensible.

The value of justice leads to the expectation that researchers will assure that subjects or participants are solicited based on the requirements of the research question being asked, and that disadvantaged people are not disproportionately selected for a study because of their availability and vulnerability to exploitation.

One outgrowth of the Belmont Report was that the US government developed regulations requiring institutions conducting research to establish **institutional review boards** (IRBs), the purpose of which is to act as ethics committees to safeguard the rights of study participants. IRBs consider the scientific merit of proposed projects, the competence of the investigators, and the suitability of all treatments and study procedures, in light of the study's potential risks and benefits. IRBs also assess the procedures for selecting and recruiting participants, for ensuring appropriate informed consent, and for maintaining confidentiality of private health care information disclosed during the study. The IRB approves the proposed design of the study from the standpoint of whether its benefits outweigh its risks, and then monitors the conduct of the study as it progresses.

In other parts of the world, these protections are less stringent or nonexistent. Some US pharmaceutical companies have recently been criticized for conducting clinical trials in third world nations, where protection of human rights in health care research is more lax.

Elements of Informed Consent for Research Study Participants

1. Purpose of the research project, or reason(s) behind the study and participant selection.

2. Procedures, or exactly what participation will involve.

3. An accurate description of the potential benefits and risks.

4. Information about available alternative procedures that do not involve participating in the study.

5. How the participant's identity will be protected in collecting, storing, and reporting of research data.

6. An assurance that participants who choose to enroll can withdraw at any time.

7. Contact information for the principal investigator of the study so that participants can ask questions to get more information.

Informed consent forms are signed by both participants and investigators, and are considered legally binding documents.

Quantitative and Qualitative Methods

In the traditional scientific worldview, hypotheses are predicated on the assumption that there is a uniform reality that can be observed, measured, and expressed in terms of numbers. There is also an assumption of linear cause and effect, for example, that a certain treatment causes a specific result in those who receive it. Methods for investigating research questions based on these assumptions are called **quantitative methods**. Their essence is the testing of hypotheses, starting from specific events and using inductive reasoning to build more general theories from these. Quantitative methods use numbers as a kind of shorthand to summarize and manage large amounts of collected information or data.

In the experimental quantitative approach, the researcher manages the treatment setting and the participants in the study, controlling the environment and participants' activities as much as possible. Quasi-experimental approaches are often used in situations where a purely experimental design is not feasible, such as in a private practice or educational setting. Elements of research design are employed to preclude rival explanations of the results so that the treatment alone can be claimed to have caused them. Statistical analysis is then used to show the probability that the results could have occurred by chance. A low probability means that the odds of the results occurring by chance alone are unlikely. Quantitative research is typically tightly designed and implemented in an attempt to isolate the cause-and-effect factors that result in a study's outcome, and a major assumption is that results obtained in one setting are reproducible under the same conditions in another setting.

Another quantitative approach is based on observation. In a quantitative observational study, the researcher observes and collects numerical data on events or participants as they naturally occur, without attempting to manage them. Observational studies frequently use existing information that has been previously collected, such as data from the US Census or state and local records. Examining the rates of lung cancer per state, and then comparing these to tobacco sales per state would be an example of this type of quantitative study. Observational studies are often used in epidemiology to determine whether a possible association between factors or outcomes exists, and whether the strength of the association merits further investigation.

In qualitative research, information or data is collected in the form of words rather than numbers. **Qualitative methods** are generally based on a different set of assumptions from quantitative methods. In the qualitative worldview there is no distinction between the observer and what is observed – each affects the other and is part of an ongoing process of change. The observer can describe what he or she observes, but there is no assumption of a uniform external reality, and any individual's description is seen as only one of several realities or perspectives that may each be equally valid. Rather than a single, linear cause and effect, there may be multiple causes or factors that influence outcomes, and these may vary from situation to situation. Each situation is considered unique. Another hallmark of qualitative research is the importance placed on observation of phenomena in their natural settings, and on the personal contact and insights of the researcher in relation to the participants in the study, rather than a more laboratory-like manipulation of the research parameters.

Reflecting these different underlying assumptions, qualitative methods consist of three types of data collection: open-ended interviews, direct observation, and documents such as personal journals, correspondence, and written answers to open-ended questionnaires and surveys. These approaches and data collection methods lend themselves to a variety of applications across many fields. For example, open-ended interviews are used in focus groups, where participants may be asked to discuss their thoughts, perceptions, and feelings about topics such as consumer products or political issues. Observations can be made along a continuum from the perspective of a complete outsider to a group or activity, as in the work of chimpanzee biologist Jane Goodall, to the perspective of a full participant, as demonstrated in Gloria Steinem's description of her career as a Playboy bunny. Documents ranging from the letters and diaries of historical figures to postings on an Internet bulletin board can all be analyzed for themes and trends.

The qualitative view is in some ways a more holistic perspective. Its essence is the desire to interpret experiences, behaviors, and points of view, to understand complex situations and multifaceted events, and to explore and pursue new paths of discovery as they emerge.

Quantitative, Qualitative, or Both?

The choice of methods in research is still somewhat contentious, although less so now compared to a generation ago. For many years a great ideological divide separated quantitative and qualitative researchers, with each touting the advantages of their preferred methodology while stressing the limitations of the others'. The quantitative paradigm still predominates in health care and medical research. The biological sciences have long tried to base their methods on the rigorous ones used in "hard" sciences like classical physics and chemistry. Recently, however, there has been a greater openness to the qualitative philosophy in health care research, particularly in nursing. Studies in the disciplines of sociology, anthropology, psychology, and education often employ qualitative methods. The incorporation of qualitative methods, and the types of knowledge gained as a result, has much to offer the study of health care.

Quantitative and qualitative studies both require careful planning and preparation in order to yield useful results. Although qualitative methods developed at least partially out of dissatisfaction with the limitations of quantitative methods, in many ways the qualitative philosophy has always been part of the foundation of science. Research hypotheses are almost always developed based on detailed description and observation from the field. It is not a simple either-or question.

Studies may use major elements of both qualitative and quantitative approaches in what is termed a mixed methods approach. Over the past decade, health care research has begun to integrate qualitative and quantitative methodologies more often than before.

For example, in an exploratory or pilot study, qualitative methods may be employed to describe and to attempt to understand phenomena – to collect more information because there is not yet enough to form a highly specific and quantifiable hypothesis. Such a study may be used to build a theory rather than to verify one. Imagine a quantitative survey of addictive behavior, where researchers might use a focus group in the development of the survey questionnaire to ensure that the questions are worded in a way that reflects the researchers' intent and is easily understood by participants. Quantitative data may also be collected as part of a qualitative study and can be used to illuminate patterns that might otherwise be overlooked. In a program evaluation of a massage therapy or acupuncture school, for example, job placement rates would be considered necessary and useful information.

The double-blind randomized clinical trial – the "gold standard" of the quantitative approach – is commonly used to assess treatment efficacy. It is usually based on a body of accumulated information, enough so that a theory has been developed and is now ready to be tested. In this type of study, qualitative data may be collected to document factors that may have influenced the results, such as the participants' reasons for dropping out of the study, or to gather additional information that could be useful in implementing the treatment in another setting.

Unusual events or unanticipated consequences can be described qualitatively and used to generate or refine new hypotheses to be tested. For example, physicians in the field reporting their observations of several pneumocystis pneumonia cases among young homosexual men in a large US city led to the identification of AIDS.[6]

Well-designed research always uses the methodology most appropriate to the question being asked. Sometimes a strategic combination of quantitative and qualitative methods is the best solution. Qualitative and quantitative methods both influence the credibility of a study based on the weight of the evidence as it is presented and interpreted. Each method requires rigorous planning and implementation; qualitative methods cannot be applied as a solution to a poorly designed quantitative study and vice versa. Even though the two methodologies are quite different in terms of their assumptions, the underlying logic used in evaluating either quantitative or qualitative studies is the same.

Much of the emphasis in upcoming chapters is placed on studies using quantitative methods, because these are still employed more extensively in health care research, particularly biomedical research. More information specific to qualitative research approaches is presented in Chapter 8, and in Chapter 9 we will examine the case report (also called the case study) as a research design that can incorporate both methodological approaches. The case report is one type of original research that is feasible for any complementary health care practitioner to conduct in the practice setting.

Weighing the Evidence

In many kinds of health care research we want to know whether a certain treatment (cause) is responsible for a particular outcome (effect). For example, does massage help premature babies gain weight? What factors (cause) contribute to developing an illness or promoting health (effect)? In critical evaluation of a journal article, we are assessing or weighing the evidence that the authors have presented. How well have they argued their case that this treatment or factor is responsible for that result? In any scientific journal article, the researchers are presenting their findings and offering their interpretation of what those findings mean. In other words, they are making a case for the reader to decide to what extent he or she accepts, accepts with reservations, or rejects the evidence presented, based on how strongly the authors have linked cause with effect.

The concept of levels of evidence refers to the idea that there are varying degrees or levels of credibility that different types of research studies can provide. It is rare that a single study demonstrates a hypothesis so conclusively that the results are beyond question. The more common scenario is that a body of knowledge accumulates, study by study, with different studies contributing different degrees and kinds of evidence.

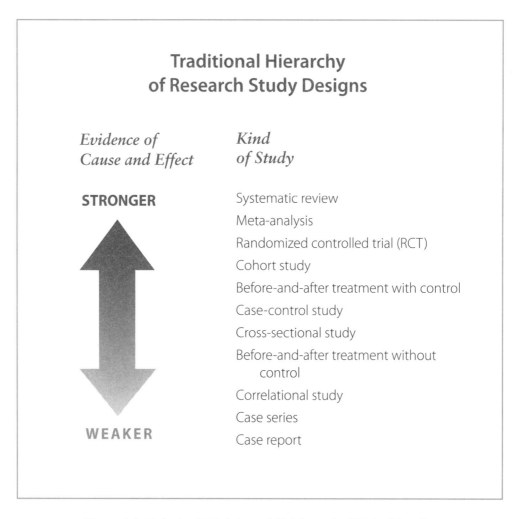

Traditional Hierarchy of Research Study Designs

Evidence of Cause and Effect

Kind of Study

STRONGER

Systematic review

Meta-analysis

Randomized controlled trial (RCT)

Cohort study

Before-and-after treatment with control

Case-control study

Cross-sectional study

Before-and-after treatment without control

Correlational study

Case series

Case report

WEAKER

Figure 1.1 Relative Weighting of Evidence in Clinical Studies

Figure 1.1 presents a visual summary of one way to look at the different types of research studies or designs in terms of their ability to link cause and effect. Within the biomedical research community, there is a traditional hierarchy of weight based on each design's ability to demonstrate this relationship. The relative strength of each design is shown schematically in this illustration by the arrow running from top to bottom, with studies that provide weaker degrees of cause and effect at the bottom and the strongest designs at the top. These different types of designs will be discussed in more detail in Chapter 4.

The studies from the case report up to the case-control study are considered descriptive or observational, meaning that the investigator is describing or observing what is naturally occurring without interfering in any way, and then reporting what he or she sees. As mentioned previously, descriptive and observational studies can be used to note associations between events and to generate hypotheses to be tested, a necessary step in developing well-designed experimental studies.

The before-and-after treatment with control, cohort study, and randomized controlled trial are examples of experimental designs. In these studies the investigator is typically actively intervening by assigning some participants to receive a treatment and comparing those participants' outcomes to the outcomes of others who receive a different intervention (or no intervention), and reporting the results. Experimental studies provide a stronger link between cause and effect; in these the investigator is systematically testing hypotheses.

Meta-analyses and systematic reviews are evaluations of groups of studies on a specific research question. By combining a number of studies and assessing their results together, the authors can evaluate the weight of the evidence as a whole on that question. These kinds of studies are considered to provide the strongest evidence of a cause-and-effect relationship between treatment and outcome.

Some methodologists prefer to classify study designs as experimental or non experimental, based on the researcher's intent to test for a cause-and-effect relationship. In both experimental and quasi-experimental designs, such as the uncontrolled before-and-after treatment study, the focus is on testing for a cause-and-effect relationship based on statistically significant differences between the groups. In this scheme, certain types of case reports and case series are considered experimental designs. Nonexperimental designs include the cross-sectional and case-control study designs, where there is less emphasis on cause-and-effect relationships among variables, and qualitative studies stand separately as a main classification of their own. All of these types of studies will be discussed in more detail in later chapters.

Evidence-Based Medicine

Research has always formed the basis of scientific thought. In health care and medicine, research began with a combination of clinical observation and empirical testing – thoughtful trial and error. A practitioner would note a certain set of symptoms, try various remedies to see which were effective, and reject those that did not seem to work. When another patient presented with the same or similar symptoms, the previously effective remedy would be tried first. For many years, most health care research consisted of observational and descriptive studies, with some before-and-after treatment studies. The widespread use of randomized controlled trials, where some kind of control or comparison group is used, is a relatively recent innovation. Credit for the modern randomized controlled trial is usually given to Sir Austin Bradford Hill.[7] The RCT, because of its design features, shows the strongest link between cause and effect using a single study.

The Centre for Evidence-Based Medicine[8] has defined **evidence-based medicine (EBM)** as "the conscientious, explicit and judicious use of current best evidence in making decisions about the care of individual patients." While many aspects of health care depend on individual preferences related to personal values and quality of life, the primary goal of EBM is to clarify the components of medical practice that can be evaluated using the scientific method and to apply that method to best predict the outcome of a given course of treatment, even as dialog about which therapies or outcomes are most desirable continues.

The growing trend toward evidence-based health care is here to stay. Both new and established treatments are now expected to demonstrate their effectiveness based on research, and insurance coverage of a treatment is increasingly likely to be linked to research supporting its use. An evidence-based focus requires the application of scientific method to the clinical practices of the health care professions. This poses a challenge for complementary and conventional practitioners alike. Many established treatments have not been tested using randomized controlled trials, and in evaluating some treatments or therapies, RCTs may not be appropriate or feasible.

Evidence-based medicine does have its critics, however. One concern raised is that EBM applies best to populations – the more that data are pooled and aggregated, the

A Brief History
of Evidence-Based Medicine

Isolated attempts to assess treatment efficacy date back several centuries, but only in the 20th century has this impetus evolved to widely impact almost all fields of health care and policy. The efforts of Dr. Archie Cochrane, a Scottish epidemiologist, through his vigorous advocacy and his book, Effectiveness and Efficiency: Random Reflections on Health Services *(1972), resulted in increasing acceptance of the concepts behind evidence-based practice. Cochrane's work was honored through the naming of centers of evidence-based medical research – Cochrane Centers – and an international organization, the Cochrane Collaboration.*

A Cochrane field group for complementary and alternative medicine research is based at the University of Maryland. The methodologies used to determine "best evidence" were largely established by the McMaster University research group led by David Sackett and Gordon Guyatt. The term "evidence-based medicine" first appeared in the medical literature in a 1992 paper by Guyatt and colleagues. It was titled "Evidence-based medicine. A new approach to teaching the practice of medicine" and was published by the Journal of the American Medical Association *(JAMA 1992;268:2420-5).*

more difficult it is to compare demographic characteristics of patients in the studies with the individual patient seen in one's practice. The most common response to this concern is that evidence-based medicine means integrating the patient's values and the experience and knowledge of the clinician with the best available external evidence based on systematic research. Other criticisms of EBM are discussed in Chapter 4.

The Evidence Circle

Another useful way to conceptualize the relative strengths and weaknesses of different research designs has been proposed by Walach et al.[9] Rather than a hierarchy, which tends to devalue designs that are at the bottom of the cause-and-effect ladder, Walach and colleagues present a circle, in which experimental designs are balanced by more observational and descriptive ones. The authors point out that the hierarchical model was founded and works well for pharmacological interventions but has since been generalized to other, more complex interventions such as physical therapy, massage, acupuncture, and surgery, for which it is usually inadequate. Instead of holding up the RCT as a gold standard against which all other designs are considered inferior, Walach's model proposes a multiplicity of methods that counterbalance the strengths and weaknesses of individual designs, and that can be considered equally rigorous, with the added benefit of greater clinical applicability. A similar model, called the *evidence house*, was previously proposed by Wayne Jonas.[10]

The Circle of Methods

Experimental methods that test specifically for efficacy (upper half of the circle in Figure 1.2) have to be complemented by observational, nonexperimental methods (lower half of the circle) that are more descriptive in nature and describe real-life effects and applicability. Shading indicates the complementarity of experimental and quasi-experimental methods.

Experts on complementary therapies, many of whom are trained as researchers and practitioners, believe that most complementary therapies are complex interventions. Factors such as intention, the patient-practitioner relationship, and complementary therapy patients' expectations, beliefs, attitudes, and preferences seem likely to be moderating variables that can influence the specific effect of an intervention or mediate the biological mechanism through which an effect is produced. The circular model offers a more helpful approach to evaluating the effectiveness of complementary therapies. This model also works well for conventional therapies such as surgery or psychotherapy, which are not pharmacological in nature.

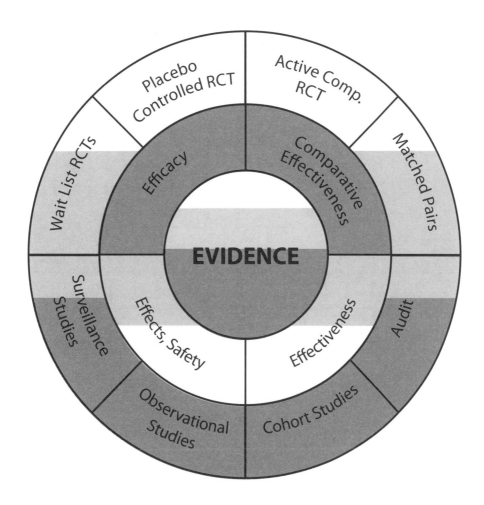

Figure 1.2 *The Circle of Methods*

from "Circular instead of hierarchical: methodological principles for the evaluation of complex interventions" Harald Walach et al, BMC Medical Research Methodology 2006;6:29

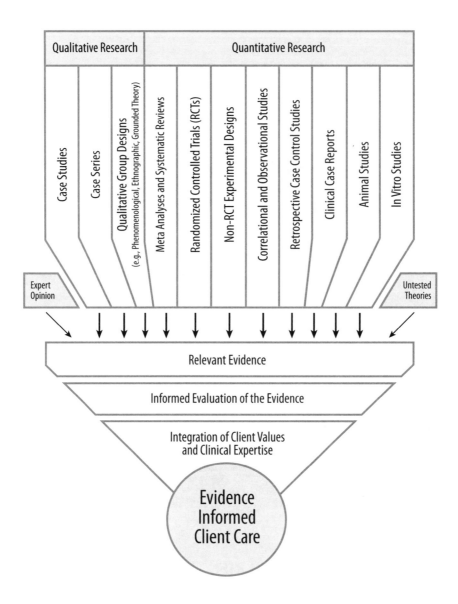

Figure 1.3 The Evidence-Based Practice Funnel

from "The evidence funnel: highlighting the importance of research literacy in the delivery of evidence informed complementary health care." Paul M. Finch, Journal of Bodywork and Movement Therapies *2007;11(1):78-81*

Evidence-Based Practice for Complementary Practitioners

Evidenced-based practice is clearly becoming the standard for health care providers, both conventional and complementary. It is also true that research literacy is a crucial component of evidence-based practice. A valuable concept that highlights the role of research literacy is the *evidence funnel*, proposed by Paul Finch.[11]

In this paradigm, the practitioner searches and sorts the available research on a given topic or question according to its relevance to a clinical case. The practitioner then prioritizes the most relevant research according to the design of the research and its alignment with the clinical question posed. For example, if the question is related to treatment effectiveness, studies with quantitative experimental designs would take precedence as best evidence. A clinical question related to patient or client experience would be better served by qualitative studies focused on the nature of that experience. Practitioners must be able to critically evaluate the weight of the research evidence to determine which studies constitute the best evidence in relation to a given clinical question.

Another appealing feature of the evidence funnel from the clinical perspective is the integration of the practitioner's expertise and the client's values with relevant research evidence. In using this model we have the best of both worlds, where appropriate research evidence informs individual clinical practice and is tempered by practitioner judgment and client preferences.

Summary

Scientific method is based on a spirit of open-minded curiosity and inquiry, using applied common sense and systematic procedures, and works best by demonstrating that a proposition is false rather than true. Knowledge is based on evidence, which accumulates over time as one study builds upon another, and as one research group replicates another's findings. Knowledge is also provisional, because new information that changes our ideas may be discovered at any time. In addition, science is a social endeavor premised upon the integrity of the individuals who design, conduct, interpret, and publish research. Health care research takes special care to protect the rights of those participating as research subjects by establishing institutional review boards (IRBs) to oversee and ensure the ethical conduct of research involving both humans and animals. The values that inform ethical research are respect for persons, beneficence, and justice.

Two major types of methodological approaches used in health care research are quantitative and qualitative; each has a different set of underlying assumptions. Although their assumptions do differ radically, the logic used to evaluate the credibility of evidence presented through published, peer-reviewed study findings is the same for both.

The hierarchical model of levels of evidence is useful in evaluating the relative strength of cause and effect in individual study designs. At the same time, the circular model of research evidence balances experimental studies with descriptive or observational ones, and has equal rigor when evaluating a group of studies on a subject. Moreover, this is a more appropriate model for weighting of evidence for the purpose of understanding complex interventions such as those common among complementary therapies. This model is also well-suited to weighing the evidence in more conventional nonpharmacological interventions such as physical therapy.

Evidence-based practice is quickly becoming the standard by which the quality of clinical health care is judged. Complementary practitioners can inform and improve their work through critical evaluation of research literature relevant to their cases combined with their professional expertise and their clients' values and preferences. Research literacy is a necessary component of evidence-informed practice.

References

1. Popper KR. *The Logic of Scientific Discovery*. New York: Basic Books; 1959.

2. Cronbach LJ. *Designing Evaluations of Educational and Social Programs*. San Francisco: Jossey-Bass; 1982.

3. Kuhn TS. *The Structure of Scientific Revolutions* (3rd edition). Chicago: University of Chicago Press; 1996.

4. Tavris C. *The Mismeasure of Woman*. New York: Simon & Schuster; 1992.

5. Gould SJ. *The Mismeasure of Man*. New York: W.W. Norton & Company; 1981.

6. CDC. Pneumocystis pneumonia – Los Angeles. June 4, 1981. *MMWR* August 30, 1996;45(34):729-733.

7. Hill AB. The clinical trial. *New England Journal of Medicine*. 1952;247:113-119.

8. Sackett DL, Rosenberg WM, Gray JA, Haynes RB, Richardson WS. Evidence based medicine: what it is and what it isn't. *BMJ*. 1996;312(7023):71-2.

9. Walach H, Falkenberg T, Fønnebø V, Lewith G, Jonas WB. Circular instead of hierarchical: methodological principles for the evaluation of complex interventions. *BMC Medical Research Methodology.* 2006;6:29.

10. Jonas WB. Building an evidence house: challenges and solutions to research in complementary and alternative medicine. *Forsch Komplementarmed Klass Naturheilkd* 2005;12(3):159-67.

11. Finch P. The evidence funnel: highlighting the importance of research literacy in the delivery of evidence informed health care. *Journal of Bodywork and Movement Therapies.* 2007;11:78-81.

Exercises

1. *How do rationalism and empiricism work together in scientific research to reinforce the validity of knowledge claims?*

2. *Explain what scientists mean by the term "falsificationism."*

3. *Describe some of the principal ways that qualitative and quantitative research methods differ from each other.*

4. *Name the two basic principles and the three core values that are the foundation for the ethical conduct of research.*

5. *Define evidence-based medicine.*

6. *Explain two different models for weighing the evidence presented in scientific research.*

7. *Using the Internet, find and read an example of an ethical dilemma in health care research. Present and discuss to the rest of the class.*

8. *A client comes to you seeking relief from frequent migraine headaches. Discuss how you would develop an evidence-informed approach to your work with this client.*

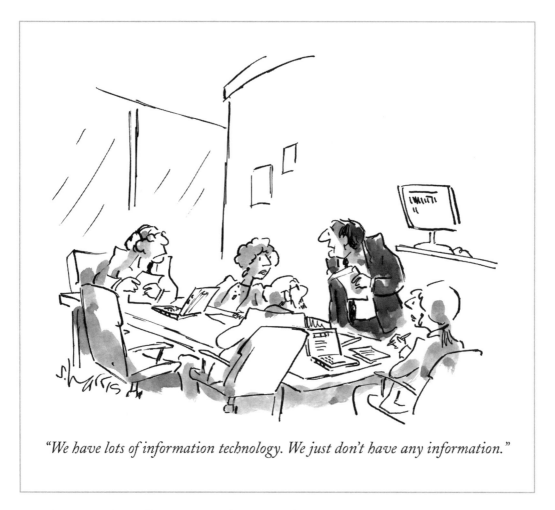

"We have lots of information technology. We just don't have any information."

Chapter 2:

Locating Journal Articles

We always need to know and understand a great deal more than we do already and to master many more skills than we now possess.

P. B. Medawar

Learning Objectives

After completing this chapter, the reader should be able to:

- Define the terms field, keywords, search strategy, and open access.

- Perform a search for journal articles using PubMed and BioMed Central.

- Save a search strategy using My NCBI.

- Create preferences with My BMC.

- Investigate other websites as additional resources for finding articles of interest.

Chapter 2: Locating Journal Articles

Before you can start reading studies to evaluate their merit, you need to be able to find them. There are numerous ways, both formal and informal, to locate journal articles or reports of research studies. For our purposes, we will concentrate on using publicly available online reference databases, as these are the most easily accessed by the largest number of readers. Two databases in particular, PubMed and BioMed Central, will be discussed in detail. PubMed is the publicly available version of MEDLINE, the reference database maintained by the National Library of Medicine in Bethesda, Maryland. BioMed Central is an independent electronic publishing house based on the principle of open access to peer-reviewed biomedical research. Both databases are very easy to use – if you can do a Google search, you can perform a search using PubMed or BioMed Central. Although we will focus on learning how to conduct a search specifically using PubMed, the same general principles apply to searching most online health care literature databases.

This chapter will make more sense if you sit down at a computer and use the information it contains to simultaneously walk through a search in real time. I have assumed minimal familiarity with online database search programs, so feel free to skip ahead if you are accustomed to using them.

Illustrations of web pages in this chapter are current as the book goes to press; however, the layout and design of websites or single web pages are subject to change. Also, the illustrations are shown using Mozilla Firefox version 2.0 as the browser. If you use a different browser, such as Microsoft Explorer or Google Chrome, pages may appear in a slightly different format but all essential features will be the same.

Reference databases provide a relatively easy way to find published articles of interest. Typically each entry, or **citation**, for an article gives its title, author(s), and publication date, and the name of the journal in which it was published, including volume and/or issue and page numbers. A short descriptive summary, or **abstract**, of the article's main points is frequently included, although older references (those prior to 1975) may not have abstracts available, or may use the first paragraph of the article as the abstract.

The title, author, journal name, publication date, and other bibliographic information are called **fields**. Searches can sometimes turn up hundreds of articles. You can use fields to narrow searches so that you are retrieving only those citations that are relevant to your purpose. Limiting or refining your search can save a great deal of time. On the other hand, to get a comprehensive view you may want to combine results from several searches to include every aspect of a topic. Whether you limit or expand your search, the particular path you select is called a **search strategy**. For example, to limit a search to articles on oncology massage for breast cancer patients, you might use the terms "massage therapy and breast cancer." For an overview of the use of alternative therapies for tension headaches, you might perform several searches using a variety of synonyms for touch therapies generally, and then combine all the results.

What If I Do Not Have a Computer?

Even if you don't have a computer at home, you may be able to use one at work or at school. Most institutions of higher learning provide students computer access. If you are unfamiliar with using a computer and browser software to access the World Wide Web, ask a reference librarian if instruction is available, or sign up for a short noncredit course at a local community college. Many public libraries offer Web access; if yours does not, ask the reference librarian for suggestions.

If you have the good fortune to live near a major research library, visit it and ask under what circumstances members of the public or health care providers who are not affiliated with the institution are allowed to use the library facilities. Some university and/or hospital-based medical libraries will allow local health care practitioners to use their services, with or without restrictions. These libraries may offer access to more specialized databases, such as AMED, the Allied and Complementary Medicine Database produced by the British Library, CINAHL, the Cumulative Index to Nursing and Allied Health Literature, PsycINFO, the primary database for the behavioral sciences, or EMBASE, a European counterpart of MEDLINE. At the very least, you will be able to use a public library computer to access PUBMED.

About PubMed

PubMed is the search service provided by the National Library of Medicine. It includes MEDLINE, the primary reference database maintained by the National Library of Medicine, along with PreMEDLINE, OLDMEDLINE, and other related health care databases, including molecular biology. PubMed contains over 17 million bibliographic citations from more than 5,200 journals covering medical, nursing, dental, veterinary medicine, life sciences, and other health care literature subjects published in more than seventy countries. Most entries are from English-language sources or have English abstracts available. The majority of citations are for articles published after 1965, although there are some dating back to 1950. PubMed is a comprehensive biomedicine database that is updated daily. In recent years, many more articles on complementary and alternative therapies have been added as these have entered the mainstream of health care literature. In fact, 'complementary therapies' is now a subset that can be searched within PubMed by using the Limits function.

Publishers who supply citations for articles and publisher sites that are linked to PubMed often allow the full text of selected articles to be viewed and printed out from your computer, although some charge various fees to nonsubscribers. Some publishers allow free full text access to articles that are older than one year, or to those that are frequently cited.

Using PubMed

Go to the PubMed website: www.ncbi.nih.nlm.gov/entrez. The page that opens on your screen should look similar to Figure 2.1. Use the bookmark function on your browser to mark this address so you won't have to retype it each time you visit the site, or you can add the PubMed icon to your toolbar in Mozilla. Look at the left margin of the screen under Entrez PubMed; click on Overview and then Help/FAQ (Frequently Asked Questions). Read these sections before proceeding further. You may want to print out the FAQ for easy reference.

If your web browser is not set to automatically accept cookies,* you will need to accept each one as it appears on the screen, or change your browser settings to accept them in order to access the widest array of PubMed features. If you would like to save your search strategy, click on the My NCBI link in the upper right-hand corner that says Register. Write down your password or tell your computer to remember it. A nice feature of My NCBI is that it will automatically update your search for any new citations added to PubMed since your last search using that strategy, and email these citations directly to you.

* A cookie is a kind of tag or label that allows the website to store and keep track of information that you provide.

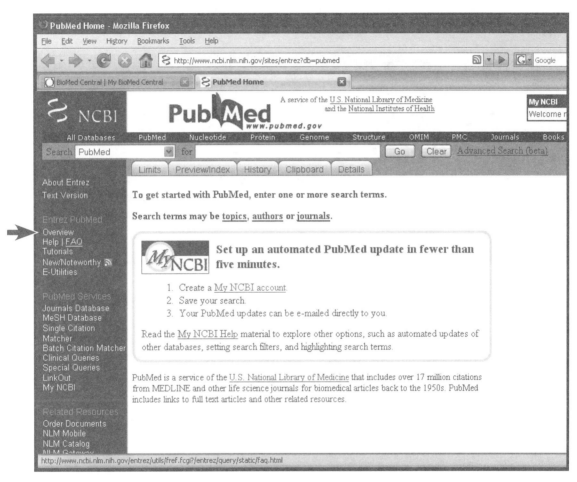

Figure 2.1 PubMed Home Page

Performing a Search

Notice the query box and toolbar just under the headline at the top of the page as seen in Figure 2.2. To perform a simple search, just type the search term in the query box and click Go.

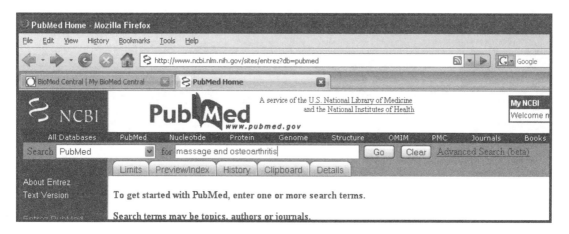

Figure 2.2 PubMed's Search Tools

A numbered list of articles with authors and titles will pop up, as in Figure 2.3. To the left of each numbered citation will be a small icon of a page.

The toolbar at the top of the page and sidebar to the left are available wherever you go in PubMed, so you can run a new search or click on other features at any point. You can use more than one term to search. For example, if you type in "massage therapy," PubMed will automatically combine the two terms, searching for "massage" and "therapy" in all the fields.

You can narrow your focus by clicking Limits in the Features bar directly below the query box. This allows you to restrict your search, say by the study participants' age or gender, or by the publication language, date or type. You can also limit your search to a particular subset of PubMed, such as AIDS-related citations, or citations in complementary medicine. Keeping the default "All" setting allows you to search for the term in all of the citation fields. In addition, you can focus the search according to title, author, keyword, or textword.

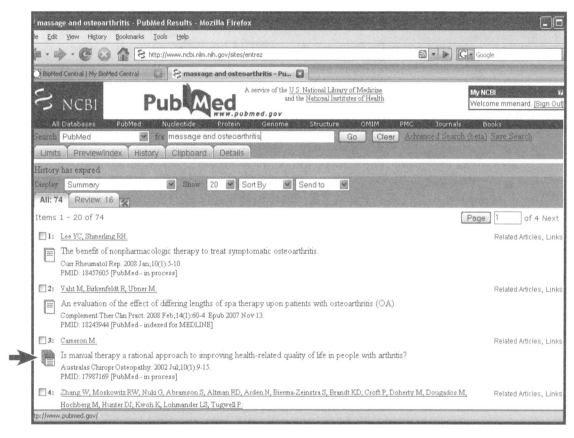

Figure 2.3 Viewing the List of Citations Found in a Search

Keywords are specific words used to index an article and provide a controlled vocabulary that employs consistent descriptive language. In both PubMed and MEDLINE, the keywords are from MeSH, which stands for Medical Subject Headings. A list of MeSH with specific terms used to identify articles on alternative and complementary medicine can be found by clicking MeSh Database from the left sidebar. If you are having trouble retrieving articles on a topic for which you know published research is available, check MeSH for keywords that might better describe your topic, or use textword to search for the term in the body of the abstract.

Textword simply means any word found in the text or body of the abstract, and is the most general way to search for relevant articles. Using textword as a search field will usually retrieve the largest number of articles.

You may also email the Reference Desk at NLM for help with search terms and strategies by clicking Write to the Help Desk at the bottom of the PubMed home page.

To preview the results of your search, click Preview. Preview allows you to see your search history all in one place with the number of results for each search. If the number of results seems excessive you may want to refine your search using what are called **Boolean operators**. These are conjunctions such as *and*, *or*, and *not*. Boolean operators allow you to restrict your search in specific ways: *and* requires that all terms be present; *or* requires that at least one of the terms be present; *not* excludes citations with that particular term. An example of a search strategy using Boolean operators might look like this: massage AND cancer OR oncology NOT prostatic massage. This strategy would retrieve articles pertaining to both massage and cancer but not those concerning massage of the prostate gland, a procedure performed by physicians.

Clicking History allows you to see all your search strategies and results in one place, as illustrated in Figure 2.4. You have to run at least one search to access History. History lists and numbers your searches in the order in which you ran them, and displays the search number, the search terms used, and the number of citations retrieved. To view the citations retrieved, click on the number of search results. This is the blue number on the far right of the page.* From either Preview or History, you can save searches, run new searches or combine results from previous searches. Be aware that unless you save it, the search history in PubMed is lost after eight hours of inactivity.

Clipboard is a feature that provides a place to collect selected citations from one or more searches. You can then print, save, or order these citations. To add a citation to Clipboard, click the check box to its left and then click Add to Clipboard. After you have added an item to Clipboard, the search record number color will turn green. If you want to keep citations you have placed in Clipboard, you must save them – items in Clipboard are lost after eight hours of inactivity.

* On the Web, text that is highlighted in blue will usually link you to another page or site.

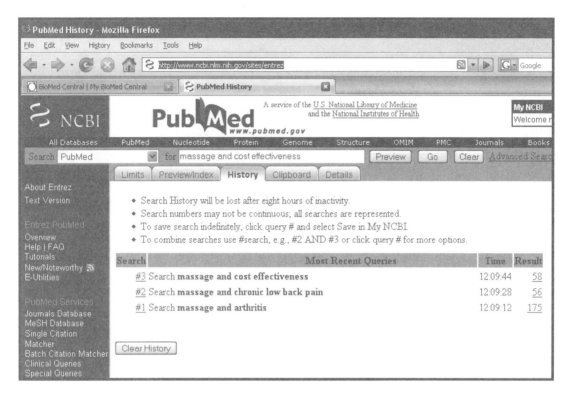

Figure 2.4 Viewing Your Search History

Viewing Search Results

PubMed displays search results in batches, usually twenty to a page. Click Display, and from the Summary drop-down menu select the Abstract format to view abstracts of the articles found in your search. Choose the MEDLINE format if you want to save citations to a bibliographic reference software program such as Reference Manager® or ProCite®. The search results page will show a group of citations listing the author, title, and journal information, organized by date with the most recent at the top. It will look similar to the page shown in Figure 2.3. Notice again the icon which looks like a page located to the left of each article. A blank page means no abstract is available; a page with lines on it indicates an abstract is present. A green stripe at the

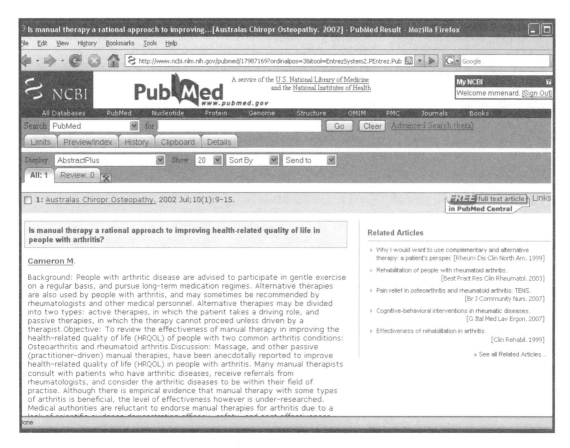

Figure 2.5 Viewing a Citation, Beginning with the Text of its Abstract

top of the icon means that the full text of the article is available for free, usually with a choice of HTML or .pdf formats. The HTML format contains electronic links to references cited in the article, while the .pdf format is a facsimile of the published article as it originally appeared in print. An orange stripe indicates that the authors' manuscript is available at no cost in PubMed Central, which provides the full text of journal articles by authors who have received NIH funding for their research.

Click on the name of the author to view the complete citation with the abstract, as shown in Figure 2.5. You will notice to the right of the citation are links to Related Articles. If you find an article that is exactly what you are looking for, Related Articles allows you to quickly go to another similar article. Links takes you to publishers' sites where you can view or print full text copies of selected articles or find other consumer health information. There may be a fee involved. A typical Links screen is shown in Figure 2.6.

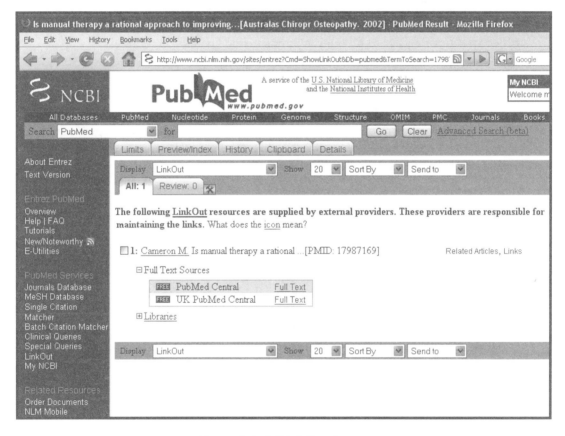

Figure 2.6 A LinkOut Screen

Use the Select Page feature (see Figure 2.4) to go to other pages containing more search results. When you want to keep search results, you can save the entire batch, which is the default setting, or you can use Add to Clipboard to save selected citations. To print citations from Clipboard, use the print function on your browser. You can also email selected citations to yourself or someone else.

Saving Search Strategies

Use My NCBI to save search strategies or view previously saved strategies. If you have not yet registered to use My NCBI (it is a free service), go to the upper right corner and click Register to fill out the online form. Then log in to access My NCBI. From your home computer you also set it to log in automatically whenever you go to PubMed. To save a search strategy, simply click Save Search at the top of the page next to the search textbox. Edit the name of your search, using a phrase that will be meaningful to you later. My NCBI will not accept numbers or dates as search names. You will also have the option to sign up for automatic email updates with new search results, and to choose how often you would like to receive them. Click on Save at the bottom of the box to save your settings.

Ordering Articles from PubMed

When you identify an article that meets your needs you often want to have a hard copy of it. Not all articles are available to be freely printed. If you have located one in a journal that is part of a university library's holdings, you may be able to make a copy of the article there. Some articles may be available with credit card payment on the Web and can be downloaded and printed directly from your computer. Some articles may be available from the publisher – if there is an icon for the publisher, click it to go to that website and access the article. If these options are not available, the National Library of Medicine (NLM) provides a document delivery service called Loansome Doc. For a small fee, you can arrange delivery through a regional medical library.

While using Loansome Doc for the first time is a much easier process than it used to be, it may still take some time to process your registration. First, from the PubMed homepage, click Order Documents from the left sidebar. An information page about the Loansome Doc system will pop up. Click Loansome Doc from the menu on the upper right. The registration portal will pop up and will look like the page in Figure 2.7. Follow the steps to search for a participating library in your area; check to see whether its services are available to the public or to unaffiliated health professionals. This screen also provides information about each library and its fees to help you choose the best one for your needs.

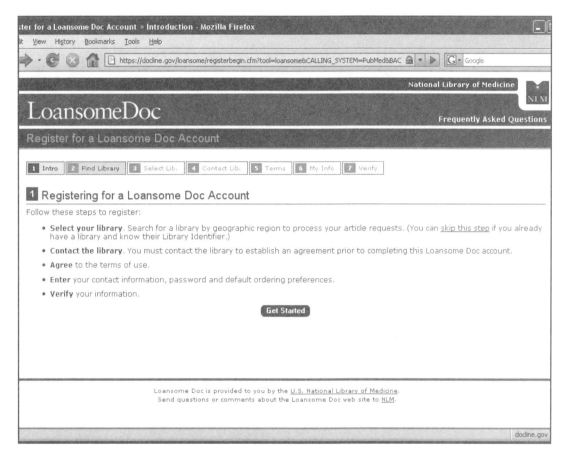

Figure 2.7 The Loansome Doc Registration Form

Each library determines its own document delivery service policies and fees. Usually these are reasonable, especially if you register as a health professional. The library I sometimes use charges $8.00 per article and mails a copy within two days of receiving my request. Faxing is quicker, but most libraries charge substantially more for this service and print quality is often poor.

Before you begin to use the Loansome Doc service to order hard copies of articles, you must agree to abide by the participating library's terms of use. You will then receive the Library Identifier number used to register for Loansome Doc. This is the second step. After you have identified a suitable library close to you, click its address (it should be highlighted in blue) and see if its agreement form is available online. If it is, print it, fill it out, and fax or mail it to the library, which will then contact you. This may take some time, but once you have the Library Identifier number you can complete the Loansome Doc registration form. After you have registered and have a Library Identifier number, it is a simple process to order an article during a PubMed search by clicking Order at the bottom of the page.

If you need more assistance or would rather speak directly to someone, in the United States call 1-800-338-7657 during normal business hours. In Canada, if your local health sciences library does not provide Loansome Doc services, you can set up an agreement with the Canada Institute for Scientific and Technical Information (CISTI), which is based in Ottawa. From the Loansome DOC Registration page, select Canada from the drop-down menu and go to the CISTI website to register. If you live outside North America, select Other Countries from the drop-down menu.

Other PubMed Features

When you are viewing any of the PubMed pages illustrated in Figures 2.1 through 2.6, look at the bottom of the left sidebar under Related Resources. Clicking Consumer Health will take you to MEDLINEplus, where, in addition to searching MEDLINE, you can access articles on various health-related topics, find locations or credentials for doctors and hospitals, and link to other organizations. You can even watch videos of common surgical procedures. Another Related Resource, called Clinical Alerts, contains the results of recent clinical trials conducted through the National Institutes of Health (NIH). In addition, ClinicalTrials.gov is a linked website that provides consumer information about the clinical trial process and a list of clinical trials currently being conducted for patients who may wish to enroll.

What if I Need More Help Using PubMed?

Click on Help – look through the menu to see if your question is listed there. You can also click on Write to Help Desk or send an email to pubmed@ncbi.nlm.nih.gov. Or you can call the NLM customer service desk at 1-888-346-3656, Monday through Friday from 8:30 a.m. to 8:45 p.m. and Saturday from 10:00 a.m. to 5:00 p.m. EST.

BioMed Central (BMC) and the Open Access Movement

The term "open access" refers to free, immediate, permanent, full-text, online access to scientific or scholarly material, primarily research articles published in peer-reviewed journals. It means that anyone, anywhere, who has Internet access may read, download, store, print, or link to the content of articles, with minimal copyright and licensing restrictions. The open access movement is international in scope, and has gained rapid momentum since the Budapest Open Access Initiative statement in February 2002, which provided the first definition of open access. You can view this document at www.soros.org/openaccess/view.cfm.

An advantage of open access is that original research is published more quickly and that articles are more widely disseminated, and therefore more likely to be read and cited by other scientists, a concept known as "research impact." Open access helps researchers as consumers of scientific research by providing access to journals not held by individual libraries, a boon to researchers in developing countries. A requirement of open access is that articles are permanently archived in a central repository using a common digital format. For example, in April 2008 the National Institutes of Health implemented a policy that requires researchers who receive federal funds to make resulting publications freely available through PubMed Central.

BioMed Central is a UK based publishing house with almost 200 peer-reviewed biomedical and scientific journals available on its website. All its biomedical journals are open access and provide the full text of each article at no charge, in HTML and .pdf format options. According to its website, the only copyright restrictions on peer-reviewed research articles appearing in any journal published by BioMed Central are that:

> The author(s) or copyright owner(s) irrevocably grant(s) to any third party, in advance and in perpetuity, the right to use, reproduce or disseminate the research article in its entirety or in part, in any format or medium, provided that no substantive errors are introduced in the process, proper attribution of authorship and correct citation details are given, and that the bibliographic details are not changed. If the article is reproduced or disseminated in part, this must be clearly and unequivocally indicated.[1]

As an example, the evidence circle diagram from the Walach article cited in Chapter 1 is from a BMC journal, *BMC Medical Research Methodology*.

Journal articles are published electronically immediately upon acceptance. BioMed Central's perspective is that open access to research is essential to ensure the rapid and efficient communication of research findings. All research articles in BioMed Central's journals receive rapid and thorough peer review. While some of its journals use traditional anonymous peer review, others, such as the medical BMC-series titles, operate using "open peer review" in which reviewers are asked to sign their remarks. In the form of a link from the published article, these journals also provide the pre-publication history of each paper, including each submitted version, with the reviewers' reports and authors' responses. Open peer review offers an interesting opportunity to see the editorial process at work, and is highly educational for those who wish to publish an article.

BioMed Central also functions as a permanent archive of published research and provides a digital archiving service called Open Repository, which can be accessed from the main list of services on the left margin. Some additional services are offered to subscribers which do require a fee.

Using BioMed Central

Go to the website at www.biomedcentral.com/. The layout is somewhat similar to PubMed, with a toolbar across the top and also down the left margin of the page. As you look at the search textbox, near the top of the left margin, notice that you can also search PubMed from this site. From the top toolbar, click About Us. Once you are on that page, look at the left margin and click on Guide to the Website under the "What We Do" heading, which you can see in Figure 2.8. This will give you a quick overview of how to use the site. If you register as a user (there is no fee), you have more search options and can perform advanced searches, then save search results and combine them. Registration also allows you to use the My BioMed Central feature, which is similar to My NCBI. My BioMed Central will search articles by subject area and send you a list of citations in those areas on a regular basis.

BioMed Central offers many different services and the website is well worth exploring. Journals on the site that publish articles on complementary therapies include *BMC Complementary and Alternative Medicine, Chinese Medicine, Chiropractic & Osteopathy*, and the *Journal of Ethnobiology and Ethnomedicine.*

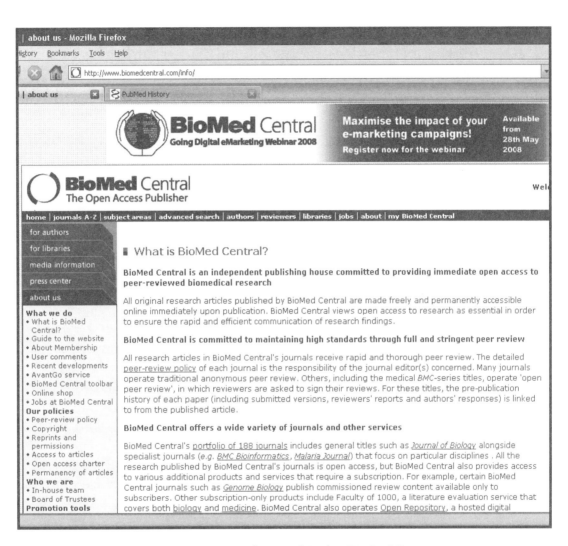

Figure 2.8 BioMed Central "What We Do" Page

Other Resources

Several medical journals publish online editions that allow access to selected articles at no charge as an incentive to visit their site and subscribe. Some of the better known journals in this category include:

Alternative Therapies in Health and Medicine
 www.alternative-therapies.com

Journal of the American Medical Association jama.ama-assn.org/issues

British Medical Journal www.bmj.com

The Lancet www.thelancet.com

New England Journal of Medicine www.nejm.org

The Townsend Letter for Doctors and Patients
 current newsletter: www.townsendletter.com/
 archives: www.tldp.com

The Physician and Sportsmedicine www.physsportsmed.com
 (access back issues search)

Direct access to current issues of several hundred full-text medical journals can be found at www.freemedicaljournals.com. Their journals are arranged in alphabetical order and by specialty. Most of the journals listed are conventional, but *Alternative Medicine Review* is available.

Another website, Alternative Health News Online (www.altmedicine.com), provides current information related to complementary therapies, including recent research studies of interest to complementary practitioners and links to several of the websites listed above. The website does not state when it was last updated, but most links appear to be functional.

A number of other sites offer access to lesser known sources of CAM journal articles, some of which can accommodate individual searches but may charge a fee. For a list of additional resources that can be searched, visit the website of the Rosenthal Center for Complementary and Alternative Medicine at Columbia University, one of ten NCCAM-funded centers in the United States. The address is www.cpmcnet.columbia.edu/dept/rosenthal. From the welcome page, click CAM Research and Information Resources, then click CAM Professional and Research Resources. This page was last updated in June 2007 and remains as an archive – it will not be updated again, so some links and information may degrade over time. The Internet Resources Grid link also contains a directory of databases with many useful links.

While you are scrolling down the Directory page, notice in particular the Cochrane Collaboration database. This is a complementary and alternative medicine field group that performs systematic reviews on CAM, based at the University of Maryland. It was mentioned briefly in Chapter 1. You can use this link, or visit the Cochrane site directly at www.cochrane.org/reviews/. Summaries of Cochrane Collaboration reviews can be viewed at no cost; however, there is a fee for full text access.

The Research Council for Complementary Medicine (RCCM), based in London, England was established in 1983 and has several features on its website. In conjunction with the University of Westminster, RCCM has created a library of comprehensive reviews on various topics and therapies called CAMEOL. Similar to the Cochrane library, these are periodically updated as new articles are published. You can visit their home page at www.rccm.org.uk.

Founded in 2004 by Marja Verhoef and Heather Boon, the Canadian Interdisciplinary Network for Complementary and Alternative Medicine Research (IN-CAM) provides networking opportunities through its website www.incamresearch.ca and hosts an annual symposium for researchers, policy makers, practitioners, and educators in CAM fields. IN-CAM also develops and maintains a database of outcomes measures of particular importance to CAM research.

Other specific therapies sources include the Consortial Center for Chiropractic Research, the Society for Acupuncture Research, and the Massage Therapy Foundation. Like the Rosenthal Center, the Consortial Center for Chiropractic Research is funded by NCCAM. The web address is www.c3r.org/home. A list of all projects currently sponsored by the Center is posted there. Additional web pages listing citations related to chiropractic research can be found at www.chiroweb.com/archives/10/04/05.html and at www.chiro.org. The website of the International Chiropractic Online Network, www.chiropage.com, contains links to a number of articles on chiropractic research and to several online journals.

The Society for Acupuncture Research (SAR) is based in Bethesda, Maryland. SAR sponsors an annual research conference and has a list of seventy clinical trials of acupuncture outcomes available for a fee; however, these are studies with positive outcomes only. SAR's website is www.acupunctureresearch.org.

The Massage Therapy Foundation has a comprehensive database of research across a variety of touch-based therapies. You can visit the Foundation's website at www.massagetherapyfoundation.org. From the menu on the left margin, click Research, then Database. The Foundation also publishes an online quarterly open access journal, the *International Journal of Therapeutic Massage and Bodywork*. It is available at www.journals.sfu.ca/ijtmb. The platform for the journal is provided through the Open Journal System of the Public Knowledge Project housed at Simon Fraser University in British Columbia, Canada. The Public Knowledge Project (www.pkp.sfu.ca/) seeks to improve the quality of academic research through developing innovative online publishing and knowledge-sharing environments.

Finally, the NIH maintains a database of federally funded research projects including those currently in progress, called Computer Retrieval of Information on Scientific Projects, or CRISP. CRISP covers a wide spectrum of scientific research funded by a variety of federal agencies – it is not limited to CAM research. This database can be used to identify specific projects or investigators, and to take note of emerging trends and research methods. To search CRISP, visit its website: www.crisp.cit.nih.gov. You can search for either current or past projects by clicking the appropriate query form on the left side of the page.

The Web offers a multitude of resources for anyone interested in learning more about finding and understanding health care research. The sites listed here are current as of July 2009 but may be subject to change. The information covered in this chapter is only a brief introduction to help you get started. Have fun exploring.

References

1.   www.biomedcentral.com/info/about/charter. Accessed May 31, 2008.

Exercises

1. *Create a search statement that is relevant to you and test it on both PubMed and BioMed Central. Follow any links resulting from your search to locate the published article or related resources.*

2. *Go to any of the other websites listed as additional resources and explore the site. Compare your findings with a fellow student.*

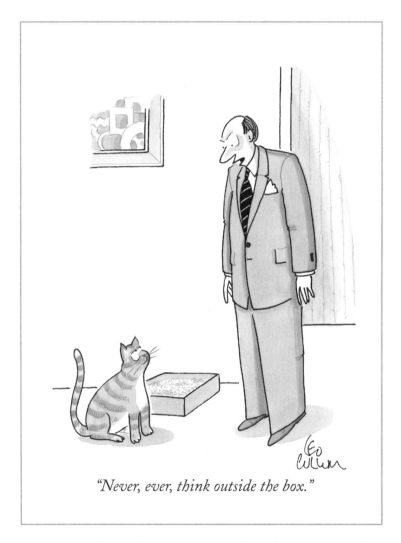

"*Never, ever, think outside the box.*"

Chapter 3:

Basic Concepts Involved in Evaluating Research

Scientific research, like other forms of exploration, is after all, a cybernetic – a steering – process, a means by which we find our way about, and try to make sense of, a bewildering and complex world.

P. B. Medawar

Learning Objectives

After completing this chapter, the reader should be able to:

- Differentiate among internal, external, and statistical validity.

- Identify four threats to internal validity.

- Differentiate between Type I and Type II error.

- Describe how design considerations such as random assignment and blinding are used to increase the internal validity of a quantitative study.

- Discuss the reasons why issues such as nonspecific response to treatment, sham treatments, and model fit validity are especially relevant in CAM research.

Chapter 3: Basic Concepts Involved in Evaluating Research

At this point, you have learned how to locate journal articles of interest and hopefully have become more intent on becoming a consumer of research that will inform your clinical practice. In order to critically evaluate scientific research, it is necessary to understand a few basic concepts before beginning to read actual studies. Readers who may be interested in pursuing health care research in more depth should pay special attention to this chapter – these same concepts are applied in designing and conducting original research. This chapter presents fundamental ideas involved in the critical evaluation of quantitative research, and discusses several special issues related to research on complementary therapies. While the main focus of this chapter is examining quantitative studies, the same type of critical thinking process can be applied to qualitative research, as will be discussed in more detail in Chapter 8.

The primary purpose of conducting a study is to be able to draw conclusions about the nature of the relationships between or among the variables studied. For example, in a quantitative study the researchers may investigate the relationship between a treatment such as massage therapy and its effect on outcomes such as pain or anxiety. It may also compare massage therapy's effectiveness with that of other treatment modalities in relation to the same outcomes. In a qualitative study the researchers may attempt to understand the process of developing a professional identity as an acupuncturist, and why some students succeed at this task while others do not.

In evaluating the general believability of any research study there are two major concerns. The first is the capacity of the findings to be generalized to a larger group than the one that participated in the study, called **generalizability**. In quantitative research, this is known as **external validity**. A common example of this concern is found in medical research involving a single group such as adult white males, which raises the question of the degree to which a particular study's results can be applied to adult males of different ethnicities, or to women or children. Also, studies that focus on a narrow range of participants or subjects may have more limited generalizability than studies that include a more diverse group. For example, a clinical trial on Type II diabetes would typically exclude participants with other medical conditions – known as **comorbidity**. If the excluded conditions actually occur frequently in people with advanced diabetes, the results of the trial would be applicable to only those with the early stage of the disease, or those without comorbid conditions, a much smaller subset of the entire population of Type II diabetics.

Qualitative research methods typically place less emphasis on the need for generalizability, depending on the particular research question. Often the goal of a qualitative study is to inform our understanding of a situation, a process, or the nature of an experience by observing and describing its unique aspects in detail, and frequently the results are intended to be applied to a specific setting or situation. While small samples are common, participants may be selected purposefully to provide differing perspectives and kinds of knowledge or experience, thus increasing the applicability of qualitative findings.

The second major concern is the capacity of the study to link cause and effect.[1] In the context of quantitative research this is known as **internal validity**. Qualitative approaches use the terms **credibility** and **trustworthiness** to refer to this concept, meaning that there is an internal cohesion and logic connecting the study's objective, methods, and results. Studies with good internal validity or credibility should exclude other hypotheses as plausible alternative explanations for their findings. For example, let's say that you are reading a study proposing that dogs are telepathic.[2] The outcome measured to demonstrate a dog's telepathic ability is the time at which the dog goes to the door to wait for its owner after he or she has decided to return home. To have good internal validity, the study's design should rule out plausible alternate explanations, for example, that the dog's seemingly telepathic behavior might be a response to a familiar routine. In Rupert Sheldrake's experiments testing this hypothesis, he gave the dog's owner a pager and signaled him or her to come home at randomly selected times, so that the designated time of return was not known by anyone until the pager went off. He used a video camera with a time stamp to verify when the dog went to the door to wait. Sheldrake also had the owner randomly vary the means of transportation home, sometimes walking or taking a subway or bus, to rule out familiar sounds such as the owner's vehicle as a cue for the dog. In a statistically significant number of cases, the dog would go to a specific spot at approximately the same time that the owner decided to go home. While many scientists find Sheldrake's experiments and results controversial, his methods are rational and replicable.

In designing or evaluating a study, there is almost always a trade-off between internal and external validity. As in the example of the clinical trial on Type II diabetes given previously, the greater the internal validity of the study, the more likely it is that the generalizability of the results will be limited to individuals who narrowly match the characteristics of the study participants. In other words, the stronger the causal link between intervention and outcome within a specific group, the less likely that the study results can be applied to other kinds of people. Conversely, the greater the generalizability of the study to the complexities of real world patients, the more difficult it becomes for the study methods to detect whether the intervention truly caused the outcomes among the various groups tested.

Threats to Internal Validity

Flaws in the design of a study can threaten its internal validity and weaken its credibility. Cook and Campbell[3] have described a number of threats to internal validity common in experimental research design. These are summarized below and should be kept in mind as you read and evaluate the study examples given later in this book. Certain types of studies are better than others at ruling out particular threats to validity; this aspect will be discussed in more detail in Chapter 4, where design features that help to promote internal validity will also be discussed.

Broadly speaking, plausible alternate explanations for the results of a quantitative study usually fall into one of three categories that are each related to the concept of internal validity: confounding, bias, or chance. Threats to internal validity are sometimes generally referred to as **confounds** and/or **sources of bias**.

A **confounding variable** blurs or masks the effect of another variable. For example, sales of ice cream and the number of burglaries in a geographic area may mirror each other closely – as one increases, so does the other, and a strong statistical association can be demonstrated. Does this mean that one causes the other? No, because both are correlated with warmer temperatures – the confounding variable in this case. Often, a confounding variable is one that is related to the baseline or the outcome variable of interest but is not measured. For example, golf is a sport that requires fine motor coordination, which tends to decrease with age. In a study where practicing tai chi is tested as an intervention to improve golf scores, participant age may affect fine motor performance as much as the intervention being tested. In this example, the researchers would want to include age as a variable, so that it could be taken into account and its effect separated from that of the tai chi in the analysis of the study data.

Bias, in the research sense, refers to a situation where there is systematic error in the measurement of a variable, such as the tendency to consistently underestimate the impact of the *placebo effect* in treatment outcomes. A well-known example of bias can be seen in the voter survey that occurred during the 1948 presidential contest between

Thomas Dewey and Harry Truman. Pollsters conducted the survey via telephone. In 1948, people who had telephones were more likely to be affluent and more likely to state that they would vote for Dewey, the Republican candidate. Truman's win was considered a great upset based on this one-sided overestimate of voters' preference. Some common examples of ways that bias may enter a study follow.

• *History*

History in this context is defined as an event that occurs during the course of the study, and influences the outcome, but is unrelated to the treatment or intervention. For example, you are reading a study testing a new treatment for depression. The participants in the study are college students at a major university. The treatment is administered over spring break. Many of the students in the study start new relationships during that time – how do you think that would affect their reports of how depressed they feel? Under such circumstances, the new treatment would likely appear to be much more effective than it actually is.

• *Maturation*

Maturation refers to events that occur naturally with the passage of time. Children get stronger and taller as they grow older; a person performing repetitions with weights becomes more fatigued the longer he or she works out during an exercise session; a surgical patient reports less pain as the incision becomes fully healed. In medicine, this is sometimes referred to as natural history or the natural course of a process or disease. A good example would be a study investigating massage therapy as a treatment for the common cold. A group of people just coming down with a cold is identified and given a daily massage for one week. At the end of that time, everyone's cold is gone. Obviously it would be a mistake for the researchers to conclude that they had found a cure for the common cold, since it is well known that most colds get better in seven days regardless of treatment. If the colds went away in two days, that might be a significant outcome. One way to rule out maturation as an explanation for a study's results is to use a comparison (control) group that does not receive the intervention or treatment.

• *Testing*

Testing refers to learned responses, such as participants becoming familiar with a process or instrument used more than once to measure an outcome of interest. The more often a test is given, the more familiar the participant can become with the correct response, or be inclined to recall particular items or mistakes when tested again. This is the reason that a test like the Scholastic Achievement Test (SAT), which is used to assess a student's academic ability, limits the number of times a person can take the test.

- *Instrumentation*

Instruments used to measure outcomes of interest should be both reliable and valid, whether the instrument is a physical device such as a blood pressure cuff or a tool like a questionnaire. **Reliability** refers to the consistency and accuracy with which an instrument measures a tangible construct, for example weight, or less tangible constructs such as anxiety or intelligence. A bathroom scale that showed you weighing 125 pounds on Monday and 159 pounds on Tuesday would not be considered reliable since it is highly improbable that anyone could gain 34 pounds overnight. **Validity** in instruments means that they measure what they purport to measure. As an example, a driving test should measure one's driving ability, not the language skills or vocabulary needed to understand the directions for taking the test.

Instrumentation can be a threat to internal validity when there is a change or problem with the degree of measurement possible with a given instrument. For example, human observers become more experienced over time and are thus able to discriminate smaller or finer differences at the end of a study compared to the beginning. Conversely, observers may become fatigued and less able to make consistent judgments. When instrumentation becomes a threat to internal validity the problem is sometimes referred to as **instrument decay**.

Another type of instrumentation problem is called a **ceiling effect** or **floor effect**, where the instrument cannot measure something above or below its scale. For example, a ceiling effect occurs when a test fails to measure the IQ of an extremely intelligent person because the test or instrument scale does not go high enough. A floor effect occurs when the lower end of the scale is artificially high, so that too many people who are being measured with the scale score zero. This is also sometimes called a **basement effect**.

- *Regression*

Many studies use some variation of the before-and-after treatment design, where participants are measured before an intervention and then again afterward. **Regression**, sometimes called **regression to the mean**, describes the tendency of very high or very low baseline or initial measurements to average out by the end of a study. For example, in studies of method effectiveness in teaching reading, groups of disadvantaged children often show marked improvement. This may attest to the degree to which they were disadvantaged at the outset rather than the efficacy of the specific teaching method. The basic idea is that extreme scores naturally tend to become less extreme given time. To give another example, if people with chronic pain enroll in a study evaluating pain relief at a time when they feel worse than they usually do, their inflated outcomes will make the new drug appear more effective than it actually is. In the context of assessing therapeutic effectiveness, this threat to validity makes the difference between the baseline measurement and the post-treatment measurement appear larger. If the instrument used to measure the outcome is unreliable, the increased amount of measurement error in the scores due to instrumentation will magnify the effect of regression to the mean.

- *Selection*

Selection bias is one of the most important and, at times, subtle threats to validity. Consider a public opinion firm that is conducting a survey to find out how extensive altruistic behavior is in urban populations, and, for the sake of convenience, polls people at a holistic health fair. The same factor that makes people interested in holistic health may also make them more likely to behave in altruistic ways, including volunteering to answer the pollster's questions. Selection bias also occurs when two groups are chosen that differ from each other in some significant way, are both given an intervention or treatment, and are then compared to each other. Any effect observed may be a result of the pre-existing difference between the groups rather than the treatment they have received. An issue common to almost all health care research is that people who volunteer to participate in research studies are likely to be different from those who choose not to participate.

- *Mortality*

Mortality in the research sense refers to attrition, or the tendency for people to drop out of or stop participating in research studies before the data collection is completed. Attrition can introduce selection bias by making the group different at the end of the data collection than it was at the beginning. For example, a new drug for depression has unpleasant side effects and the people with the most severe depression, who have less tolerance of additional unpleasantness, tend to drop out of the study at a higher rate than those with less severe symptoms. Consequently, the remaining people seem to demonstrate miraculous improvement as compared to the group baseline because their symptoms were milder to begin with and the drug thus appears to be more effective than it really is. Attrition can be a serious problem in long-term studies. The longer a study continues the more opportunities there are for participants to drop out or be lost to follow-up.

Statistical Validity

Another concern that can arise when evaluating a study is its **statistical validity**. Statistical validity is closely related to internal validity. It generally refers to the "number-crunching" aspects of a research study – whether the numbers and the formulas used in the statistical analysis of the study data were properly selected, computed, justified, and explained in order to rule out chance as an explanation for the results. Chance is one of the plausible explanations that always needs to be considered when evaluating a study's findings. Chance can be considered as a kind of random confounding error, as opposed to the systematic error of bias. Problems that can occur with the statistical validity of a research study include multiple comparisons and low statistical power.

In many of our examples of threats to internal validity, the result is that a treatment appears to have an effect when it actually does not. Falsely concluding that a genuine effect exists is a **Type I error**. Statistical tests are routinely performed on research data to rule out the possibility that seemingly meaningful results are actually due to chance. However, the more comparisons or statistical tests that are run on a given set of data, especially when several outcomes are measured, the greater the possibility that some differences will show up as statistically meaningful just by chance alone. Some statistical tests are designed to be used in cases where only one outcome is measured, while others are designed for the analysis of multiple outcomes. The type of statistical analysis used should make sense given the hypothesis being tested and the number of outcomes measured. More detailed information on recognizing issues related to statistical validity will be presented in Chapter 7.

Another problem arises when there are not enough participants in a quantitative study, also known as **small sample size**. A small number of participants means low **statistical power**. Power in this context refers to the ability of the statistical test to detect a genuine effect and is based on both the number of participants and the number of outcomes to be measured. Generally speaking, the more participants who complete their role in a study and the fewer the outcomes measured, the greater the statistical power to detect a true effect. In which survey of high school students voting in a student council election would you have more confidence, one that asked 10 students or one that asked 100 students?

If the statistical power of a study is low, a true effect may be operating that cannot be demonstrated by the data. Falsely concluding that no effect is present is a **Type II error**. Another way to think of Type II error is reflected in a common saying in science, "absence of evidence is not evidence of absence."

Yet another problem related to statistical validity can occur when there is a lack of treatment standardization. If a treatment is implemented in several different ways or formats by various research personnel, this can reduce the general effectiveness of the treatment or make it more difficult to measure accurately. Quantitative studies, and the interpretation of their results, must be based on the assumption that the treatment intervention is the same for everyone. Lack of standardization usually introduces a larger amount of variation in the data collected that can be considered as measurement error. For example, imagine a pharmaceutical study where some participants received different amounts of the same medication than the rest of the study group, with a few participants receiving an additional drug as well. These departures from the study protocol would muddy the waters and make interpretation of the data more difficult. This consideration is especially relevant to research in complementary medicine and will be discussed in more detail in Chapter 6. The crucial issues are the degree to which the intervention as defined for the purposes of the study can be standardized, and whether the degree of standardization is appropriate to the research question asked.

Other Design Considerations in Evaluating Research

Other design issues relevant to health care research include random assignment, blinding, placebo or nonspecific response, sham treatment, and model fit validity.

- *Random Assignment*

Random assignment to group is used in studies to reduce the potential effect of influences over which the investigator has no control, and also to avoid potential researcher bias in choosing who to place in which group. Random assignment ensures that each participant has an equal chance of being assigned to a treatment group or to another group that will be compared with the treatment group. This second group is called a **control group** or **comparison group**, and a study that uses a control or comparison group is referred to as a **controlled study**. The control group receives no intervention, or a different intervention, but its members are similar in all other important respects to the other participants in the study.

Treatment effect is measured by subtracting the mean or average of the control group from that of the treatment group (i.e., treatment group mean minus control group mean). If a large enough pool of participants is randomly divided into treatment and control groups, chance variations in demographic factors, the treatment environment, or lifestyle factors – the within group variation – should be equal between the two groups, thus canceling each other out. Generally, random assignment to treatment increases the internal validity of a study because it is very effective at ruling out other plausible explanations, even those that the researcher cannot anticipate.

In randomized controlled studies that use more than one comparison group, or **arm**, random assignment to group effectively makes the different study arms equivalent and helps to eliminate selection bias as an alternate explanation for the study's results. For example, a study might compare a new therapy with both the current standard of care and with no treatment. Waiting list control groups are often used as the "no treatment" control because these participants receive attention and have positive expectations of receiving future treatment. This helps control for the effects of the patient's positive expectation and attention received, which should be equal among all the groups. The no treatment group additionally controls for the effect of maturation. However, random assignment to group is not possible in every situation for both practical and ethical reasons.

Imagine a research study where participants were randomly assigned to receive a treatment suspected or known to be harmful, or to have a beneficial treatment withheld. No research ethics review committee or IRB would approve it. This is one reason that there will never be a randomized controlled trial of whether cigarette smoking induces lung cancer.

While the use of random assignment avoids many threats to internal validity, it is not a panacea for increasing the trustworthiness of a study. Random assignment does not address what are called **reactivity issues** in studies, which occur when participants react to the obtrusiveness of the study's data collection methods or when the normal conditions of the study are disrupted in some way, usually because participants figure out which group they are in at some point prior to completion of the data collection. For example, **diffusion of treatment** may occur when people in the comparison group realize that they are not receiving the active treatment and attempt to obtain it on their own. Or participants in a placebo control group may change, for example by becoming depressed, when they realize that they are receiving a less desirable treatment. Each situation could potentially affect the outcomes being measured, in the first case by artificially inflating the results of the comparison group and in the second by reducing them.

At other times randomization may fail during the course of a study. For example, participants might communicate with each other and compare notes, or systematic attrition within one group might occur because one treatment is less desirable. Participants may seek out other treatments in addition to the study intervention and use these during the study without informing the researcher.

Random assignment may not be appropriate when practitioner intention or client expectation are a defined component of the treatment, or when individualization of treatment, learning, or choice are necessary for maximum effectiveness, as in studies that evaluate educational or psychotherapeutic interventions. The complex nature of many complementary therapies makes the issue of random assignment one that needs to be considered carefully in evaluating its appropriateness to the research question.

In some studies, the randomization procedure used may be faulty. It is standard practice in research to base assignment to group on a table of random numbers. Methods such as flipping a coin or alternating participant assignment to group may not be truly random, especially when sample size is smaller. As a measure of the integrity of a study, baseline and/or demographic data is typically reported to show that the groups of participants are indeed comparable to one another. This information provides one of the best ways of checking to make sure that the randomization procedure worked.

- *Blinding*

Blinding refers to concealing the group assignment from the participants, the researchers, or both. It is used to rule out expectation as an alternate explanation for a treatment effect. Blinding is often used in conjunction with a sham treatment, which is usually referred to as a **placebo**. Without participants knowing which treatment they are receiving – active or placebo – expectation should be equal in both groups. When only the participants or the researcher is blinded, it is referred to as a **single blind study**; when neither the researcher nor the participants knows which group is receiving the active treatment, it is called a **double blind study**. Blinding poses an obvious challenge for complementary modalities that involve manual skills, or for conventional treatments such as surgery or physical therapy. In such cases, participants can sometimes be blinded depending on the specific intervention, but the practitioners cannot.

Although it may be impossible to use double blinding in some studies of hands-on therapies, the person who collects or assesses the data can and should be blinded. For example, if blood or saliva tests are done as part of an evaluation of treatment effectiveness, the technician need not be informed about which participants are in which groups. Statisticians who analyze study data are routinely blinded.

Just as random assignment can sometimes fail during a study, blinding can too. An investigator should check to see if blinding procedures worked throughout the course of the study or if participants were able to guess which group they were in. Depending on the study question and intervention tested, this can be accomplished at some middle point during the study or through the use of a brief exit interview or survey of participants at the conclusion of the data collection.

Informed consent requirements can also pose a challenge for blinding, in terms of following IRB mandates while simultaneously avoiding potential bias as a result of revealing too much information about the specific purpose of the study or its procedures. While deception is not permitted, researchers are allowed to conceal from participants whether they are receiving a specific or nonspecific intervention, as long as they have been told that they may be assigned to one of X number of groups.

Whether to inform prospective participants that they may be assigned to receive a placebo is a controversial issue in designing studies. Some argue that telling people they might receive a placebo creates a negative expectation that could bias the results, while others feel strongly that withholding such information is unethical. Most IRBs now require informing participants about placebo use if the study employs a two group, treatment versus placebo design, particularly in research related to serious or life-threatening conditions. In studies with the objective of identifying mechanisms of action in CAM therapies, especially those involving stable or chronic conditions, some concealment may be justified, particularly if those who receive a placebo also have a subsequent opportunity to receive the genuine treatment. For example, in a randomized controlled trial of reflexology for PMS that used a sham intervention as a comparison, the informed consent document stated that participants would be assigned to one of two treatment groups, both of which were potentially beneficial.

This was a truthful statement – the positive effects of expectation frequently do result in the improvement of symptoms such as pain and anxiety – yet it avoided telling participants that they had an equal chance of receiving a placebo. At the study's conclusion, participants who received the sham treatment reported that they found it pleasant and relaxing, and believed they had received the genuine treatment. Their symptoms improved somewhat but significantly less than those who received the true reflexology.

• *Placebo Response and Nonspecific Treatment Effects*

Traditionally, a placebo is a pharmacologically inert substance such as a sugar pill, or a treatment that is presumed to have no specific effect on the outcome of interest. As you might guess, placebos were first used in drug studies. However, early researchers were surprised to learn that some participants responded to the inactive sugar pill as though they had been given the actual drug, apparently from their expectation alone that they were receiving a drug that would help. The use of a placebo group is another way to control for participant expectation. Much has been written about placebo response in medicine; some authors estimate that it may account for 30-80% of response to any treatment.[4]

Another term that is sometimes used synonymously with placebo response is **nonspecific response**, or **nonspecific treatment effect**. These are more accurate and less contentious terms than placebo response. Nonspecific responses result from pervasive aspects of health care interventions such as patient and practitioner beliefs, attitudes and expectations, the nature and quality of the therapeutic relationship, or the degree and kind of patient social support. Because the nature of the healing relationship is that patients expect to be helped and practitioners intend to help them, nonspecific treatment elements are present and embedded to some degree in any treatment. Paterson and Dieppe[5] have argued that the biomedical model of splitting a treatment into specific and nonspecific effects does not work for the complex interventions found in many complementary therapies such as acupuncture, massage, and other nonpharmacological interventions such as physical therapy. They note that elements considered to be nonspecific in the biomedical model may be defined as specific or characteristic in different theoretical models, a concept we will come back to.

Nonspecific response is a physiologically active treatment in and of itself – it is not "all in one's head." In other words, it can produce tangible and measureable biological effects and from a clinical perspective (including the patient's), it is often quite desirable. However, it has a negative connotation in research because it is usually viewed as an alternative explanation to be ruled out, rather than as an intrinsic aspect of every treatment; it is considered "noise" rather than "signal." Nonspecific response presents a thorny problem in health care research for a variety of reasons, among them the surprisingly persistent idea that mind and body are separate entities. Recent research has demonstrated through the use of real-time brain imaging that the biological effects of nonspecific response are psychologically mediated.[6]

There is an extensive literature on nonspecific response that cannot be summarized in such a brief introduction to this fascinating topic. Interested readers wanting more information on the history and current state of the research on placebo response in health care may wish to peruse any of the several papers on this topic by Ted Kaptchuk and colleagues; for a neurobiological perspective, see the work of Fabrizio Benedetti. However, it is important to emphasize several points about the use of controls for nonspecific response. According to many psychologists and neurobiologists, patient expectation and learned responses do more to explain nonspecific effects of treatment than the belief that only certain types of people are likely to respond to a placebo. For example, research summarized by Patrick Wall[7] shows that nonspecific responses are stronger and more frequent in studies where the participants know that potent narcotics such as morphine are being tested as compared to non-narcotic medications like aspirin. In studies using a crossover design* the placebo effect is stronger when the placebo is given second rather than first, again suggesting learned behavior by patients. In addition, research has determined that those who are likely to respond strongly to nonspecific aspects of treatment are most easily identified by asking what their expectations are rather than by assessing their personality traits.

The traditional assumption of placebo as noise rather than signal assumes that there is a true therapeutic effect that can be separated out. This may not always be possible because all active substances or treatments have their own nonspecific components. Teasing out the relative contributions of specific and nonspecific effects can be difficult. Wall makes a strong case that participants in trials are quite sensitive to subtle cues from researchers or data collectors who may be blinded as to group but still have a general knowledge of what the study is investigating (as likely do the

---

* In a crossover design, two groups are used and each receives a different treatment. At some point during the study the two groups switch treatments ('cross over') and the results of each treatment are compared before and after the switch.

participants, based on their informed consent to participate in the study). As a result blind trials are rarely truly blind, and nonspecific treatment effects are not always independent of "true" treatment effect.

In some cases, a placebo control group is not the best comparison group in evaluating the clinical effectiveness of a treatment. If a "gold standard" treatment exists for a particular condition, a trial comparing a new intervention to the standard treatment is more useful from a clinical perspective and the standpoint of cost effectiveness. This design also avoids the ethical issue of blinding and concealment of placebo allocation discussed earlier.

A related issue is the **nocebo** effect, or the effect of negative expectations. Anticipatory nausea and vomiting in patients undergoing chemotherapy is one example of nocebo effect. Another can occur when practitioners give subtle cues indicating their own distress to participants in a research study when they are asked to perform a treatment which they believe to be ineffective.

Rather than discounting or dismissing the nonspecific components of complementary therapies, these could instead be measured or assessed to determine their relative contribution to the effectiveness of the treatment as a whole. A recent study by Kaptchuk and colleagues[8] did just that by comparing two types of placebo acupuncture interventions with a wait list control group. Their design used the three groups to separate placebo effects into three additive components: assessment and observation in the wait-listed group, a limited therapeutic ritual consisting of sham acupuncture alone, and sham acupuncture augmented with a supportive patient-practitioner relationship. Each group showed improvement in all outcome measures along a progressive dose-response curve, with the relationship group demonstrating the most improvement.

An important implication of this study is that nonspecific aspects of treatment, and the therapeutic relationship connection in particular, have merit because these can be used to improve the clinical success of other types of conventional medical treatments as well as being valuable in their own right. Massage therapy, like other complementary therapies, has many elements that promote nonspecific response, including an emphasis on therapeutic relationship. Consider, for example, that massage is a popular therapy used by many people with cancer. In hospital-based oncology programs that incorporate massage therapy, patients report reductions in symptom severity of 50% or more, sometimes after only five to fifteen minutes of foot massage.[9] Treatments that produce their results primarily from nonspecific effects should not be immediately regarded as lacking effectiveness, particularly if they reliably produce a positive clinical outcome at a lower cost with little or no risk of adverse effects compared to medication or surgery.

• *Sham Treatment*

Sham treatments are a variation of the placebo control designed to separate the specific effect of a treatment from nonspecific effects. They are considered somewhat controversial among many complementary researchers and practitioners. When a sham treatment is given the assumption is made that there is no specific effect being produced. Yet in order for the sham treatment to be credible to the participant it must closely mimic the real thing, thus running the risk that some specific effect may indeed be produced. A comparison is really being made between two treatments, one that is less active versus one that is more active, but the degree to which one is less active than the other is often unknown. If both treatments are active to a similar degree, then there will be no difference in the outcome between the two groups, leading to the erroneous conclusion that the active treatment is not effective when in fact it is.

This situation is a variation of the "efficacy paradox" described by Walach and colleagues[10] in which two treatments, X and Y, are both compared with control treatments (see Figure 3.1). In the diagram, notice the relative sizes of the specific and nonspecific treatment components. Treatment X has a small specific effect and both it and its control treatment have a large nonspecific effect. Treatment Y has a much larger specific effect, but both it and its control treatment have a small nonspecific effect when compared to X. The total specific and nonspecific effect combined of Treatment Y are smaller than the total specific and nonspecific effects together of Treatment X. Treatment X is actually more effective overall than Treatment Y, but Treatment Y will appear to be more effective, when only the specific effects are compared in the data analysis.

It is fairly easy to devise sham treatments for medical devices such as electrical stimulation. The treatment can be made credible if the machine lights up, makes noise, or otherwise appears to be active even though no current is being delivered. Acupuncture provides some excellent examples of the difficulty with sham treatment. The act of needling a point, even if it is not one that is relevant for the condition being treated, may have a specific effect in itself that could influence the outcome. In addition, patients who have received genuine acupuncture quickly learn from the sensation of the needle whether the acupuncturist has hit the point or not, so that

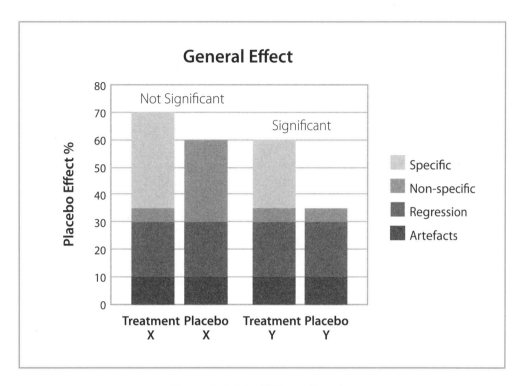

Figure 3.1 The Efficacy Paradox

from "Circular instead of hierarchical: methodological principles for the evaluation of complex interventions" Harald Walach et al,
BMC Medical Research Methodology *2006;6:29*

experienced patients who are assigned to a sham treatment group are not likely to remain blinded for very long.

Therapies such as massage and other forms of bodywork pose a considerable challenge to efforts to create credible yet sufficiently inactive forms of sham treatment. Social touch, such as parent/baby contact, has been used as a control for the nonspecific effects of touch in some studies of massage with premature infants.[11] Other strategies might involve using a type of touch that is either too light or too heavy to produce the intended result, or, as in the acupuncture example, the treatment might be applied to an area of the body that should have no effect on the outcome being measured.

These strategies can also be combined – using both the wrong pressure and the wrong location. This procedure has in fact been used in a novel randomized controlled trial (RCT) discussed previously in this chapter that tested reflexology in relieving symptoms of PMS.[12]

Sham treatments also present the ethical issue mentioned previously of either providing an ineffective treatment to people needing help or withholding a treatment that the practitioner believes to be beneficial. The latter was a real concern mentioned by the practitioners involved in the reflexology study just cited, although the blinded participants who received the sham intervention found it relaxing and showed some small improvement.

The problem with each situation presented in this discussion is again: an active treatment is being compared with one that is assumed to be less active, but how much less active is unknown. Blinding and ethical issues may also require consideration. Thus, the use of sham treatment is not always an ideal solution when attempting to separate specific from nonspecific effects. Readers should thoughtfully consider the use of control groups in terms of whether they are appropriate to the study hypothesis tested and whether the type of control procedures employed, or the manner in which they are implemented, provides a plausible alternate explanation for the study results.

• Model Fit Validity

Model fit validity is a design consideration first discussed by Claire Cassidy[13] and more recently by Walach and colleagues.[10] It refers to the idea that the underlying assumptions or model of the research methods being used should match those of the therapy being studied. This concept is an issue in much of the research on complementary therapies.

Cassidy contends that lack of model fit is like using the rules of baseball to understand or explain football. For instance, in many complementary therapies patients/clients are encouraged to be active participants in their care and treatment is individualized to meet each person's needs – the treatment, which can often vary from session to session, is tailored to each person so that it is as effective as possible for that individual at that time. These two ideas run counter to the assumption in most quantitative health care research that patients are relatively passive and interchangeable recipients of treatment for the purposes of a study. A one-size-fits-all approach works to some extent for pharmaceutical interventions, but this model does not translate well to most complementary therapies. Rather than maximizing clinical effectiveness, the lack of standardized treatment in complementary therapies is perceived as a source of measurement error from the biomedical perspective. If a complementary treatment is significantly altered to fit the assumptions of a study's research model or if it is not allowed to be performed as it is defined by its practitioners, then the study is not a valid assessment of the treatment. It is only a valid assessment of the specific protocol used and not the complex intervention as it is practiced in the real world.

For example, in many studies of massage therapy, the term "massage therapy" is not explicitly defined from a theoretical perspective. In the United States, historical definitions from both the American Massage Therapy Association[14] and the National Certification Board for Therapeutic Massage and Bodywork[15] state that a healing relationship is an essential component of the practice of massage therapy. Rarely, however, does the massage intervention in research studies include or imply "healing relationship" as a necessary element of the treatment. In many of the early studies on massage therapy, treatment was provided by individuals (often nurses) without specific massage therapy training or experience, using standardized protocols that bear little resemblance to the way massage is clinically practiced. It is not surprising that many of these studies showed ambiguous results that were difficult to interpret.

Model fit validity is closely related to a concept known as **ecological validity**. If a health care study has ecological validity, then its setting, participants, methods, and procedures should resemble the clinical situation under investigation. When a study has good ecological validity, it is likely to have more generalizability as well. Studies that use isolated components of a whole system and do not employ treatments as they are clinically practiced, either explicitly or implicitly, tend to ignore crucial aspects of the treatment and its theoretical model. They are reductionist and are not an honest test of the treatment or intervention under investigation. This is another example of the tension between internal and external validity, and the usefulness of the circle of methods model.

Summary

This chapter has presented fundamental concepts necessary to understanding the logic that supports the design of quantitative studies. While qualitative research employs different approaches based on the analysis of language rather than numbers, the same standard of common sense can be applied. In critically evaluating health care research, the three most likely categories of alternate explanations for a study's results are chance, bias, and confounding. By becoming familiar with common threats to internal and statistical validity, and with the principles of random assignment and blinding, readers will be able to spot problems in a study that render it less plausible. In evaluating research on complementary therapies, special attention should be paid to issues such as the use of placebo or sham treatments and model fit validity. Well-designed CAM research employs procedures appropriate to the study's research question and is consistent with both the theoretical model and customary clinical practice of the intervention examined.

References

1. Krathwohl DR. *Methods of Educational and Social Science Research*. New York: Longman Publishing Group; 1993.

2. Sheldrake R. *Dogs That Know When Their Owners are Coming Home*. New York: Three Rivers Press; 1999.

3. Cook TD, Campbell DT. *Quasi-experimentation: Design and Analysis for Field Settings*. Boston: Houghton Mifflin Company; 1979.

4. Moerman D et al. Placebo effects and research in alternative and conventional medicine. *Chinese Journal of Integrated Traditional and Western Medicine*. 1996;2(2):141-148.

5. Paterson C, Dieppe P. Characteristic and incidental (placebo) effects in complex interventions such as acupuncture. *BMJ*. 2005 May 21;330(7501):1202-5.

6. Enck P, Benedetti F, Schedlowski M. New insights into the placebo and nocebo responses. *Neuron*. 2008 Jul 31;59(2):195-206.

7. Wall P. The placebo and placebo response. In: Wall P, Melzack R, editors, *Textbook of Pain*. Edinburgh: Churchill Livingstone; 1994. pp. 1297-1308.

8. Kaptchuk TJ, Kelley JM, Conboy LA, Davis RB, Kerr CE, Jacobson EE, Kirsch I, Schyner RN, Nam BH, Nguyen LT, Park M, Rivers AL, McManus C, Kokkotou E, Drossman DA, Goldman P, Lembo AJ. Components of placebo effect: randomised controlled trial in patients with irritable bowel syndrome. *BMJ*. 2008 May 3;336(7651):999-1003. Epub 2008 Apr 3.

9. Cassileth BR, Vickers AJ. Massage therapy for symptom control: outcome study at a major cancer center. *Journal of Pain and Symptom Management*. 2004 Sep;28(3):244-9.

10. Walach H, Falkenberg T, Fønnebø V, Lewith G, Jonas WB. Circular instead of hierarchical: methodological principles for the evaluation of complex interventions. *BMC Medical Research Methodology*. 2006;6:29.

11. Scafidi F et al. Massage stimulates growth in preterm infants: a replication. *Infant Behavior and Development*. 1990;13:167-188.

12. Oleson T, Flocco W. Randomized controlled study of premenstrual symptoms treated with ear, hand, and foot reflexology. *Obstetrics and Gynecology* 1993;82:906-11.

13. Cassidy C. Unraveling the ball of string: reality, paradigms and the study of alternative medicine. Advances, *Journal of Mind-Body Medicine*. 1994;10:5-31.

14. American Massage Therapy Association. Evanston: The Association; 2008. AMTA Definition of Massage Therapy. *www.amtamassage.org/about/definition.html*.

15. National Certification Board for Therapeutic Massage and Bodywork, *Background Information for NCBTMB's New Exam Content*. McLean, Virginia: National Certification Board for Therapeutic Massage and Bodywork; 1997.

Exercises

1. Define internal and external validity, and explain why increasing one tends to decrease the other.

2. Think about a study you have previously read or heard summarized in the media, and describe any threat to internal validity it contained.

3. Discuss the difference between Type I and Type II error.

4. In studies of manual therapies such as massage therapy or physical therapy, who is it possible to blind regarding group assignment? Which study personnel should always be blinded?

5. Explain how random assignment increases the internal validity of a quantitative study.

6. Why is model fit validity necessary in CAM research?

7. Discuss factors in your practice that could enhance a client's nonspecific response to your work.

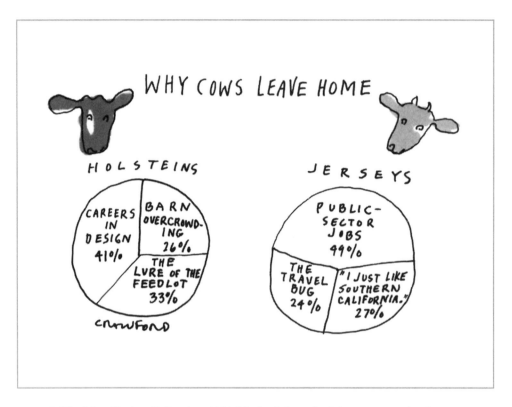

WHY COWS LEAVE HOME

HOLSTEINS

CAREERS IN DESIGN 41%
BARN OVERCROWDING 26%
THE LURE OF THE FEEDLOT 33%

CRAWFORD

JERSEYS

PUBLIC-SECTOR JOBS 49%
THE TRAVEL BUG 24%
"I JUST LIKE SOUTHERN CALIFORNIA." 27%

Types of Journal Articles and Study Designs

*Observation is a critical and purposive process; there is
a scientific reason for making one observation
rather than another . . . Experimentation, too, is a
critical process, one that discriminates between possibilities
and gives direction to further thought.*

P. B. Medawar

Learning Objectives

After completing this chapter,
the reader should be able to:

- Describe three general types of articles found in peer-reviewed journals.

- Identify five types of clinical research designs.

- Explain the strengths and weaknesses of these designs in providing evidence of cause and effect.

Chapter 4: Types of Journal Articles and Study Designs

When we think of health care research and the journals in which such research is published, we usually think first of reports of experimental studies. In this chapter and the next, we will look at the structure of experimental studies and other types of clinical research in more detail. We will also consider the relative strengths of each type of study design in judging whether cause-and-effect relationships exist among the study variables. Recognizing and understanding study design types alerts you to the potential strengths and weaknesses you are likely to encounter as you read and evaluate a given study.

A major consideration when evaluating a study is to what extent the research design and methods used are a good fit with the study question. The research question may be clearly articulated and highly significant, but if the design and/or methods are poorly suited to answer it, the findings can be inconclusive, misleading, or not interpretable. Particularly in complementary therapy research, the appropriateness of the treatment protocol to the question should be thoughtfully examined. As discussed previously, this issue of model fit validity is important for several reasons. Many of the complementary disciplines do not have large bodies of research, so that even one or two poorly conceived studies can have a negative impact on understanding a therapy's efficacy or practices. A protocol that is inappropriate to the study question also diminishes the usefulness of that research to practitioners, and makes translating research into practice more difficult.

Reports of experimental studies are not the only published writings you will come across as you read. Before we begin our focus on clinically related research, we will consider other categories of articles that are found in peer-reviewed journals. Two of these that are especially useful to practitioners and other research consumers are letters to the editor and literature reviews.

Letters to the Editor

Letters to the editor are often profitable to read. They can provide commentary on previous articles, share clinical situations that the author has encountered, or contribute new data in the form of brief reports or observations. Because these are not peer-reviewed, one should be cautious about giving one opinion too much weight. Letters that offer critiques of the methods used in previously published articles can be especially helpful. Such critiques can bring to our attention issues that we had not previously considered. Depending on the persuasiveness of the author's argument, a letter can change our opinion. Some letters will also cite other articles to back up the author's arguments, and following up on these references can add to the reader's understanding of the issues. References listed in letters can sometimes provide a source of more obscure or hard-to-find citations from other published studies.

Literature Reviews

Literature reviews can be an invaluable resource. They provide an overview of a particular research question and identify key studies in that area. Although review articles will show up in a general search, they can also be searched for specifically by using "review" or "meta-analysis" as keywords. Literature reviews fall into three categories:

- the narrative review or survey of the literature

- the meta-analysis

- a more specialized type of meta-analysis, the systematic review

Bibliographies of review articles are also a good source of related studies. For someone looking for a synopsis of current thinking on a research question, a recent literature review is an excellent place to start. It can tell you, among other things, which articles are worth your time reading in their entirety.

• *Narrative Reviews*

The **narrative review** examines a group of studies in a particular subject area and, as all literature reviews do, attempts to come to some conclusion based on a synthesis of the group as a whole. The author determines which studies are selected to form the group – this feature can be both a strength and a weakness. The primary strength of the narrative review is that the author can discuss the methods and conclusions of important studies in detail, and give an opinion about their relative merits. A major weakness of narrative reviews is the risk associated with author selection; in some cases, the author may be unaware of or unable to access all the relevant studies. Poorer quality studies may be included and treated as equal to better quality studies. The author may also choose to ignore studies with outcomes that are not consistent with the hypothesis presented, although this practice is not considered acceptable and is (one hopes) not common.

There are several examples of narrative reviews that are pertinent to the field of massage therapy. A well known and excellent example is the review of research on touch compiled by anthropologist Ashley Montague in his book *Touching*.[1] Montague integrates research from several fields, including biology, psychology, anthropology, and sociology, and makes a compelling case for his argument that touch is a biological necessity for human survival and optimal well-being.

A narrative review that attempts to document the psychological and physiological effects of massage was done in 1998 by Tiffany Field.[2] This review is noteworthy for its interesting discussion of possible mechanisms that might explain the effects in the studies listed. However, a weakness of the review is that it does not consider studies that produced negative results, and few studies other than those conducted by the Touch Research Institute, with which she is associated, are included. A more balanced example is a review written by a practitioner, Phyllis Keenan. It is a compilation of studies on the benefits of massage and use of a doula during labor and birth.[3] This review presents both positive and negative study results, for instance noting that while perineal massage performed during pregnancy reduces the rates of tearing and caesarean section, perineal massage performed during labor shows no benefit.

• *Meta-analyses*

The **meta-analysis**, developed as a way to improve upon the weaknesses of the narrative review, has increasingly gained respect as a form of literature review. Meta-analysis is possible as a result of the development of computerized databases, which make locating studies much easier. This review format is more necessary than ever before in health care due to the expanding volume of research studies.

In a meta-analysis, studies on a particular question are grouped according to pre-established criteria and a literature search using one or more major online databases is conducted to locate the articles that meet those criteria. This practice is analogous to specifying eligibility criteria for clinical study participants prior to their recruitment into the study. Defining the criteria for inclusion in advance reduces the potential for selection bias on the part of the investigator.

Results of the studies that meet the stated criteria are then pooled, that is, combined so that the statistical power of the group of studies is much greater than each individual study alone. Meta-analysis is often used to estimate the size of a treatment effect or to settle a question when there are several contradictory or inconclusive studies with small numbers of participants. An important consideration in evaluating a meta-analysis is whether the studies that have been pooled are similar enough in terms of their hypotheses tested and outcomes measured. One criticism of this method is that while it can be an improvement over the more subjective narrative review, meta-analysis can sometimes pool such disparate studies that the authors are in effect combining apples and oranges. If the research question is about fruit salad, so to speak, there is no problem. If not, the results can be misleading. This is a particular risk in fields like massage therapy where the specific combinations of modalities used in an individual treatment session can vary so widely.

Another concern with meta-analysis is that **publication bias** has the potential to skew the results. Publication bias refers to the tendency for journals to reject studies with negative or inconclusive results and to be more likely to publish those with positive results. Because it is therefore probable that studies with negative findings are less likely to be included in any subsequent analysis, their absence can prejudice the results, for example by making an intervention appear more effective than it really is.

• *Systematic Reviews*

The **systematic review** is a more refined version of the meta-analysis. It attempts to compensate for publication bias by making additional efforts, such as locating dissertations, hand searching journals that are not indexed in online databases, and personally communicating with authors of unpublished studies to identify every relevant study on a given research question. These are then usually weighted in terms of the strength and quality of the evidence presented. For example, a study employing random assignment of participants to an intervention or a control group would be weighted more heavily than one without these design features. Standardized methods are used for weighting studies based on internal validity and appropriateness of their statistical analysis methods. Randomized controlled trials are usually given more weight in a systematic review because of their greater capacity to link cause and effect, which places them higher on the hierarchical model of levels of evidence.

• *The Cochrane Collaboration*

Systematic reviews have been popularized by the Cochrane Collaboration, a voluntary group of health care providers, consumers, and scientists whose name commemorates the late British physician and epidemiologist Archie Cochrane. Dr. Cochrane was a pioneer of the evidence-based medicine movement who strongly believed in the importance of systematic reviews in shifting medical care towards practice based on research evidence. For more information on the Cochrane Collaboration, including abstracts of systematic reviews, visit their website: www.cochrane.org. A related group, the Chalmers Research Group based at the University of Ottawa, develops high quality systematic reviews and health technology assessments. Dr. David Moher, who is the director of the CRG, also leads the Cochrane Collaboration's Bias Methods Groups, which deals with problems of bias in systematic reviews.

Since its inception in 1993, the Cochrane Collaboration has completed over 600 reviews, and another 600 are planned. A working group interested in complementary medicine has been formed and a surprisingly large number of systematic reviews has been conducted. An early review, on the use of massage for premature infants, was last updated in 2004.[4] An abstract of this study can be viewed at the Cochrane website.

Another Cochrane review has been conducted on the use of massage for low back pain.[5] This study uses a slightly different method of systematic review called **best evidence synthesis**.[6] Best evidence synthesis developed as a way to combine the quantitative features of meta-analysis with the advantages of the qualitative narrative review. It is used when the studies that are located turn out to be too different from one another or lack sufficient data to be pooled in the manner done in a traditional meta-analysis. Instead, reviewers evaluate the selected studies by carefully considering the evidence presented in each one, and then draw an overall conclusion about where the weight of the evidence lies. Systematic reviews can be expected to continue to gain popularity as a way to synthesize a large quantity of research on disputed questions and render verdicts.

Clinically Related Health Care Research

Now let us turn to clinically related health care research, which comprises the bulk of the studies in which we are likely to be interested. While there are several different ways to classify research studies, for our purposes we will use an epidemiological approach, which is used primarily to classify quantitative health care research.

Guidelines for Evaluating Literature Reviews

In-depth evaluation of literature reviews is a detailed and technically challenging process whose methods continue to be refined. Nonetheless, several general guidelines can be applied to assess the quality of a review:[7]

1. *The research question addressed by the review should be specific and clearly defined. If possible, check out the background and expertise of the reviewers, who should represent a balanced and comprehensive team suitable to conducting a review on the subject in question. A statistician familiar with systematic review procedures is a necessity.*

2. *The methods used to locate studies should be described, along with the criteria for inclusion or exclusion of studies from the review.*

3. *If studies are ranked or weighted, the internal validity of the studies included should be assessed according to objective and reproducible methods, and the weighting methods should be described.*

4. *If a meta-analysis was performed, the pooled data should be combined appropriately (apples with apples). A table that lists the individual studies with brief summaries describing the participants, methods, and results of each study helps the reader to judge similarities.*

5. *Just as in any research study, the reviewers' conclusions should be supported by the data presented.*

Epidemiologists are scientists who study the causes of disease. Although the principles of research design are the same in every discipline, the field of epidemiology has specialized methods to determine whether a relationship exists between a particular cause and a disease, and if so, to assess the strength of that relationship. The terms that epidemiologists prefer to use, rather than cause and disease, are **exposure** and **outcome**. An exposure can refer to a factor such as smoking that predisposes someone to develop an outcome like heart disease or cancer, or it can refer to a protective factor such as exercise that reduces the risk of developing the condition. An outcome can refer to development of a disease or to any clinical endpoint of interest such as heart rate, urinary cortisol level, or quality of life. Given its role in preventing and controlling the spread of infectious disease, it is understandable that epidemiological research places a major emphasis on determining whether a cause-and-effect relationship exists between an exposure and an outcome.

Classification of Studies

Epidemiologists have developed several ways of classifying the various types of studies and the terminology used to describe them. No matter what methods or design strategies are used to answer a research question, the goal of almost all clinically related research is to describe or explain events. As a result, studies can be grouped into two broad categories: **descriptive** and **explanatory**.

Descriptive studies do just that: they provide a record or description of events or activities. Explanatory studies seek to elucidate connections between events or variables and can be further divided into **observational** and **experimental** studies. In an observational study, the researcher attempts to explain a connection between naturally occurring events, such as exposure to a risk factor or predictor and the subsequent development of an outcome, without influencing or intervening in those events. In an experimental study, the researcher directs events, for example, by giving a treatment and then assessing its effects. Figure 4.1 illustrates these different types of studies. Explanations and examples of the various kinds of descriptive, observational, and experimental studies follow.

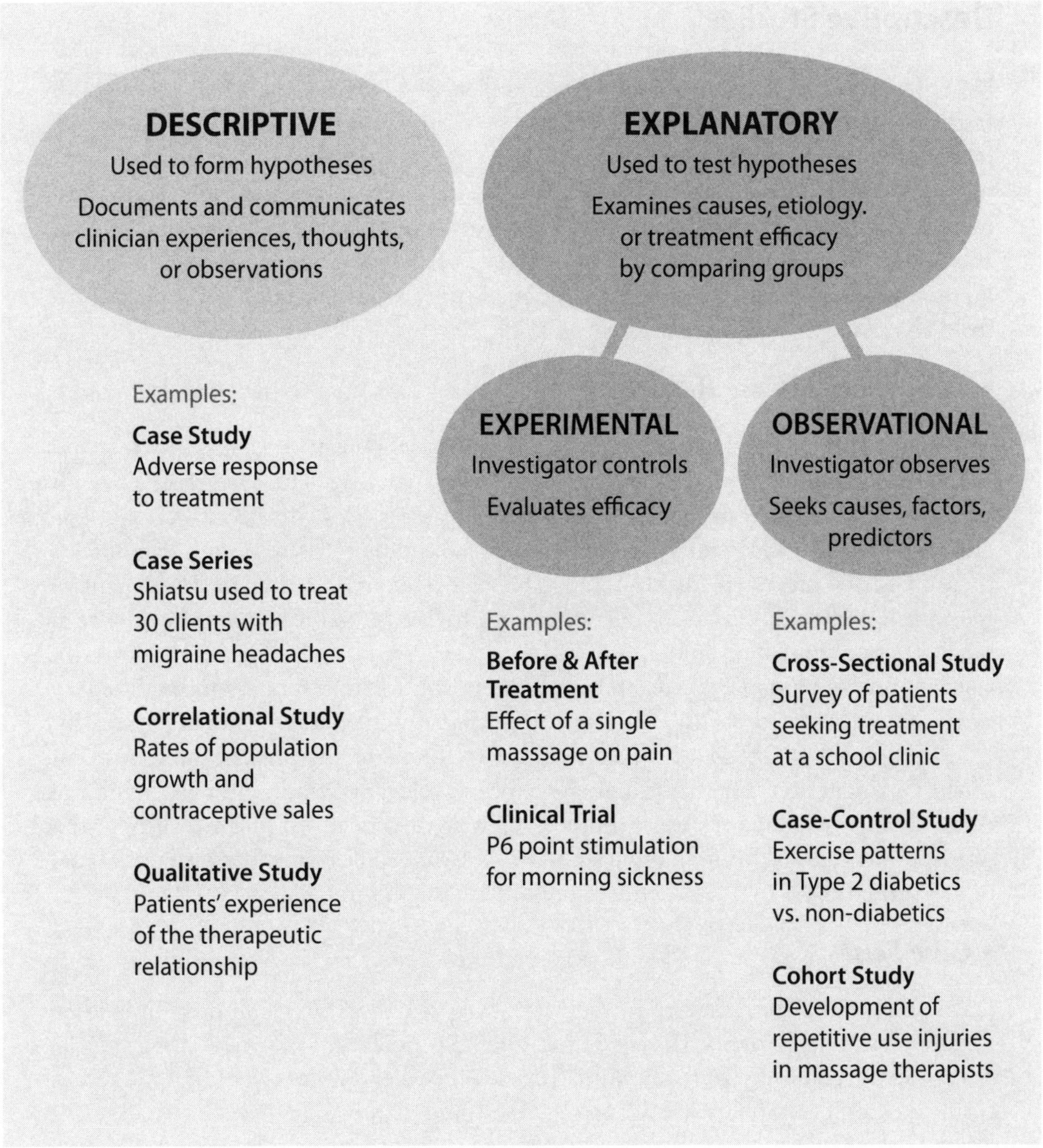

DESCRIPTIVE
Used to form hypotheses

Documents and communicates clinician experiences, thoughts, or observations

EXPLANATORY
Used to test hypotheses

Examines causes, etiology. or treatment efficacy by comparing groups

Examples:

Case Study
Adverse response to treatment

Case Series
Shiatsu used to treat 30 clients with migraine headaches

Correlational Study
Rates of population growth and contraceptive sales

Qualitative Study
Patients' experience of the therapeutic relationship

EXPERIMENTAL
Investigator controls

Evaluates efficacy

OBSERVATIONAL
Investigator observes

Seeks causes, factors, predictors

Examples:

Before & After Treatment
Effect of a single masssage on pain

Clinical Trial
P6 point stimulation for morning sickness

Examples:

Cross-Sectional Study
Survey of patients seeking treatment at a school clinic

Case-Control Study
Exercise patterns in Type 2 diabetics vs. non-diabetics

Cohort Study
Development of repetitive use injuries in massage therapists

Figure 4.1 Types of Study Designs

Descriptive Studies

Descriptive studies are considered weaker evidence of a cause-and-effect relationship largely because they lack a control or comparison group, a necessary feature for increasing internal validity. However, they can suggest further hypotheses to be tested, provide detailed information to help refine the design of an explanatory study, and, in combination with consistent results from observational or experimental studies, can add to the cumulative weight of evidence on a given question. Some kinds of qualitative research, such a phenomenological study, would be considered descriptive from an epidemiological perspective.

• *Case Studies (Case Reports)*

The simplest form of descriptive study is the **case study** or **case report**, which describes the events related to the care of a single patient. The case report usually features some unusual aspect of health history, assessment, or effect of treatment, although it will occasionally be used to present a typical or textbook example of a case and its successful resolution, or to report an innovation in assessment or treatment. Although the case report does not provide the same weight of evidence as a randomized controlled trial, it is valuable as a basis for developing new hypotheses. Case reports or studies may also be used to report adverse responses to treatment or to document unusual events, thus alerting other practitioners. What separates the case study from an anecdote is a compelling rationale for its presentation, a review of the pertinent literature, thorough description, relevant detail, and a discussion of contradictory evidence or observations along with directions for future investigations or recommendations for managing similar cases. A specific type of experimental case report, called the *n-of-1 trial*, will be presented in detail in Chapter 9.

• *Case Series*

Case series take the case study method a step further by combining individual studies of similar patients; they are often the first indication of a new disease or an adverse effect resulting from a new procedure. A good example is the July 1981 report from the Centers for Disease Control[8] describing an unusual number of cases of Kaposi's sarcoma among young, previously healthy gay men at a time when this form of cancer was typically seen in the elderly. This case series was one of several reports that heralded the beginning of the AIDS epidemic. Case studies and case series raise potential research questions but alone cannot usually provide evidence of a valid association or causal relationship.

Guidelines for Evaluating
Case Reports and Case Series

1. *Is the research objective or question clearly stated?*

2. *Is the subject interesting or relevant to your practice?*

3. *Is there a clear statement of the clinical importance of the case(s)? Are references provided?*

4. *Is all relevant patient data or history reported in sufficient detail?*

5. *Is any assessment done or treatment provided described adequately? Could you replicate it?*

6. *Are other plausible explanations for the results considered?*

7. *Are the strengths and weaknesses, implications, and relevance to other similar cases or studies discussed?*

8. *Are directions for future studies in this area or the management of similar cases discussed?*

These considerations used in evaluating case reports and studies are the same ones used to design or construct a case report, and will be discussed in more depth in Chapter 9.

• Correlational Studies

The **correlational study**, or *population survey*, uses existing aggregated group data from large populations. These studies are very useful as a quick way to see whether an association between an exposure and outcome exists. For example, a well-known correlational study first described patterns of death from coronary heart disease in 1960 in relationship to per capita cigarette sales across the United States.[9] As sales of cigarettes (exposure) increased during that time, so did death rates (outcome). Correlational studies are often a next step in testing a new hypothesis because they are relatively low cost, simple, and quick to conduct using previously collected data available from public agencies.

A correlational study describes or demonstrates a statistical association between an exposure and an outcome, but does not explain it. One cannot assume from correlation alone that a causal relationship exists between the exposure and the outcome. Other factors may be involved. For example, as the number of churches in a city increases, so does the number of alcoholics.* It would be a mistake to conclude on this evidence alone that going to church causes alcoholism. Numbers of churches and alcoholics are both functions of population increase; if you compare a small city with a large one, you will find that the large city has more churches and more alcoholics since it has more people. It is also not clear which came first, more churches or more alcoholics. Thus, correlation alone does not indicate causation. Such a spurious relationship between an exposure and an outcome due to the effects of a related factor is another example of confounding. Confounding as an alternative explanation needs to be considered by the reader in almost all types of clinical studies, including experimental ones.

Conversely, lack of correlation does not guarantee that a causal relationship does not exist. Rather than jumping to conclusions about causation, the key issue in evaluating a correlational study is the strength of the evidence presented in demonstrating that an association exists.

• Qualitative Studies

Although they are not usually considered in epidemiology texts, qualitative studies deserve a special mention as another type of descriptive study. As discussed in Chapter 1, qualitative methods are preferred when investigating topics about which

---

* *I am indebted to UVA statistics professor Don Ball for this example.*

little is known. In recent years, more qualitative studies are being performed within health care research, particularly in the field of nursing. They are often utilized as a way to gain insight into the experiences, choices, and behaviors of patients and providers.[10] Such research is valuable in its own right as a part of evidence-based health care, and also provides important information that can be used to improve the design of quantitative studies. Because of the complex nature of many CAM therapies and the importance of the therapeutic relationship between client and practitioner, the field of integrative medicine can benefit greatly from more qualitative research. We will explore qualitative methodology and evaluation in more depth in Chapter 8.

Explanatory Studies

Explanatory studies seek to test hypotheses, clarify or establish cause-and-effect relationships, and ideally to provide evidence about questions such as disease prevalence and treatment efficacy. As was mentioned earlier, this broad category of studies is divided into observational and experimental subgroups.

1. Observational Studies

Observational studies attempt to explain the relationship between exposure and outcome by observing the natural course of events, collecting information about the people or events involved, and then sorting them into groups based on that data. By comparing the groups, an investigator hopes to draw conclusions about the relationship between exposure and outcome. An example of this kind of study would be one that shows a correlation between levels of education in the general population and the degree to which people use complementary therapies. Observational studies are sometimes referred to as analytical studies. Types of observational studies include:

- cross-sectional studies
- case-control studies
- cohort studies

• *Cross-Sectional Studies*

One way to classify the different kinds of observational studies is based on the time at which exposures and outcomes are measured. In a **cross-sectional study**, data regarding the exposure and outcome are simultaneously collected across a population at a particular point in time, then sorted and compared. This design provides a snapshot of a situation, specific to a moment or period of time, or to some significant marker whose effects or characteristics can vary from person to person. Examples would be admission to a professional training program or the birth of a first child. Surveys are a familiar example of the cross-sectional study.

Cross-sectional studies are frequently used to identify predictive or causal factors or to determine the **prevalence*** of a problem or a specific occurrence. For example, in a prevalence study researchers might catalog the kinds of health problems reported among clients who are seeking treatment at a student clinic in an acupuncture school.

Demographic data,** together with different types of health problems occurring in the group, might then be analyzed to see who is using the clinic, and what health problems are most common among them. Some types of people might report certain conditions more frequently; for example, there may be a high number of older men with osteoarthritis, or of young women and infants with HIV. Knowing the demographics of clinic users and the more frequently seen conditions would be helpful for educators planning coursework to prepare students to work in the clinic.

Cross-sectional studies can also be used to predict risk factors linked to an outcome. Early studies of the AIDS epidemic showed that the disease was more prevalent among gay men and individuals who had received blood transfusions compared to others without these exposures.

Cross-sectional studies are generally used in the early stages of an investigation to "map out the territory." They provide a great deal of descriptive information and can often be conducted quickly and cheaply by using existing data. However, there is a significant limitation with this design. Because exposure and outcome are assessed at the same time, it may be impossible to determine which came first. If people with osteoarthritis tend to be overweight, is it because their joint problems prevented them from getting enough exercise to keep their weight down? Or did the excess weight increase the amount of wear and tear on their joints in the first place?

* *Prevalence is defined as the number of cases of existing disease or outcome per population at risk; basically, how common is it at this point in time?*

** *Includes characteristics such as age, sex or gender, educational level, regional location, ethnicity, annual income, socio-economic status, or others that can be used to describe or classify groups.*

• Case-Control Studies

In the **case-control design**, the second type of observational study, both the outcome and the exposure have already occurred, and selection is made based on whether individuals do or do not have the outcome of interest. Investigators identify a group with a disease (cases) and then compare them to another group without the disease (controls). Case-control studies are sometimes referred to as *retrospective studies*. Predictive factors are analyzed by looking backwards in time and examining the kinds and degrees of exposures between the two groups. This type of study has become more widespread during the past 50 years as epidemiology has focused more on the risk factors associated with chronic illnesses.

This design has the advantage of allowing the researcher to explore many different exposures along with the possibility of interrelationships among them. The disadvantage is that because both the exposure and the outcome have already happened by the time participants are selected for the study, two potential sources of bias are introduced. Bias can enter either from the way in which cases and controls are defined and selected, or from a lack of accuracy or completeness in the data collected regarding the exposure. To avoid bias, the disease or outcome should be clearly defined and diagnostic criteria specified prior to the selection of individual cases and controls; cases and controls must truly be comparable to each other in everything except their exposure. Patients documented as having a general reproductive cancer diagnosis, for example, may have different specific types of uterine and ovarian cancer, each with different risk factors or causes. In another example, patients selected from a tertiary care hospital that provides more specialized care may differ in significant ways from patients with the same diagnosis seen in a community-based hospital; patients with the same diagnosis in the former are more likely to be more seriously ill, and co-morbidities that are less frequent in a general hospital population may appear more often.

It is more difficult to avoid bias in collecting data from participants regarding amount or degree of exposure. Participants may not remember events accurately or may be reluctant to disclose information about their habits, a phenomenon sometimes referred to as **recall bias**. A case-control study setting out to examine the role of diet in the development of cancer might depend upon participants remembering how often they ate red meat historically or being willing to reveal the quantity of alcohol they consumed daily. Also, the same "chicken-or-egg" problem regarding the temporal relationship of exposure to outcome seen in the cross-sectional study can occur with the case-control design. It may not always be clear whether the exposure precedes the outcome or is a consequence of it.

For the reader evaluating a case-control study, it is important to notice whether the authors have acknowledged these potential sources of bias. A well-designed study will discuss and/or estimate the role of any possible sources of bias that cannot be eliminated by the study's design.

• *Cohort Studies*

In the third type of observational study, the **cohort study**, the outcome has not yet occurred. A group, or **cohort**, is defined based on the presence or absence of their exposure to a risk factor, and the members of the group are followed over a span of time to see which ones develop the outcome. For this reason, cohort studies are sometimes called *longitudinal*, *follow-up*, or *prospective* studies.

Cohort studies avoid the problems of selection and recall bias related to case-control studies and demonstrate stronger evidence that a cause-and-effect relationship exists than either cross-sectional or case-control designs. However, attrition of participants is a major issue with cohort studies because studies using this design may follow participants for months, years, or even decades. Associated with this problem is the fact that people can change their habits or lifestyle – they take up exercise, stop drinking coffee, or get a new and more stressful job. Well-designed cohort studies regularly contact participants to appraise such changes.

A good example of an ongoing cohort study is the Nurses' Health Study, which enrolled 120,000 married female registered nurses in the United States after initial surveys were mailed out during the mid 1970s. A baseline questionnaire was used to collect information regarding medical history along with demographic, reproductive, and lifestyle variables. Every two years since, participants have provided follow-up information on the baseline variables, on new variables that have been added, and on the development of outcomes. Comparing women who have been exposed to risk factors such as hormone use or a family history of disease with those who have not has provided considerable data about the relationship of such factors to the subsequent development of cardiovascular disease and cancer. This study, among other epidemiological studies, raised serious questions regarding the risks and benefits of hormone replacement therapy, and led to the Women's Health Initiative Randomized Control Trial that showed an association between HRT and breast cancer risk.

In the next chapter we will look at a study using data from the Nurses' Health Study as an example; it examines whether caffeinated beverages act as a risk factor for breast cancer.

Observational study designs provide stronger evidence of a valid association between exposure and outcome than do descriptive studies. Both cross-sectional and case-control designs can be problematic in terms of determining whether the exposure precedes the outcome. Cohort designs, which provide the strongest evidence, avoid this problem but pose their own challenges, and are expensive as well as time-consuming to conduct.

Traditional Hierarchy of Research Study Designs

STRONGER Evidence of Cause and Effect

Systematic review
Meta-analysis
Randomized controlled trial (RCT)
Cohort study
Before-and-after treatment with control
Case-control study
Cross-sectional study
Before-and-after treatment without control
Correlational study
Case series
Case report

WEAKER Evidence of Cause and Effect

Figure 4.2 Weighting Evidence in Clinical Studies

2. Experimental Studies

There are several key differences between experimental studies and other kinds of research studies. The primary difference is the active intervention of the researcher. He or she assigns the exposure, for example a treatment of some kind, to the participants. Ethical considerations are also a primary concern. Investigators are not allowed to offer an intervention that appears to be harmful to participants or to withhold one that appears beneficial; there must be sufficient doubt in either direction to justify the experiment.

Participants in clinical studies must provide informed consent. The investigator is required to explain in understandable language the procedures and treatments to be performed on the individual should he or she choose to participate in the study, as well as the potential risks and benefits of the intervention, so that the individual can make an informed decision.

We will consider two kinds of experimental studies:

- before-and-after treatment designs
- clinical trials

Experimental studies provide the most direct evidence of a valid cause and effect relationship between treatment and outcome, with the clinical trial providing the strongest indication.

• *Before-and-After Treatment Studies*

The **before-and-after treatment design** is frequently used by complementary practitioners conducting research into their own practices. A former director of the Office of Alternative Medicine (the predecessor to NCCAM), Wayne Jonas, has advocated this design as a useful and practical way to measure the effectiveness of complementary and alternative therapies. Basically, the before-and-after treatment design can be considered as a kind of case series. The practitioner defines a hypothesis, specifies eligibility criteria and methods to be used, collects pertinent baseline data, provides the treatment, and measures the after-treatment outcomes for a series of patients.

The primary weakness of the before-and-after treatment design is that it typically lacks a control group for comparison purposes and, according to Schneider and Jonas,[11] has the potential to overestimate the true size of any treatment effect by up to 40 percent, as in our previous example of the common cold study. In addition, if the practitioner who provides the treatment also collects subjective data directly, there is the possibility that his or her patients may tend to report what they think the practitioner wants to hear. Despite these limitations, the before-and-after treatment, when done well, remains a useful type of design that can contribute valuable information to clinical practice and to the development of more rigorous studies.

When evaluating before-and-after studies, notice whether the hypothesis is simply and clearly defined. As with any study, a vague research question will not produce useful information. Is it clear that the analysis was planned before the data was collected? Choosing the method of analysis after data collection leaves open the possibility that the analysis was either an afterthought or tailored to produce the desired results, rather than having been planned in advance as the most appropriate method for the study. To minimize bias, careful measurement of baseline data and outcomes is especially important, as well as the issue of who performs the data collection. When reading this type of study, consider whether any arguments presented for generalizing the results beyond the study group are reasonable. The use of a control group, if possible, greatly increases the strength of this design.

• *Clinical Trials*

The **clinical trial**, sometimes called an *intervention study*, a *randomized trial*, or a *randomized controlled trial (RCT)*, provides the most direct evidence of a cause-and-effect relationship between an exposure and an outcome. It is considered the gold standard of health care research design. What makes this design so powerful is the random assignment of participants to either an intervention group or to some kind of control or comparison group. As discussed in Chapter 3, when properly implemented with sufficient numbers of participants, random assignment controls not only for known factors that could influence the outcome but also for those not anticipated at the outset, a boon to the clinical researcher who often cannot fully control the research setting. Incorporation of features such as blinding or using a placebo control increases the strength of the design.

Characteristics of Clinical Trials

There are several important questions to bear in mind when evaluating a clinical trial:

1. How is the study population defined: what are the criteria for entry into or exclusion from the study?

2. How were participants assigned to group(s)?

3. How well were treatment and data collection protocols described and adhered to?

4. How is the problem of attrition handled?

While these issues are helpful to keep in mind generally when evaluating any kind of research study, they assume greater importance in clinical trials because of the greater evidentiary weight normally given to this type of study.

• *The Study Population*

The term "population" can have several different meanings in health care literature. There is the **reference population**, which is the larger group to which a study's findings can (hopefully) be generalized; the **experimental population**, which is the group of possible study participants, including those who decide not to participate; and the **study population** itself, the actual group of participants who are eligible, willing and able to take part in the study. It is important to keep in mind that the study population is a subset of the total experimental population – its members are likely to be different from eligible candidates not willing or able for various reasons to participate in the study.*

• *Sampling*

Because it is generally impossible to collect data from the total experimental population, researchers must select a smaller portion or sample of the total population to represent it. This is known as **sampling** – a familiar example of the importance of sampling can be seen in opinion surveys. The key issue in sampling is that the study population should be representative of the total population. There

---

* *Researchers across many different fields have found that people who volunteer to be part of a study are more likely to be female, older, better educated, and have higher socioeconomic status compared to those who choose not to volunteer. Almost all of these factors have been linked with better health status and outcomes.*

are a number of ways to accomplish this goal. **Random sampling,** or **probability sampling,** requires that every member of the total population has an equal chance of being included as the best way to ensure that the results of the study reflect the total population. In national opinion surveys this goal is feasible. Much is known about the demographics of the total population of most countries, and it is relatively easy for a researcher to randomly select an equivalent percentage of the sample for each demographic group. In this way, a small sample of 1000-2000 people can accurately represent the opinions of an entire country, because the proportions of the sample are equal to the composition of the total population.

In clinical research, however, it is much harder and often impossible to have true random sampling. The reader will therefore have to determine, through a close reading of the description of the methods used in such a study, just how representative the study group is of the reference population and to what extent the results can be generalized as a whole or to one's practice. The example of drawing patients from a tertiary care hospital compared to a community-based hospital again applies.

• Eligibility Criteria

Researchers are expected to define their eligibility criteria clearly using objective standards. Not doing so will introduce confusion and possible bias because participants have not been classified accurately. Criteria should be based on acceptable definitions of the disease or condition being studied, and any techniques or measures used to make a diagnosis or assessment should be reasonably available to other comparable practitioners. As a hypothetical example, let us say that a study evaluating the effectiveness of massage therapy for runners classified participants based on the number of fast twitch fibers relative to slow twitch fibers in their quadriceps muscles, as measured by a biopsy. Positive results were found only for those runners with a high number of fast twitch fibers. Because massage therapists cannot perform muscle biopsies in their workplaces, the practical application of the results would be severely limited, as would the reproducibility of the study.

• Allocation of Participants

Selection and allocation of participants to groups within a study is another issue to be considered when evaluating a clinical trial. Participants in the control or comparison group should as a matter of course be drawn from the same population as those who receive the intervention. Each group needs to be comparable in terms of risk factors and circumstances that might affect the outcome under study.

• Random Assignment

When random assignment has been used, it is important for the reader to determine exactly how it was carried out. It is not random to assign study participants based on odd or even days of the week, on the flip of a coin, or on the convenience of their being in the right place at the right time. The crucial issue is whether all participants have an equal chance of being assigned to any of the study groups. Preferably, this has been achieved through the use of a randomly generated table of numbers. Participants in a study are generally given an ID number. An existing number such as their SSN or SIN may be used, or one is arbitrarily assigned. These numbers are matched to the table of random numbers to determine group assignment.

Only when random assignment is properly carried out can selection bias that might create inter-group differences be avoided. Prudent investigators check the data on relevant group characteristics to verify that randomization was successfully applied and balance among the groups was accomplished. Typically, this is one of the first tables of results presented in a published study; it usually contains demographic and baseline data across all study groups. If there are imbalances among groups with respect to known confounding variables after randomization, this can be compensated for during the statistical analysis of the study data through the use of a technique called *analysis of covariance*, abbreviated *ANCOVA* (explained in Chapter 6). This technique takes the confounding variable, for example age, into account as part of the analysis and in effect removes it from the results.

• Adherence to Protocols

Compliance is the term used to describe how faithfully a study's participants adhere to the requirements the study asks of them. Lack of compliance is a potential source of bias, especially when treatments or their measurements are difficult, demanding, or unpleasant for participants. For example, they may fail to follow procedures because the medicine has disagreeable side effects or because keeping the daily food diary is too much trouble. A treatment may appear ineffective because the participants did not receive it as defined in the study protocol or because the measurement of outcome data is incomplete. As discussed in Chapter 3, unbeknownst to the investigator participants may seek out additional treatments or substitute other treatments as co-interventions. A co-intervention can be blatant, as in the use of herbal supplements that may interact with the medication being studied, or it may be something as subtle as extra attention from an assistant collecting the data. Distributed unevenly among groups as they tend to be, co-interventions can result in significant bias.

A related issue posing obvious risks of introducing bias is how systematically investigators carried out the study procedures or protocol. The discussion of threats to internal validity in Chapter 3 considered the issue of bias resulting from unequal observation or measurement of outcomes by researchers and participants.

• *Attrition*

Finally, there is the problem of attrition. Participants may drop out of a trial or be lost to follow-up for a variety of reasons. While there are statistical techniques for estimating missing data, the question of whether the attrition is a result of the treatment remains. As in the example from Chapter 1 of the antidepressant with unpleasant side effects, this type of attrition is selective and occurs more in a specific treatment group than in the control group or in groups receiving other types of treatment. Thus, bias enters into the study. This is another reason why practical steps to ensure participant compliance and the collection of complete follow-up information are so important. Of course, if an intervention is so unpleasant or a treatment too complicated for a significant number of participants to follow, the intervention and the study may not be realistic to begin with.

Statistical procedures for estimating missing data should always be described. Many epidemiologists believe that investigators should always analyze clinical trial data using a principle known as **intention to treat**, meaning that all study participants are included in the analysis whether or not they complete the course of treatment. In the Chapter 1 example, rates of clinical depression at the study endpoint among patients receiving the antidepressant with the unpleasant side effects would vary depending on whether dropouts were included or excluded from the analysis. An easy way to remember this idea is "once randomized, always analyzed."[12] Analysis by intention to treat is the only way to reap the full benefit of random assignment in estimating the true effect of an intervention.

Criticisms of Clinical Trials and Systematic Reviews

The high degree of internal validity found in clinical trials usually translates into reduced generalizability – the results can only be applied to individuals with the same characteristics as those in the trial. Yet RCTs form the basis of systematic reviews, which, in the era of evidence-based medicine, are now considered the last word on efficacy. Efficacy and effectiveness are two different things.

In epidemiological terms, "efficacy" is the impact of an intervention in a clinical trial, whereas "effectiveness" speaks to the impact in real world situations. Sounds like internal and external validity again, doesn't it? An intervention may be demonstrated to be clinically effective in what is called a **pragmatic trial**, yet the specific mechanism by which the intervention produces its results may not be known. A pragmatic trial is a test of an intervention in a real-world setting under routine conditions that are likely to be encountered by clinicians. While it can be very useful to know the specific mechanism through which an intervention produces its result, it is not a necessity in demonstrating effectiveness. Aspirin is a good example. Widely used in clinical practice since the early 1900s, the discovery of the specific mechanism by which acetylsalicylic acid works to reduce inflammation on a molecular level did not occur for another 70 years.

Although RCTs, and now systematic reviews, have become regarded as the gold standard for clinical practice and treatment guidelines, there are several reasons why many current medical and surgical practices do not have a strong literature base supporting them. As we mentioned earlier, RCTs would be considered unethical for most surgical procedures; observational studies may be the only option. As well, groups such as women, minorities, and people with co-morbid conditions have been historically under-researched and so there are fewer studies with adequate numbers. Two other issues are that: (1) randomized, double-blind placebo-controlled trials are usually expensive, so that funding source priorities play a role in what gets investigated – governmental agencies may tend to fund preventive medicine studies to improve public health as a whole, while pharmaceutical companies are more interested in funding studies that demonstrate the efficacy and safety of particular (proprietary) drugs; (2) studies found in medical journals may not be representative of all the studies that are completed on a given topic (published and unpublished) or may be misleading due to publication bias. It can be difficult and certainly time-consuming to locate articles published in non-indexed journals or to contact investigators with unpublished results.

A particular issue for complementary therapies is that well-designed RCTs have yet to be conducted in many cases, and the number of existing RCTs is small. Poorly designed RCTs run the risk of asking the wrong research question, or of using methods that are inappropriate to the question asked. In a small group of available studies, a misleading one can have significant impact.

Complementary therapies, with the possible exception of homeopathic preparations, generally do not lend themselves to investigation in the same way as a pharmaceutical intervention. In the case of massage therapy for various conditions, several systematic reviews have found that there are simply not enough high quality studies to evaluate and that they cannot reach a conclusion – not enough evidence. Too often lack of evidence is confused with lack of benefit. In addition, systematic reviews give scant weight to qualitative studies. Most complementary therapies depend to some extent on nonspecific effects, as discussed previously. It seems likely that psychosocial factors such as the quality of attention or relationship between patient and practitioner could moderate specific physiological effects. Also, single components of systems such as Traditional Chinese Medicine or naturopathy can have synergistic effects when combined, and these possibilities should be taken into account in study design.

A growing number of researchers are calling for a "whole systems" approach[13,14,15] to complementary and alternative therapies. **Whole systems research** takes the perspective that because the individual components of most whole systems are inseparable, complement one another, and are likely synergistic, valid studies should not focus only on the "active" ingredients of a system. Important issues such as treatment individualization, problems of diagnosis, patient-practitioner interaction, varying therapeutic contexts, and patient-determined outcome values need to be considered carefully. This approach also has the potential to enrich the current methods used in designing RCTs. Whole systems research incorporates qualitative approaches, encourages the use of mixed methods, and fits well with the concept of the evidence circle (see Chapter 1). One of the appeals of the evidence circle is that this model balances quantitative and qualitative approaches, and combines internal with external validity, providing a more complete and more rigorous evaluation of an intervention.

Summary

In health care research, each type of study has its own merits, its own advantages and disadvantages, its own appropriate applications, and the potential to contribute to scientific knowledge. Each provides a certain type of evidence. The important questions for the reader to consider are whether the design is consistent with the hypothesis being tested and whether the study conclusions are justified by the weight and kind of evidence presented. The reader who can identify study designs and understand the relative strengths and weaknesses of each type is alert to the key issues to be examined when evaluating published studies.

It is important to remember that no study is perfect. Scrutinized closely enough, any study will reveal flaws and limitations. The crucial issue is whether and to what extent a flaw in the design or conduct of a study is so great that it provides a plausible alternative explanation (such as chance, bias, or confounding) for its findings, casting reasonable doubt on the authors' conclusions.

References

1. Montague A. *Touching: The Significance of the Human Skin*. 2nd edition. New York: Harper Books; 1978.

2. Field T. Massage therapy effects. *American Psychologist*. 1998;53(12):1270-1281.

3. Keenan P. Benefits of massage therapy and use of a doula during labor and childbirth. *Alternative Therapies in Health and Medicine*. 2000;6(1):66-74.

4. Vickers A, Ohlsson A, Lacy JB, Horsley A. Massage for promoting growth and development of preterm and/or low birth-weight infants. *Cochrane Database of Systematic Reviews*. 2004; Issue 1. Art. No.: CD000390. DOI: 10.1002/14651858. CD000390.pub2.

5. Furlan AD, Brosseau L, Imamura M, Irvin E. Massage for low-back pain. *Cochrane Database of Systematic Reviews*. 2002; Issue 1. Art. No.: CD001929. DOI: 10.1002/14651858.

6. Slavin RE. Best evidence synthesis: an intelligent alternative to meta-analysis. *Journal of Clinical Epidemiology*. 1995;48(1):9-18.

7. Hutchinson B. Critical appraisal of review articles. *Canadian Family Physician*. 1993;39:1097-1102.

8. Centers for Disease Control. Kaposi's sarcoma and pneumocystis pneumonia among homosexual men – New York City and California. *Morbidity and Mortality Weekly Report*. Jul 3 1981;30(25):305-308.

9. Friedman GD. Cigarette smoking and geographic variation in coronary heart disease mortality in the United States. *Journal of Chronic Diseases*. 1967;20(10):769-779.

10. Morse JM, Field PA. *Qualitative Research Methods for Health Professionals*. Thousand Oaks, CA: Sage Publications; 1995.

11. Schneider C, Jonas W. Are alternative treatments effective? issues and methods involved in measuring effectiveness of alternative treatments. *Subtle Energies*. 1994;5(1):69-92.

12. Hennekens CH, Buring JE. *Epidemiology in Medicine*. Boston: Little, Brown and Company; 1987.

13. Ritenbaugh C, Verhoef M, Fleishman S, Boon H, Leis A. Whole systems research: a discipline for studying complementary and alternative medicine. *Alternative Therapies in Health and Medicine*. 2003 Jul-Aug;9(4):32-6.

14. Verhoef MJ, Lewith G, Ritenbaugh C, Boon H, Fleishman S, Leis A. Complementary and alternative medicine whole systems research: beyond identification of inadequacies of the RCT. *Complementary Therapies in Medicine*. 2005 Sep;13(3):206-12.

15. Elder C, Aickin M, Bell IR, Fønnebø V, Lewith GT, Ritenbaugh C, Verhoef M. Methodological challenges in whole systems research. *Journal of Alternative and Complementary Medicine*. 2006 Nov;12(9):843-50.

Exercises

1. *Find an example of a narrative review and a systematic review in your own discipline. Present both to your class for discussion, comparing and contrasting their similarities and differences.*

2. *Describe the differences among a correlational study, a case-control study, and a cohort study. Use these as search terms in PubMed to locate an example of each kind of study.*

3. *What issues need to be considered in evaluating a clinical trial?*

4. *How can you tell whether participants in a clinical trial were randomly assigned to group(s)?*

5. *In any study, careful reading will discover limitations or flaws. What is the crucial issue in deciding whether a study is too seriously flawed to be useful as a basis for informing clinical practice?*

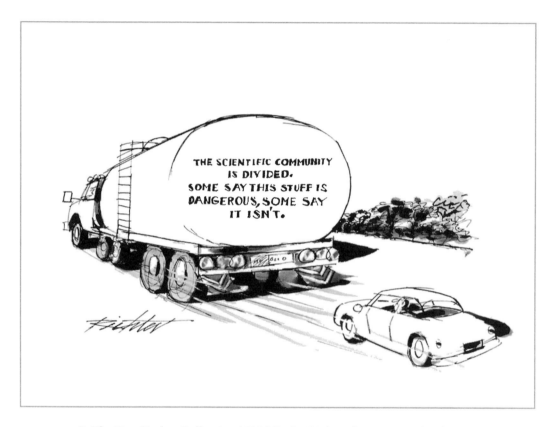

The Anatomy of an Original Research Article

A good tutor taught the whole of his subject and not just that part of it in which he himself happened to be especially interested or proficient; to "teach" did not, of course, mean to "impart factual information," a relatively unimportant consideration, but rather to guide thought and reading and encourage reflection.

P. B. Medawar

Learning Objectives

After completing this chapter,
the reader should be able to:

· *Name the six sections of an original research article.*

· *Describe two primary functions of each section.*

· *Recognize the essential component(s) of each section.*

Chapter 5: The Anatomy of an Original Research Article

Just as the practice of the health care professions requires a working knowledge of the anatomy and physiology of the human body, critical examination of a research article requires identification and study of its various components. Having clarified the logic and basic concepts that form the foundation of scientific thinking and investigation, and broadly discussed various aspects of health care research design, we will now focus more specifically on examining the elements that are common to any clinical research article.

A typical journal article has six sections:

- the abstract
- the introduction
- the methods
- the results
- the discussion or conclusion
- the references

Two related elements that are common to most articles are the author/article information, that is, the description of the institutional affiliations of the authors and sources of financial support for the study, and the acknowledgements, where the authors thank individuals who have assisted them during the study itself or in preparing the manuscript for submission to a peer-reviewed journal.

This chapter provides an overview of the structure and function of each research article component. In this instance, a study using a prospective cohort design will be used as the example, while in subsequent chapters we will scrutinize clinical trials, qualitative studies and case reports. The questions in this chapter are intended as food for thought as you read – do not be concerned about being able to answer them in detail. At this point, the goal is to simply get you to start thinking critically. A step-by-step protocol for analyzing research articles will be laid out in the chapters that follow, providing a road map for more detailed examination.

We begin the process, then, by looking at an observational study based on data from the Nurses' Health Study, which is one of the largest and longest inquiries using a prospective cohort design conducted in the United States. Our study uses classic epidemiological methods to investigate whether consumption of coffee, tea, and caffeine creates risk factors or exposures for developing breast cancer as a subsequent outcome. The results of this type of large-scale study are frequently reported in the popular media, which is one reason why we have chosen to use it as an example. Several of the terms and concepts in the article were covered in Chapter 4; you may feel the need to go back and review some items as you are reading.

The Abstract

The **abstract** is the first section of a journal article. It functions as an executive summary of the article's contents, containing the core information on which the article is reporting. Ideally, it uses an abbreviated format and includes:

- a statement of the background or context of the study
- the purpose of the study or the research objective
- a simple description of the research design
- a description of the methodology, or how the research was carried out
- the results
- the conclusion(s) of the authors

Each topic is normally summarized in one or two sentences. In some fields of study, for example in the social sciences, abstracts may be written in a more narrative format or may be a repetition of the first paragraph of the article. An abstract should always be a single page or less in length, yet it should convey enough information for the reader to determine whether he or she is interested in reading the full text of the article. The length and format of an abstract also varies according to the specific requirements of the journal in which it is published.

In recent years, many authors of quantitative health care literature have adopted what is known as a standardized abstract, using headings such as "Background," "Participants," "Design," "Outcome Measures," and so forth. Standardized abstracts provide core information in a consistent manner, making it easier to quickly identify essential information (such as the type of study design or the outcome measures used) and to compare information across different articles. Our sample study, which was published electronically prior to its appearance in print, uses a narrative abstract.

Author and Article Information

Author and article information is an addendum to the article – it is usually found on the first page with the abstract. The credentials and organizational or institutional affiliations of the author(s) are described, and contact information is provided for those wishing to request reprints of the article or to correspond with the lead author. Almost all peer-reviewed journals now require authors to disclose all sources of funding for the study as well, so that readers can decide whether the sources of money that supported the study may have influenced the results, and similarly, the organizations or institutions that employ the authors.

As you read this sample abstract, consider the following questions:

1. Do you think the authors have provided a brief summary that is complete and to the point?

2. Have they provided enough pertinent detail to capture your interest and lead you to read the full text?

3. Who are the authors, what is their institutional affiliation, and what organizations provided the funding for the study?

Coffee, Tea, Caffeine and Risk of Breast Cancer: A 22-Year Follow-Up

Davaasambuu Ganmaa[1*], Walter C. Willett[1,2,3], Tricia Y. Li[1], Diane Feskanich[3], Rob M. van Dam[1], Esther Lopez-Garcia[1], David J. Hunter[1,2], Michelle D. Holmes[3]

[1]Department of Nutrition, Harvard School of Public Health, Boston, MA

[2]Department of Epidemiology, Harvard School of Public Health, Boston, MA

[3]Channing Laboratory, Department of Medicine, Brigham and Women's Hospital and Harvard Medical School, Boston, MA

Grant Sponsor: National Cancer Institute; Grant Number CA050385-16.
Grant Sponsors: National Institutes of Health and Breast Cancer Research Foundation.
*Correspondence to: Department of Nutrition, Harvard School of Public Health, 665 Huntington Avenue, Boston, MA 02115 USA.
Fax: +617-432-2435. E-mail: gdavaasa@hsph.harvard.edu
Received 7 August 2007; Accepted after revision 29 October 2007
DOI 10.1002/ijc/23336
Published online 8 January 2008 in Wiley InterScience (www.interscience.wiley.com)

The relation between consumption of coffee, tea and caffeine and risk of breast cancer remains unsettled. We examined data from a large, long-term cohort study to evaluate whether high intake of coffee and caffeine is associated with increased risk of breast cancer. This was a prospective cohort study with 85,987 female participants in the Nurses' Health Study. Consumption of coffee, tea and caffeine consumption was assessed in 1980, 1984, 1986, 1990, 1994, 1998 and the follow-up continued through 2002. We documented 5,272 cases of invasive breast cancer during 1,715,230 person-years. The multivariate relative risks (RRs) of breast cancer across categories of caffeinated coffee consumption were: 1.0 for <1cup/month (reference category), 1.01 (95% confidence interval: 0.92–1.12) for 1 month to 4.9 week, 0.92 (0.84–1.01) for 5 week to 1.9 days, 0.93 (0.85–1.02) for 2–3.9 days, 0.92 (0.82–1.03) for ≥4cups per day (p for trend = 0.14). Intakes of tea and decaffeinated coffee were also not significantly associated with risk of breast cancer. RRs (95% CI) for increasing quintiles of caffeine intake were 1.00, 0.98 (0.90–1.07), 0.92 (0.84–1.00), 0.94 (0.87–1.03) and 0.93 (0.85–1.01) (p for trend = 0.06). A significant inverse association of caffeine intake with breast cancers was observed among postmenopausal women; for the highest quintile of intake compared to the lowest RR 0.88 (95% CI = 0.79–0.97, p for trend = 0.03). We observed no substantial association between caffeinated and decaffeinated coffee and tea consumption and risk of breast cancer in the overall cohort. However, our results suggested a weak inverse association between caffeine-containing beverages and risk of postmenopausal breast cancer.

Keywords: *breast cancer; dietary practices; coffee; tea; caffeine*

In this abstract, the authors have provided a great deal of information, particularly regarding the results of the study. Their conclusion, based on an extremely large sample of women, is that there is little associated risk of developing breast cancer from consumption of caffeine; furthermore, there appears to be a mild protective benefit to postmenopausal women. The authors are affiliated with the Harvard University schools of public health and medicine, and the study was funded by grants from the National Cancer Institute, the National Institutes of Health, and the Breast Cancer Research Foundation.

The Introduction

An article's introduction states the general purpose for conducting the research study and the specific research question that the study has attempted to answer. In addition, it should include a discussion of previous literature pertinent to the question, referred to as a **review of the literature**. A good review places the current study into the context of prior related research and provides the rationale for pursuing this study at this time. Notice that of the 53 citations listed in the study references, the first 38 occur in this section. Gaps in the previous literature can be identified as a support for the study rationale. A well-written introduction answers the question, "Why should anyone care?" In other words, why should anyone bother to study this particular research question, and why should anyone else be interested in the results?

As you read the study's introduction, reflect on these questions:

1. Have the authors stated the purpose of the study clearly?

2. Is a review of the literature contained in the introduction?

3. How well do you think the authors make their case for the importance of conducting this study?

Coffee and tea consumption have been hypothesized both to increase and to decrease the risk of developing breast cancer. Caffeine is a naturally occurring plant alkaloid found in coffee, tea, cocoa and as an additive in many soft drinks and medications. It belongs to a group of purine-based compounds collectively referred to as methylxanthines.[1] Speculation that caffeine may increase breast cancer risk followed reports that women with benign breast disease experienced symptom relief after eliminating methylxanthines from their diet.[2-4] Animal studies have indicated that caffeine can both stimulate and suppress mammary tumors, depending on the rodent species and strain as well as the tumorigenic phase (initiation/promotion) at the caffeine administration.[5,6] Caffeine-rich foods such as tea, coffee and chocolate were suggested to be carcinogenic in 1970s and 1980s.[7,8]

Coffee and tea are also rich in phenolic compounds including substantial amounts of several lignans.[9] These lignans can be converted into enterolactone and enterodiol which have antiestrogenic properties and can potentially reduce the risk of certain cancers.[10] In addition, in vitro evidence indicates beverages high in phenolic compounds have antioxidant activity and can also protect mammalian cells against genotoxic effects, inhibit cell-replication enzymes and prevent cancer growth through antiestrogenic pathways or mitochondrial toxicity.[11–13] Coffee is the major source of the phenol chlorogenic acid,[14] and a major contributor to the total antioxidant capacity of the diet in several populations.[15,16] The primary antioxidant potential of tea is attributed to its catechins, chief among them, epigallocatechin gallate (EGCG) for which green tea has a higher concentration than black tea.[17] In various studies, rats with breast tumors that were given green tea had reductions in tumor size and tumor growth.[18,19] Some human case-control studies suggest protective effects of polyphenols against breast cancer specifically.[20] These findings, coupled with observations of lower rates of breast cancer in countries where green tea is consumed daily, suggest that green tea may protect against human breast cancer.

International comparative studies have shown a positive association between coffee and breast cancer incidence and mortality.[21,22] The association between coffee and breast cancer, however, has been inconsistent in observational studies, with reports of no association,[23–31] inverse association[32–36] and positive association.[37,38] The associations between coffee consumption and breast cancer may be confounded by other aspects of diet or by the lack of appropriate control for nondietary confounding factors. Another concern is that tea consumption in countries that traditionally consume coffee may reflect noncoffee consumption, and the effect attributed to tea may be in fact because of the absence of coffee.

To address the relationship of caffeinated and decaffeinated coffee and tea consumption to breast cancer risk in women, we examined this association prospectively in a large population of women with long follow-up and repeated measures of intake.

The introduction, which does review the pertinent literature on the study question, is admirably succinct and lays out the rationale for the study quite clearly. Because previous studies have found conflicting evidence, one compelling reason for conducting such a large-scale, prospective study is to determine both the extent and the direction of any association between consumption of caffeine and a subsequent risk of developing breast cancer.

Methods and Procedures

The methods section of an article describes in detail exactly how the study was carried out. This section is one of the most important in terms of gauging the possibility that chance, bias, or confounding have affected the study's results. Careful reading should reveal whether other plausible explanations for the study results are possible. In particular, the reader should closely examine details about how participants were selected, how random assignment to group (if used) was performed, how abstract concepts such as anxiety, intelligence or patriotism were defined in terms of observable and measurable behaviors, and exactly what procedures were followed to implement any treatment that was given. For studies that test or evaluate the effectiveness of complementary therapies, the protocol for the treatment should be considered in terms of its appropriateness to the study's research question. The qualifications of the study personnel providing the treatment are also relevant.

With surveys and interviews, the way in which questions are worded and the order in which they are asked can make a great deal of difference to how participants respond. While print journal space rarely permits the full text of a scripted interview or questionnaire to be included, authors may disclose the wording of particular questions, especially if the results are surprising or controversial, to demonstrate that they have not tried to manipulate the responses. One advantage of electronic publication is that there are no space limitations – questionnaires, interview questions and prompts, or other instruments used may be included as an appendix to the article.

Another issue to consider is this: to what degree is the sample of survey respondents representative of the entire population to which the results will be generalized? In most countries, sufficient demographic information exists so that researchers can select a sample that will duplicate these characteristics accurately and proportionally. The nonresponse rate is also important to consider, since those who complete the surveys (respondents) can and often do differ from those who do not (nonrespondents) in ways that affect the survey results and their interpretation. If only 40% of a sample actually complete the survey, the findings may not prove useful because the other 60% of the sample may have a different response to the questions asked. Generally speaking, surveys with less than a 50% response rate should be viewed with caution. A reasonable response rate for a mailed survey is 60% or more; telephone surveys often have higher rates of response, as much as 75% to 90%.[1]

In surveys and studies where participants are interviewed face-to-face and are asked to self-report regarding their lifestyle, or behaviors such as diet, social acceptability may affect the answers participants are willing to give directly to interviewers. Mailed surveys and anonymous surveys are more likely to get an accurate estimate regarding self-reported activities such as exercise, drinking, or extramarital sexual relationships. Memory may also play a role when participants are asked to recall information such as how much or how often they eat a specific food group.

In the Nurses' Health Study, which was established in 1976, 121,700 female registered nurses aged 30 to 55 who resided in the 11 most populous US states completed a mailed questionnaire regarding their medical history and lifestyle factors. This is an ongoing study; participants are asked to complete the questionnaire again every two years, and new items may be added. Questions on food frequency consumption were added in 1980, and are repeated every four years.

In the study methods section of the case example described here (by Ganmaa et al.), note the degree of detail used to describe the methods and procedures that were followed in conducting the study. If a term is used that you don't understand, first see if you can figure it out from the context in which it is used, then look it up. Don't worry too much about the description of how the statistical analysis was performed – we'll go into more detail on this topic in the next two chapters.

The primary focus of the study is to determine whether a high intake of caffeine is associated with an increased risk of developing breast cancer. It uses a method common in epidemiological studies called the **relative risk** (**RR**). The relative risk estimates the size of the association between an exposure and an outcome, and also indicates the likelihood of developing the outcome in the exposed group relative to those not exposed.

As you read this section, consider your answers to the following questions:

1. What do you think of the authors' description of the study participants and why they were included or excluded?

2. What do you think of the description of the study questionnaire?

3. Why do you think it might be important to include the types of breast cancer diagnoses?

4. What can you tell about the statistical analysis, based on your current knowledge? What information would be helpful to better understand, in general terms, what was involved in performing the statistical analysis?

Material and methods

Study population

The Nurses' Health Study cohort was established in 1976 when 121,700 female registered nurses, 30–55 years of age and from 11 states in the USA, answered a mailed questionnaire on risk factors for cancer and lifestyles. Further details have been published elsewhere.[39] We excluded women who did not complete more than 10 items on the 1980 dietary questionnaire, had extreme scores for total daily intake of energy (<500 or >3,500 kcal), or who had greatly increased or decreased their coffee intake over the past 10 years to reduce measurement error and to capture a measure of long-term intake. We excluded women who had a prior history of cancer (except nonmelanoma skin cancer), or in situ breast cancer, leaving 85,987 women who were followed from 1980 to 2002.

Exposure assessment

In 1980, diet was assessed with a 60-item food frequency questionnaire (FFQ) which included the following caffeine-containing foods and beverages: coffee with caffeine, tea, cola and other carbonated beverages with caffeine, and chocolate. For each food, participants were asked if their use had greatly increased or decreased over the past 10 years. Decaffeinated coffee was added to an expanded FFQ (~130 foods) in 1984, 1986, 1990, 1994 and 1998. For each item, participants were asked how often, on average, they had consumed a specified amount of each beverage or food over the past year. The participants could choose from nine frequency categories (never, 1–3 per month, 1 per week, 2–4 per week, 5–6 per week, 1 per day, 2–3 per day, 4–5 per day and 6 or more per day). Intakes of nutrients and caffeine were calculated using US Department of Agriculture food composition sources. In these calculations, we assumed the content of caffeine was 137 mg per 8 oz cup of coffee, 47 mg per 8 oz cup of tea, 46 mg per 12 oz can or bottle of cola or other caffeinated carbonated beverage, and 7 mg per 1 oz serving of chocolate candy. We assessed the total intake of caffeine by summing the caffeine content for the specified amount of each food multiplied by a weight proportional to the frequency of its use. In a validation among a subsample of our cohort, we obtained high correlations between intake of caffeinated coffee and other caffeinated beverages from the FFQ and four 1-week diet records (coffee, r = 0.78; tea, r = 0.93; and caffeinated sodas, r = 0.85).[40,41] For the present analysis, caffeinated or decaffeinated coffee and tea consumption were categorized into 5 groups: less than 1 cup/month, 1 cup/month to 4.9 cups/week, 5 cups/week to 1.9 cups/day, 2–3.9 cups/day, and 4 or more cups/day. Caffeine intake was divided into 5 categories with equal number of participants.

Identification of breast cancer cases

In each biennial questionnaire, participants were asked whether they had been diagnosed as having breast cancer in the previous 2 years, and we attempted to interview nonrespondents by telephone. The response rates were ~90% for each questionnaire. Deaths were identified by a report from a family member, the postal service or the National Death Index. When a case of breast cancer was reported, we asked the participant (or next of kin if she had died) for permission to obtain medical records. Since self-reports have been confirmed by pathology reports in 98% of instances, we included the few-self reported cases for whom we could not obtain medical records in the analysis. Pathology reports were also reviewed to obtain information on estrogen receptor (ER) and progesterone receptor (PR) status. Seventy-four percent of the cases had receptor status information (51% were estrogen and progesterone receptor positive breast cancer, 23% were estrogen and PR negative breast cancer). Cases of carcinoma in situ were not included in the analysis.

Assessment of medical history, anthropometric data and other lifestyle factors

On the 1976 baseline questionnaires, we requested information about age, weight and height, smoking status, family history of breast cancer, use of hormone therapy and personal history of other diseases. This information (except height) has been updated on the biennial follow-up questionnaires. Body mass index (BMI) was calculated as weight in kilograms divided by the square of height in meters. Alcohol intake was assessed on the FFQ from consumption of beer, wine and liquor. Other covariates included were age at menarche, parity, age at first birth, age at menopause, history of benign breast disease, physical activity, weight change after age 18.

Statistical analysis

For each participant, we calculated person-months of follow-up from the date of return of the 1980 baseline questionnaire to the date of breast cancer, other cancer except nonmelanoma skin cancer, death, or June 1, 2002, whichever came first. Participants were classified according to levels of coffee, tea and caffeine consumption. We used Cox proportional hazard regression models to examine the association between dietary exposures and incidence of breast cancer. Hazard ratios were calculated to estimate relative-risks (RRs) and 95% confidence intervals (CIs) using the lowest category of intake as the reference.

To reduce within-subject variation and best represent long-term effect for diet, we used the cumulative average of coffee, tea and caffeine intakes from all available dietary questionnaires up to the start of each 2-year follow-up interval.[42] For example, the coffee intake from the 1980 FFQ was used to characterize follow-up between 1980 and 1984, the average of the 1980 and 1984 intakes was used for the follow-up between 1984 and 1986, the average of the 1980, 1984 and 1986 intakes was used for the follow-up between 1986 and 1990, etc.

In alternative analyses, we used simple updating (the most recent dietary information) to study the short-term effects of caffeinated coffee, tea and caffeine on breast cancer. We also compared the results of the analysis using cumulatively averaged and updated consumption with those obtained when we stopped updating the consumption at the beginning of a time interval in which individuals developed hypertension, hypercholesterolemia, type 2 diabetes mellitus, or cardiovascular diseases. The diagnosis of these endpoints may alter intake of coffee or tea. In additional analyses, we examined various latency periods between caffeine exposure and breast cancer diagnosis using the multiple questionnaires to maximize power. For example, in analyses with a latency period of 4–7.9 years, the 1980 diet was used for cases from 1984 to 1988, the 1984 diet was used to follow-up from 1988–1990, the 1986 diet was used to follow-up from 1990–1994, and the 1990 diet was used to follow-up from 1994 to 1998, and so on.

Models were first adjusted for age, smoking status (never, past and current 1–14, 15–24 and ≥25 cigarettes/day), and BMI (<18.5, 18.5–24.9, 25.0–29.9, 30.0–34.9, ≥35.0 kg/m²). Physical activity, history of benign breast disease, family history of breast cancer, height, weight change since age 18, age at menarche, parity, age at first birth, alcohol intake, total energy intake, age at menopause and postmenopausal hormone use were added in multivariable proportional hazard models. To test for linear trends across exposure categories, we used the median of each category as a continuous variable. SAS PROC PHREG with SAS version 8.2 was used for all analyses.

Results

The results section is exactly that, a description of the analysis of the study data. The description can be either qualitative or quantitative and is presented as objectively as possible, neither supporting nor dismissing the hypothesis or study purpose. The results section is generally divided into two parts. The first part contains a descriptive analysis of the study participants' demographic data. In studies where groups of participants are compared to each other, analysis of the demographic data allows the reader to determine how comparable participants were to one another at the beginning of the study and whether there were any preexisting differences among the participants that might have influenced the results. In the current study, baseline data for the whole group of study participants regarding caffeine consumption, demographic factors such as age, and other medical history such as smoking and family history of breast cancer are described first.

The second part usually contains an analysis of the outcome data. This analysis may be presented in a variety of formats, such as tables, charts or graphs, along with a written description. Visual presentation of the outcome data allows the reader to see at a glance whether any statistically significant differences among groups of participants are present, and is often easier to grasp immediately than the written description. Ideally, any visual presentation or display functions as a quantitative summary of the study's information, and should be clearly labeled and easy to understand. As you are practicing how to read this section of an article, you may find it helpful to look at the tables first in order to get a general picture of the overall results. Then read the written explanation of results in the text. Go back to the tables again and see if they are now clearer to you.

In the Ganmaa study, a brief written summary of the results precedes each table. The primary outcome reported is the relative risk of developing breast cancer based on caffeine consumption. This risk calculation is adjusted for other risk factors, such as age, menopause status, smoking and body mass index, by taking these factors into account as part of the statistical analysis. A relative risk of 1 means that there is no difference in risk between the groups compared; a number higher or lower than 1 means that the risk is respectively larger or smaller. So a relative risk of 2 means the probable risk is twice as large, and a relative risk of 0.5 means the risk is cut in half – not a risk at all but likely a protective factor. Because participants in the study were followed for different amounts of time, based on when they entered and exited the study due to date of cancer diagnosis, death, or the end of the study period, the authors used person-time units (person-years and person-months) to make time measures equivalent across the entire group, instead of relying on number of people alone or amount of time alone, so that a valid comparison among all the participants could be made.

As you continue reading the Ganmaa study, consider the following:

1. How would you rate the tables in this section in terms of clarity? Even though you may not understand exactly what a Cox proportional hazard regression model is, can you pick out the number of cases of breast cancer across each category of amount of caffeine consumed?

2. Which do you find easier to understand at first glance, the tables or the written explanation in the text?

3. What was the total number of women included in this study and, of those, how many cases of breast cancer were diagnosed?

4. Do the data suggest that caffeine is a high risk factor for developing breast cancer?

Results

During the 22 years of follow-up we documented 6,552 cases of incident invasive breast cancer in the cohort who completed the 1980 dietary questionnaire. Cases were excluded for the following reasons: diagnosis before baseline (667) or after end of follow-up (93), previous diagnosis of another cancer except nonmelanoma skin cancer (495) and missing date of diagnosis (n = 25). This left 5,272 incident cases of invasive breast cancer among 85,987 women for this analysis.

Characteristics of the population according to caffeinated coffee consumption in 1980 are presented in Table I. Frequent coffee consumption was strongly associated with smoking. In addition, women who drank more coffee were more likely to drink alcohol, less likely to drink tea, and less likely to use postmenopausal hormones than those who drank little coffee. Coffee drinkers were less likely to gain weight, though current BMI was not related to coffee intake.

TABLE I – Baseline Characteristics by Levels of Coffee Consumption among Participants in the Nurses' Health Study

	Coffee consumption, cups in women in NHS (1980 Baseline)				
	<1 month	1 month to 4 week	5 week to 1.9 days	2–3.9 days	>4 days
Participants, n	19,462	5,223	11,676	28,178	21,448
Caffeine (mg/day)	116	134	219	419	794
Tea (cups/day)	1.3	1.1	0.9	0.8	0.6
Age (years)	45.5	45.3	46.6	46.6	46.3
Current smoker (%)	19.0	20.0	20.0	28.0	46.0
BMI (kg/m^2)	24.8	24.5	24.5	24.3	24.2
Physical exercise (hr/week)	4.0	4.0	3.9	3.9	3.7
Age at menarche (years)	12.4	12.4	12.5	12.4	12.4
Age at first birth (years)[1]	24.4	24.5	24.6	24.4	24.2
Parity[1]	2.9	2.8	2.9	3.0	3.0
Postmenopausal (%)	33.0	33.0	32.0	33.0	33.0
Postmenopausal hormone use (%)[2]	22.0	22.0	22.0	21.0	18.0
Age at menopause	44.9	45.2	45.7	45.8	45.4
Duration of PMH use (years)[3]	2.1	2.0	2.4	2.2	2.0
History of benign breast disease (%)	25.0	24.0	23.0	24.0	25.0
Family history of breast cancer (%)	6.0	6.0	6.0	6.0	6.0
Alcohol (gram/day)	4.4	5.2	5.8	7.5	7.2
Weight change since age of 18 (kg)	9.6	9.1	9.2	7.9	6.5
Height (inches)	64.5	64.5	64.4	64.5	64.6

NHS, nurses' health study; BMI, body mass index.
Values are means unless otherwise indicated. Data were directly standardized to the age distribution in the study population.
[1]Among parous women only.
[2]Among postmenopausal women only.
[3]Among current post menopausal hormone users only.

In age-adjusted analysis, we found a weak inverse association between the cumulative average caffeinated coffee consumption and the risk of the breast cancer (Table II). Compared with women who drank <1 cup of caffeinated coffee/month, the relative risk for women who drank ≥4 cups/day was 0.91 (95% CI 0.82–1.01) and the p-value for the linear trend across all categories was 0.04. After multivariate adjustment, the RRs were somewhat attenuated and the linear trend was not significant. For tea, the multivariate relative risk and 95% confidence interval was 0.94 (0.77–1.14) for the women consuming ≥4 cups/day compared to the women consuming less than 1 cup/month. Caffeinated coffee and tea consumption were mutually adjusted in these multivariate analyses.

TABLE II – Multivariate RR and 95% CI of Breast Cancer According to Cumulatively Averaged and Updated Consumption of Coffee and Tea in Relation to Risk of Breast Cancer in All Women

	Coffee and tea consumption, cups					
	<1 month	1 month to 4.9 weeks	5 weeks to 1.9 days	2–3.9 days	≥4 days	p-value for trend[1]
Coffee						
Person-years	286,165	207,883	403,471	567,032	250,650	
Cases, no	837	745	1,335	1,718	637	
Age-adjusted	1.0	1.06 (0.96–1.17)	0.97 (0.88–1.05)	0.96 (0.88–1.04)	0.91 (0.82–1.01)	0.04
Multivariate[2]	1.0	1.01 (0.92–1.12)	0.92 (0.84–1.01)	0.93 (0.85–1.02)	0.92 (0.82–1.03)	0.14
Tea						
Person-years	386,876	707,013	393,506	183,582	44,225	
Cases, no		1,165	2,284	1,201	514	108
Age-adjusted	1.0	0.98 (0.91–1.05)	0.95 (0.88–1.04)	0.97 (0.88–1.08)	0.94 (0.77–1.14)	0.27
Multivariate	1.0	0.95 (0.89–1.02)	0.94 (0.86–1.02)	0.96 (0.86–1.07)	0.94 (0.77–1.14)	0.25
Decaf coffee[3]						
Person-years	462,124	355,046	256,056	128,400	21,133	
Cases, no		1,504	1,259	979	422	70
Age-adjusted	1.00	1.00 (0.93–1.08)	1.07 (0.98–1.16)	0.97 (0.87–1.08)	1.07 (0.84–1.36)	0.81
Multivariate	1.00	0.97 (0.90–1.05)	1.01 (0.93–1.10)	0.90 (0.80–1.01)	1.03 (0.81–1.31)	0.26

[1]p-values for trend calculated using continuous values.
[2]Adjusted for: age months, smoking status (never, past and current 1–14, 15–24 and ≥25 cigarettes/day), body mass index (<18.5, 18.5–24.9, 25.0–29.9, 30.0–34.9, ≥35.0 kg/m2), physical activity (quintiles of hr/week <1.0, 1.0–1.9, 2.0–3.9, 4.0–6.9, ≥7.0 hr/week), height (<63, 63–63.9, 64–65.9, ≥66 inches), alcohol intake (never, 0.1–4.9, 5.0–14.9, ≥15.0 g/days), family history of breast cancer in mother or a sister (yes, no), history of benign breast disease (yes, no), menopausal status, age at menopause, use of hormone therapy (postmenopausal <48 never, postmenopausal <48 past, postmenopausal <48 current <5 year, postmenopausal <48 current >5 years, postmenopausal 48–52 never, postmenopausal 48–52 past, postmenopausal 48–52 current <5 year, postmenopausal 48–52 current ≥5year, postmenopausal 53+ never, postmenopausal 53+ past, postmenopausal 53+ current <5year, postmenopausal 53+ current ≥5year), age at menarche (≤12, 13, ≥14years), parity and age at first birth (nulliparous, parity ≤2 and age at first birth <25years, parity ≤2 and age at first birth 25–30 years, parity ≤2 and age at first birth ≥30 years, parity 3–4 and age at first birth <25years, parity 3–4 and age at first birth 25–30 years, parity 3–4 and age at first birth ≥30, parity ≥5 and age at first birth <25, and parity ≥5 and age at first birth 25–30), weight change after 18 (loss >4 kg, stable, gain 4.1–10 kg, gain 10.1–20 kg, gain 20.1–40 kg, gain 40.1 kg and above) and duration of postmenopausal hormone use (continuous). Coffee and tea intake mutually adjusted for each other.
[3]Follow-up from 1984, additionally adjusted for coffee intake.

There was no association between decaffeinated coffee intake (Table II) and breast cancer risk either after adjustment for age, caffeinated coffee and multiple breast cancer risk factors. There was also no apparent association between intakes of caffeinated soft drinks and chocolates, which contribute to caffeine intake, and breast cancer occurrence (data not shown).

Analyses stratified by BMI did not reveal any statistically significant difference in the association between caffeinated coffee consumption and breast cancer in obese participants as compared with normal and overweight participants. (p for interaction = 0.72) (Table III). The relationship also did not differ significantly between premenopausal and postmenopausal women; the multivariable RRs for ≥4 cups/day were 1.00 (95% CI = 0.80–1.27, p for trend = 0.79) and 0.89 (95% CI = 0.78–1.02, p for trend = 0.08), respectively. Given the known variation in the BMI-breast cancer relationship by menopausal status, we conducted further analyses stratified by baseline BMI status restricted to postmenopausal women only. The results did not show any statistically significant difference (data not shown).

TABLE III – Multivariate RR and 95% CI of Breast Cancer According to Cumulatively Averaged and Updated Coffee Consumption Stratified by BMI

	Coffee consumption, cups						
	<1 month	1 month to 4.9 week	5 week to 1.9 days	2–3.9 days	≥4 days	p value for trend	p value for interaction
BMI < 25 kg/m²							
Person-years	150,186	106,140	207,014	309,513	145,524	0.43	
Cases, no	421	363	656	892	353		
Multivariate[1]	1.0	1.00 (0.86–1.15)	0.93 (0.82–1.06)	0.94 (0.83–1.06)	0.93 (0.80–1.08)		
BMI 25–29.9							
Person-years	79,896	61,403	123,467	170,149	71,118	0.06	
Cases, no	246	239	449	545	187		
Multivariate	1.0	1.09 (0.91–1.31)	0.98 (0.83–1.15)	0.94 (0.81–1.11)	0.87 (0.71–1.07)		
BMI ≥30							
Person-years	55,357	39,978	72,299	86,609	33,466	0.52	
Cases, no	170	142	229	277	95		
Multivariate	1.0	0.98 (0.78–1.24)	0.88 (0.71–1.08)	0.97 (0.79–1.19)	1.02 (0.78–1.33)		0.72

Models, RR (95% CI).
[1]Adjusted for the same covariates as in Table 2, except for BMI.

To address the issue that low consumers of coffee tend to be higher drinkers of tea and vice versa we cross-classified coffee and tea drinkers with the reference category being low consumption of both coffee and tea (i.e., <1 cup/month). We found no significant association between risk of breast cancer and high tea consumption (i.e., 4+ cups/day) among women with low coffee intake (RR = 0.98, CI = 0.87–1.10) or high coffee consumption among women with low tea intake (RR = 1.02, 95% CI = 0.91–1.15).

We observed a weak, but statistically significant inverse relation between caffeine intake and risk of breast cancer in the age-adjusted analysis; the RRs comparing the highest with the lowest quintile were 0.91 (95% CI = 0.83–0.99 for trend = 0.01). In the multivariate analysis the trend was a slightly attenuated, but lower risk remained for the highest compared with the lowest quintile (RR 0.93, 95% CI 0.85–1.01) (Table IV). We also categorized total caffeine intakes into deciles. No additional benefit was apparent in comparisons of the highest and lowest deciles of intake. The multivariate RRs for the uppermost versus lowermost deciles of intake were 0.99 (95% CI = 0.87–1.12) for total caffeine.

The association between caffeine and breast cancer was stronger among postmenopausal women; for the highest quintile of intake compared to lowest RR = 0.88 (95% CI = 0.79–0.97 for = 0.03) than among premenopausal women (RR 1.09, 95% CI = 0.87–1.37 for = 0.77).

When breast cancers were classified by estrogen and progesterone receptor status, we observed a statistically significant inverse association of caffeine intake with breast cancers that had positive estrogen and progesterone receptors (p for = 0.01) (Table IV). Results were similar for ER negative and PR negative cases. However, perhaps due to lower power the linear trend was not statistically significant.

The association between caffeine and breast cancer was stronger among postmenopausal women with estrogen-receptor and progesterone-receptor positive breast cancer (RR = 0.81, 95% CI = 0.70–0.95 for trend = 0.006) than those with estrogen-receptor and progesterone-receptor negative breast cancer (RR 0.94, 95% CI = 0.70–1.26 for trend = 0.97).

TABLE IV – Multivariate RR and 95% CI of Breast Cancer (Total, ER+/PR+ and ER-/PR-)
According to Quintiles of Cumulatively Averaged and Updated Caffeine

	Caffeine Quintile					p value for trend
	1 (lowest)	2	3	4	5 (highest)	
Median intake (range), mg/d	51 (0–139)	191 (140–336)	363 (337–404)	501 (405–692)	816 (≥693)	
All cases						0.06
Person-years	336,496	342,156	347,356	344,680	344,541	
Cases, No	1,085	1,101	1,059	1,048	979	
Multivariate[1]	1.00	0.98 (0.90–1.07)	0.92 (0.84–1.00)	0.94 (0.87–1.03)	0.93 (0.85–1.01)	
Premenopausal women						
Person-years	91,365	93,756	90,427	91,367	91,045	0.77
Cases, no	157	202	172	162	173	
Multivariate	1.0	1.28 (1.04–1.58)	1.07 (0.85–1.33)	1.02 (0.81–1.28)	1.09 (0.87–1.37)	
Postmenopausal women						
Person-years	208,178	214,244	221,842	215,627	209,067	0.03
Cases, no	844	810	800	797	698	
Multivariate	1.0	0.91 (0.83–1.01)	0.87 (0.79–0.96)	0.92 (0.83–1.02)	0.88 (0.79–0.97)	
Receptor status						
Cases, no	500	533	463	474	432	0.01
ER+/PR+	1.0	1.01 (0.90–1.15)	0.85 (0.75–0.97)	0.90 (0.79–1.03)	0.88 (0.77–1.00)	
Cases, No	153	142	163	141	132	0.33
ER-/PR-	1.0	0.90 (0.72–1.14)	1.02 (0.82–1.28)	0.89 (0.71–1.13)	0.88 (0.69–1.12)	

Models, RR (95% CI).
[1]Adjusted for the same covariates as in Table 2.

Alternative analyses using the most recent caffeine intake before diagnosis of breast cancer showed no association (multivariate RRs for increasing quintiles of caffeine consumption were 0.99, 0.99, 1.00 and 0.96 (95% CI = 0.87–1.05). In our main analysis, caffeine intake was calculated as cumulative averages of the diet data collected during follow-up. However, it is possible that earlier diet plays more critical role in the etiology of breast cancer. We used the repeated questionnaires to assess the temporal relationship between caffeine intake and breast cancer risk (Table V). No significant association was observed with a longer latency interval.

TABLE V – Multivariate RR and 95% CI of Breast Cancer According to Caffeine Intake with Various Lag Times Between Diet Assessment and Follow-Up Among Participants in the NHS

Latency (years)	N of cases	Caffeine Quintile					p for trend
		1	2	3	4	5	
4–7.9	4,642	1.0	0.91 (0.84–1.00)	0.91 (0.83–1.00)	0.94 (0.86–1.03)	0.86 (0.78–0.95)	0.01
8–11.9	4,032	1.0	0.90 (0.82–0.99)	0.89 (0.81–0.98)	0.97 (0.88–1.07)	0.88 (0.79–0.97)	0.12
12–15.9	2,816	1.0	0.84 (0.74–0.94)	0.87 (0.78–0.98)	0.95 (0.85–1.06)	0.82 (0.72–0.92)	0.05
16–19.9	1,791	1.0	0.98 (0.84–1.14)	1.08 (0.94–1.25)	1.00 (0.86–1.16)	0.97 (0.83–1.13)	0.75

Adjusted for the same covariates as in Table 2.

Discussion of Results or Conclusion

This section answers the question, "So what do these results mean in terms of the research question?" The conclusion of an article is often the most interesting, and just like a mystery novel, many readers skip ahead and peek to see how the story ends. It is important to remember, however, that this section is based on the authors' interpretation and opinion of what the data mean. Ideally, this opinion is informed and supported by the results just presented. Citations to other studies that are consistent with the study's findings are also helpful in bolstering the authors' case.

As you read the Ganmaa study example, note that the authors have focused on a discussion of the reasons for negative or null findings in studies generally, and their arguments against other explanations for the observed results of their analyses. This is usually a good indication that the authors have given thought to the strength of the association between the exposure (caffeine, in this study) and the observed outcome (the relative risk of developing breast cancer). The authors also return to the point made in the introduction regarding previous inconsistent findings in earlier studies on caffeine and breast cancer. They then go on to provide explanations for their conclusions, based on their methods and data.

Following the discussion/conclusion section of an article, authors may also include acknowledgements. This extremely brief section typically consists of a sentence or two in which the authors thank or acknowledge the assistance of others, such as research assistants who helped carry out the study or colleagues who critiqued the manuscript. In some cases, the relative contribution of each author is also described.

Consider the following questions as you continue to read:

1. What do you think of the authors' discussion of the study's strengths?

2. Do you agree with the authors' rationale for why previous studies reached a different conclusion from theirs?

3. Do the authors cite other evidence to support their conclusion?

4. If you were to go back and reread the results section after having read the conclusion, would you have a clearer understanding of the results?

5. Do you agree with their conclusions overall?

Discussion

In this large cohort of women, we observed no substantial association between caffeinated or decaffeinated coffee and tea consumption and risk of breast cancer during 22 years of follow-up. We found no evidence of an effect of either recent or long-term average consumption. We observed a weak overall inverse association with caffeine intake, and this association was stronger in postmenopausal women compared to premenopausal women.

Possible explanations for null findings include a narrow range of exposure, low statistical power, or measurement error. The current study had a wide range of coffee and tea intakes with the upper categories of 4 or more cups/day. The study included 5,272 cases and 1.8 million person-years, thus CI were narrow and statistical power was not a major problem. The use of repeated measures in the analysis not only accounts for changes in coffee use over time but also decreases measurement error.[43] Also, current coffee and caffeine intake had high correlations with estimates from four 1-week diet records.[40,41] Many biases inherent in case-control studies are avoided by a cohort design with nearly complete follow-up. Unmeasured confounding is still possible, although we adjusted for many breast cancer risk factors.

Results from other cohort studies of coffee, caffeine and risk of breast cancer generally have been inconsistent. The preliminary results from the Nurses' Health Study by Hunter et al., showed an inverse dose-related association of caffeine with breast cancer incidence.[32] Michels et al., assessed coffee consumption in relation to breast cancer cases in Swedish women[24] and reported that women who drank 4 or more cups of coffee/day had a covariate-adjusted hazard ratio of breast cancer of 0.94 [95% confidence interval (CI) 0.75–1.28] compared to women who reported drinking 1 cup a week or less. The corresponding hazard ratio for tea consumption was 1.13 (95% CI 0.91–1.40). Similarly, women in the highest quintile of self-reported caffeine intake had a hazard ratio of beast cancer of 1.04 (95% CI 0.87–1.24) compared to women in the lowest quintile. Folsom et al., assessed coffee intake prospectively in postmenopausal women; and found no apparent association between daily intake of coffee and risk of breast cancer.[26] The results of the study by Vatten et al., in 14,593 Norwegian women suggested that coffee consumption reduces the risk of breast cancer in lean women, whereas coffee might have the opposite effect in relatively obese women.[37] In the lean women, drinking 5 cups or more per day had an age-adjusted IRR of 0.5 (95% CI, 0.3 and 0.9) compared to women who had 2 cups or less. In more obese women there was a positive relation between coffee intake and breast cancer risk; the age-adjusted IRR was 2.1 (95% CI, 0.8 and 5.2). The reason for discrepancy between their findings and ours is not clear although the majority of the cases from the Norwegian cohort were premenopausal at the diagnosis of breast cancer, and most were certainly premenopausal at initiation phase. However, in the present study when we analyzed the coffee and breast cancer incidence stratified by menopausal status, among our premenopausal women we did not observe a significant association.

We also found caffeine to be associated with a lower risk of postmenopausal breast cancer than with premenopausal breast cancers; and this association was stronger with estrogen-receptor positive and progesterone-receptor positive breast cancer than with receptor negative breast cancer, suggesting a possible mechanistic role involving steroid hormones. Our results suggest that caffeine may be inversely associated with postmenopausal breast cancer risk, particularly in a low-estrogen environment. An inhibitory effect of caffeine on hormone-induced rat breast cancer has been reported by Petrek et al.,[44] who examined the effect of 2 caffeine doses in rats,[45] with and without diethylstilbestrol (DES). With DES, increasing caffeine dosage lengthened the time to first cancer, decreased the number of rats that developed cancers, and reduced the number of cancers overall. The inverse association observed for caffeine also may reflect beneficial effects of components of coffee and tea other than caffeine. Higher coffee consumption (or caffeine intake) has been directly associated with plasma estradiol, estrone and sex-binding globulin levels.[46,47] Jernstrom et al.,[48] reported that coffee consumption was the second most important lifestyle factor associated with increased plasma 2-OHE/16a-OHE ratio, and in some studies a relatively high 2-OHE/16a-OHE ratio has been associated with low rate of breast cancer.[49,50] 2-hydroxyestrone (OHE) is catalyzed by the cytochrome P450 (CYP) 1A2[51] and caffeine in turn appears to be an inducer of CYP1A2 activity.[52] Nkondock et al., reported that women with BRCA1 or BRCA2 mutations who consumed at least 6 cups of coffee per day to have a statistically significant reduction in breast cancer risk (OR = 0.31, 95% CI 0.13–0.71) compared to BRCA mutation carriers who have never drunk coffee.[53]

In conclusion, no substantial association was observed between consumption of caffeinated or decaffeinated coffee and tea and risk of breast cancer for the overall cohort. Higher consumption of caffeine-containing beverages may modestly reduce risk of postmenopausal breast cancer, and this relation needs to be examined further.

Acknowledgement

The authors thank Dr. Frank Hu for his technical support and valuable advice.

References

The reference section of an article establishes whether and how well the author has considered the work of other researchers and scholars. The formatting of the references will vary according to the publishing journal's chosen style, but sufficient information is always provided so that the reader could locate the original source of the citation. The list of citations should be current in relation to the article's publication date and content. For example, if the majority of citations in an article on acupuncture and immune function are more than 15 years old, the article's concepts are likely to have been superceded because immunology is such a rapidly expanding field. The obvious exception is an article that is primarily historical in nature, or one that is describing the course of development in an area.

A bonus feature of many electronically published articles is that the HTML version will often have an embedded direct link to each individual citation, so that you can click on the link and go right to the full text of the cited article.

Ideally, a reference section is both relevant and succinct. Look out for the brief article with more references than text – the authors may be trying to impress you with quantity rather than quality. Equally suspicious is the speculative article with little grounding in previous studies that is notable for its lack of citations. Reference lists also provide a good resource for further exploration of a topic.

As you become knowledgeable about the literature in a given area, you will also begin to notice whether references with which you are familiar are being used appropriately. Does the cited article really support the author's statement? For example, an author may assert that 75% of complementary practitioners have more than 1000 hours of training in their specialty, and references another article as the basis for this statement. Is the cited article a well-designed and carefully conducted survey published in a peer-reviewed journal, or is it an editorial in a popular magazine?

1. In the Ganmaa study, are there any references that you would want to seek out and read for more information?

References

1. *Wolfrom D, Welsch CW. Caffeine and the development of normal, benign and carcinomatous human breast tissue: a relationship? J Med 1990;21:225–50.*

2. *Minton JP, Foecking M, Webster D, Matthews RH. Caffeine, cyclic nucleotodes with breast disease. Surgery 1979;86:105–9.*

3. *Minton JP, Foecking M, Webster D, Matthews RH. Response of fibrocystic disease to caffeine withdrawal and correlation of cyclic nucleotides with breast disease. Am J Obstet Gynecol 1979;135:157–8.*

4. *Holmes MD, Willett WC. Does diet affect breast cancer risk? Breast Cancer Res 2004;6:170–8.*

5. Welsch CW. Caffeine and the development of the normal and neoplastic mammary gland. Proc Soc Exp Biol Med 1994;207:1–12.

6. VanderPloeg LC, Wolfrom DM, Rao AR, Braselton WE, Welsch CW. Caffeine, theophylline, theobromine, and developmental growth of the mouse mammary gland. J Environ Pathol Toxicol Oncol 1992;11:177–89.

7. James JE, Stirling KP. Caffeine: a survey of some of the known and suspected deleterious effects of habitual use. Br J Addict 1983;78:251–8.

8. Tarka SM. The toxicology of cocoa and methylxanthines: a review of the literature. Crit Rev Toxicol 1982;9:275–312.

9. Milder IE, Arts IC, van de Putte B, Venema DP, Hollman PC. Lignan contents of Dutch plant foods: a database including lariciresinol, pinoresinol, secoisolariciresinol and matairesinol. Br J Nutr 2005;93:393–402.

10. Galati G, O' Brien JP. Potential toxicity of flavonoids and other dietary phenolics: signi.cance for their chemopreventive and anticancer properties. Free Radic Biol Med 2004;37:287–303.

11. Le Bail JC, Varnat F, Nicolas JC, Habrioux G. Estrogenic and antiproliferative activities on MCF-7 human breast cancer cells by flavonoids. Cancer Lett 1998;130:209–16.

12. Williams RJ, Spencer JP, Rice-Evans C. Flavonoids: antioxidants or signaling molecules? Free Radic Biol Med 2004;36:838–49.

13. Abraham SK, Stopper H. Anti-genotoxicity of coffee against Nmethyl-N-nitro-N-nitrosoguanidine in mouse lymphoma cells. Mutat Res 2004;561:23–33.

14. Clifford MN. Chlorogenic acids and other cinnamates–nature, occurrence, dietary burden, absorption and metabolism. J Sci Food Agric 1999;79:362–372.

15. Svilaas A, Sakhi AK, Andersen LF, Svilaas T, Ström EC, Jacobs DR, Ose L, Blomhoff R. Intakes of antioxidants in coffee, wine, and vegetables are correlated with plasma carotenoids in humans. J Nutr 2004;134:562–7.

16. Pulido R, Hernandez-Garcia M, Saura-Calixto F. Contribution of beverages to the intake of lipophilic and hydrophilic antioxidants in the Spanish diet. Eur J Clin Nutr 2003;57:1275–82.

17. Kavanagh KT, Hafer LJ, Kim DW, Mann KK, Sherr DH, Rogers AE, Sonenshein GE. Green tea extracts decrease carcinogen-induced mammary tumor burden in rats and rate of breast cancer cell proliferation in culture. J Cell Biochem 2001;82:387–98.

18. Hirose M, Hoshiya T, Akagi K, Futakuchi M, Ito N. Inhibition of mammary gland carcinogenesis by green tea catechins and other naturally occurring antioxidants in female Sprague-Dawley rats pretreated with 7,12-dimethylbenzaanthracene. Cancer Lett 1994;83:149–56.

19. Tanaka H, Hirose M, Kawabe M, Sano M, Takesada Y, Hagiwara A, Shirai T. Post-initiation inhibitory effects of green tea catechins on 7,12-dimethylbenz[a] anthracene-induced mammary gland carcinogenesis in female Sprague-Dawley rats. Cancer Lett 1997;116:47–52.

20. Wu AH, Yu MC, Tseng CC, Hankin J, Pike MC. Green tea and risk of breast cancer in Asian Americans. Int J Cancer 2003;106:574–9.

21. Rose DP, Boyar AP, Wynder EL. International comparisons of mortality rates for cancer of the breast, ovary, prostate, and colon, and per capita food consumption. Cancer 1986;58:2363–71.

22. Ganmaa D, Sato A. The possible role of female sex hormones in milk from pregnant cows in the development of breast, ovarian and corpus uteri cancers. Med Hypotheses 2005;65:1028–37.

23. Ewertz M. Breast cancer in Denmark. Incidence, risk factors, and characteristics of survival. Acta Oncol 1993;32:595–615.

24. Michels KB, Holmberg L, Bergkvist L, Wolk A. Coffee, tea, and caffeine consumption and breast cancer incidence in a cohort of Swedish women. Ann Epidemiol 2002;12:21–6.

25. Ewertz M, Gill C. Dietary factors and breast cancer risk in Denmark. Int J Cancer 1990;46:779–84.

26. Folsom AR, McKenzie DR, Bisgard KM, Kushi LH, Sellers TA. No association between caffeine intake and postmenopausal breast cancer incidence in the Iowa Women's Health Study. Am J Epidemiol 1993;138:380–3.

27. Tavani A, Pregnolato A, La Vecchia C, Favero A, Franceschi S. Coffee consumption and the risk of breast cancer. Eur J Cancer Prev 1998;7:77–82.

28. Rohan TE, McMichael AJ. Methylxanthines & breast cancer. Int J Cancer 1988;41:390–3.

29. Jacobsen BK, Bjelke E, Kvale G, Heuch I. Coffee drinking, mortality, and cancer incidence: results from a Norwegian prospective study. J Natl Cancer Inst 1986;76:823–31.

30. Rosenberg L, Miller DR, Helmrich SP, Kaufman DW, Schottenfeld D, Stolley PD, Shapiro S. Breast cancer and the consumption of coffee. Am J Epidemiol 1985;122:391–9.

31. Lawson DH, Jick H, Rothman KJ. Coffee and tea consumption and breast disease. Surgery 1981;90:801–3.

32. Hunter DJ, Manson JE, Stampfer MJ, Colditz GA, Rosner B, Hennekens CH, Speizer FE, Willett WC. A prospective study of caffeine, coffee, tea, and breast cancer. Am J Epidemiol 1992;136:1000–1 (Abstract).

33. Franceschi S, Favero A, La Vecchia C, Negri E, Dal Maso L, Salvini S, Decarli A, Giacosa A. Influence of food groups and food diversity on breast cancer risk in Italy. Int J Cancer 1995;63:785–9.

34. Lubin F, Ron E, Wax Y, Modan B. *Coffee and methylxanthines and breast cancer: a case-control study. J Natl Cancer Inst 1985;74:569–73.*

35. Männistö S, Pietinen P, Virtanen M, Kataja V, Uusitupa M. *Diet and the risk of breast cancer in a case-control study: does the threat of disease have an influence on recall bias? J Clin Epidemiol 1999;52:429–39.*

36. Lê MG. *Coffee consumption, benign breast disease, and breast cancer. Am J Epidemiol 1985;122:721.*

37. Vatten LJ, Solvoll K, Løken EB. *Coffee consumption and the risk of breast cancer. A prospective study of 14,593 Norwegian women. Br J Cancer 1990;62:267–70.*

38. Mansel RE, Webster DJT, Burr M, St. Leger S. *Is there a relationship between coffee consumption and breast disease? Br J Surg 1982;69:295–6 (Abstract).*

39. Willett WC, Green A, Stampfer MJ, Speizer FE, Colditz GA, Rosner B, Monson RR, Stason W, Hennekens CH. *Relative and absolute excess risks of coronary heart disease among women who smoke cigarettes. N Engl J Med 1987;317:1303–9.*

40. Salvini S, Hunter DJ, Sampson L, Stampfer MJ, Colditz GA, Rosner B, Willett WC. *Food-based validation of a dietary questionnaire: the effects of week-to-week variation in food consumption. Int J Epidemiol 1989;18:858–67.*

41. Willett WC, Sampson L, Stampfer MJ, Sampson L, Rosner B, Hennekens CH, Speizer FE. *Reproducibility and validity of a semiquantitative food frequency questionnaire. Am J Epidemiol 1985;122:51–65.*

42. Hu FB, Stampfer MJ, Rimm E, Ascherio A, Rosner BA, Spiegelman D, Willett WC. *Dietary fat and coronary heart disease: a comparison of approaches for adjusting for total energy intake and modeling repeated dietary measurements. Am J Epidemiol 1999;149:531–40.*

43. Willett WC, Sampson L, Browne ML, Stampfer MJ, Rosner B, Hennekens CH, Speizer FE. *The use of a self-administered questionnaire to assess diet four years in the past. Am J Epidemiol 1988;127:188–99.*

44. Petrek JA, Sandberg WA, Cole MN, Silberman MS, Collins DC. *The inhibitory effect of caffeine on hormone-induced rat breast cancer. Cancer 1985;56:1977–81.*

45. *Inbred and genetically defined strains of laboratory animals. In: Altman PL, Katz DD, eds. Inbred strains: rat. Bethesda Maryland: Federation of American Societies for Experimental Biology, 1979. 238–9.*

46. Nagata C, Kabuto M, Shimizu H. *Association of coffee, green tea, and caffeine intakes with serum concentrations of estradiol and sex-hormone binding globulin in premenopausal Japanese women. Nutr Cancer 1998;30:21–4.*

47. Ferrini RL, Barrett-Connor E. *Caffeine intake and endogenous sex steroid levels in postmenopausal women. The Rancho Bernardo Study. Am J Epidemiol 1996;144:642–4.*

48. Jernstrom H, Klug TL, Sepkovic DW, Bradlow HL, Narod SA. *Predictors of the plasma ratio of 2-hydroxyestrone to 16a-hydroxyestrone among pre-menopausal, nulliparous women from four ethnic groups. Carcinogenesis 2003;24:991–1005.*

49. Meilahn EN, De Stavola B, Allen DS, Fentiman I, Bradlow HL, Sepkovic DW, Kuller LH. *Do urinary oestrogen metabolites predict breast cancer? Guernsey III cohort follow-up. Br J Cancer 1998;78:1250–5.*

50. Muti P, Bradlow HL, Micheli A, Krogh V, Freudenheim JL, Schunemann HJ, Stanulla M, Yang J, Sepkovic DW, Trevisan M, Berrino F. *Estrogen metabolism and risk of breast cancer: a prospective study of the 2:16a-hydroxyestrone ratio in premenopausal and postmenopausal women. Epidemiology 2000;11:635–40.*

51. Bradlow HL, Telang NT, Sepkovic DW, Osborne MP. *2-hydroxyestrone: the 'good' estrogen. J Endocrinol 1996;150(Suppl):S259–S265.*

52. Kotsopoulos J, Ghadirian P, El-Sohemy A, Lynch HT, Snyder C, Daly M, Domchek S, Randall S, Karlan B, Zhang P, Zhang S, Sun P, et al. *The CYP1A2 genotype modifies the association between coffee consumption and breast cancer risk among BRCA1 mutation carriers. Cancer Epidemiol Biomarkers Prev 2007;16:912–6.*

53. Nkondjock A, Ghadirian P, Kotsopoulos J, Lubinski J, Lynch H, Kim-Sing C, Horsman D, Rosen B, Isaacs C, Weber B, Foulkes W, Ainsworth P, et al. *Coffee consumption and breast cancer risk among BRCA1 and BRCA2 mutation carriers. Int J Cancer 2006;118:103–7.*

Summary

Each section of an original research article helps to create its overall structure and serves a specific function. These include: the abstract, which summarizes the article; the introduction, which states the research question and provides a review of the relevant literature; the methods and procedures, where the exact steps used to carry out the study are described in detail; the results, which contain a visual summary and written description of the statistical analyses of the study data; the discussion or conclusion, where the authors discuss their interpretation of what the results mean; and the references, which provide complete citations to other published works. Familiarity with each section of an article and its purpose is a necessary and useful step in critical evaluation.

Reference

1. Dillman DA. Mail and Telephone Surveys: The Total Design Method. New York: John Wiley and Sons; 1978.

Exercise

1. *Write a paragraph or two presenting your opinion of the strengths and weaknesses of the sample study by Ganmaa et al. Think about the structure and purpose of each section of a research article, and use the questions in the chapter text as a resource and guide for your discussion.*

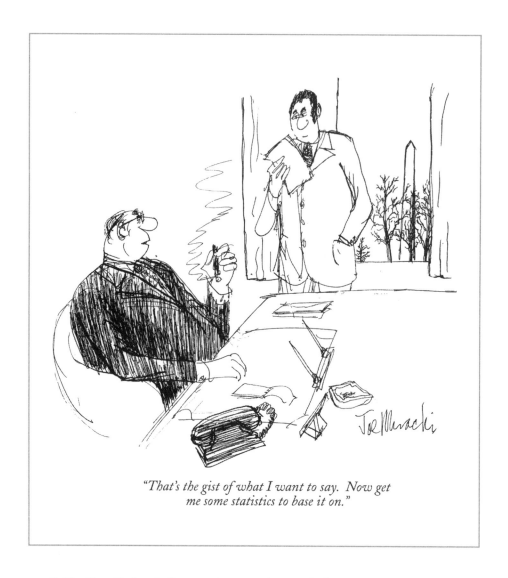

"That's the gist of what I want to say. Now get
me some statistics to base it on."

Chapter 6:

Making Sense of Statistics

Common sense one cannot do without.

P. B. Medawar

Learning Objectives

**After completing this chapter,
the reader should be able to:**

- Define probability.

- Name two common misconceptions about probability.

- Explain the difference between descriptive and inferential statistics.

- Discuss the differences among the mean, median, and mode.

- Describe the null hypothesis.

- Define statistical power.

- Define the four classes of variables.

- Explain two differences between parametric and nonparametric statistics.

- Identify one misuse of any common statistical test.

Chapter 6: Making Sense of Statistics

Statistics in Everyday Life

The word *statistics* comes from the Latin root "status" or the state of a thing. It suggests that statistics might be useful in describing the status of how things are. We all use statistical concepts in our day-to-day lives, often without a second thought. When we check the weather forecast to decide whether to take an umbrella with us, we are thinking statistically. Advertisements that say four out of five dentists recommend a certain toothpaste are relying on our tendency to think statistically. When we check a baseball player's batting average, we are thinking statistically. And if we play a hand of poker or are deciding whether or not to buy lottery tickets, we stand to make a better decision if we are thinking statistically. The best way to begin our education is to understand the basics of probability.

Probability

When mathematicians talk about **probability**, what they mean is: the chances of a particular outcome occurring as a result of a random process. A random process is one that varies in a random way, usually within certain limits. Think of a coin that may be tossed to give heads or tails, or of a die that can be cast to land on any one of its six sides. The individual outcome of each toss or cast will always be free to vary within the limits of the total number of outcomes possible – in the case of the coin, one out of two, or in the case of the die, one out of six. Every probability can be expressed as a number between 0 and 1, or as a percentage, a fraction of 100. With the coin, the probability is 1 divided by two, or 50%. The probability of any face coming up when the die is cast is 1 divided by 6, or 16.7%. A probability of 0% means the outcome will never happen, and a probability of 100% means that it is always certain to happen – a sure thing. And the sum of the probabilities of all possible outcomes always adds up to 1, or 100%.

To take this idea a little further, imagine that you want to know the probability of one outcome that is part of a larger set, say, the chances that you will roll an even number on a cast of a single die. You add together the probabilities of rolling a 2, a 4, and a 6, so that $1/6 + 1/6 + 1/6 = 3/6 = \frac{1}{2}$, which equals 50%.

The **complement** of an event is all the possible outcomes except those that make up the event. In other words, if A is an outcome whose probability of happening is 1 out 10, then the probability that A will not happen is 9 out of 10, or 90%. Another way to say this is that the odds against A are 9 to 1. We will come back to the idea of odds a bit later, in terms of gambling and in terms of research results. In many instances, it is simpler to arrive at the probability of an event by figuring out the complement instead of adding together all the possible probabilities.

Probability Myths

Sometimes, probabilities can be counterintuitive. We may think that a situation has only two possible outcomes, so the probability of either of the two outcomes occurring must be 50%, just like the toss of a fair coin described previously. However, in many situations there is a higher probability of one outcome over the other. Think of baseball players. It would seem that the chances of a player hitting the ball are 50-50, since they either hit the ball or they don't, but the chances are 50-50 only if the player's batting average is .500, or 50%, over many, many attempts. It is much more likely, since a great batting average starts at around .300, that the physical and psychological challenges involved make the chances lower than 50%.

There are three other misconceptions that are important to keep in mind when considering probabilities:

1. Probability is effective when predicting long-term behavior but much less so in the case of short-term behavior. You may know that an event will occur at some point, and you may be able to tell how roughly long you might have to wait for it to happen, but you can't predict exactly *when* it will happen. For example, you may know that the newspaper is predicting rain later in the week, but it is unlikely the report indicates that showers will begin at 4:56 p.m. on Friday.

2. In gambling, there is no such thing as being "on a roll." Probability, cards and dice have no memory, so if a process is being repeated under the same conditions over and over again, the probability is always the same for each repetition. Related to this idea is the fact that sequences of outcomes that look random often have the same probability as a group of sequences that appear to be less random, say, the sequences

of heads and tails in a group of coin tosses. Which sequence do you think is more likely to happen: HHTTTTHH, or HTTHHTHT? Each sequence has the same probability, because each contains four heads and four tails, and the order in which they occur doesn't matter.

3. We tend to rate the probability of a rare event differently depending whether we see it as good or bad. Most of us would rather bet on our chances of winning the lottery ("It's got to be somebody and it might be me!"), compared to the chances of being struck by lightning in our house during a thunderstorm. In the same way, we tend to systematically underestimate the probability of dying from a chronic health condition such as heart disease, and instead worry more about more distressing events that are statistically much less likely to occur, such as dying in an airplane crash.

We may be more familiar with the use of probabilities to calculate the payout in gambling or in games of chance, with more favorable odds paying smaller amounts than the long shots. Think of poker, where the ranking of winning hands is based on the probability of drawing them – a royal flush beats a pair, because the probability of drawing a royal flush is much lower than that of drawing a pair. In organized gambling the odds always favor the house by a small edge. In roulette, for example, the amount of money you could theoretically win by betting on black or red (even odds, or odds of 1 to 1) would be much less than the amount you could win by betting on a specific number, because the odds of landing on any given number are 37 to 1. Why 37 to 1, when there are 36 numbers on the wheel? The slots on the wheel are numbered 0 to 36, and players bet only on the numbers 1 through 36, with the house paying off based on that probability. Because nobody bets on 0, this gives the house an edge of 1/37, or 2.7%, on every bet made.

It is a small edge but over a long enough period of time the odds will always favor the house. This is why, if you ever win big at a casino, you should pocket your winnings and walk away – the longer you stay, the more likely that the house will win back the money from you. You may have noticed, if you have ever been in a casino, that the décor is deliberately designed to encourage patrons to lose track of time. There are no clocks on the wall and no windows. Similarly, if you invest in the stock market, the commission you pay on each transaction is just like the house advantage – the more trades you make, the harder it is to get ahead. If you are interested in learning more about how to bet intelligently across a number of common situations, read the classic book by John D. McGervey, called *Probabilities in Everyday Life*.[1] Another classic and quite entertaining work is titled *How to Lie With Statistics*, by Darrell Huff.[2] In spite of its tongue-in-cheek title, this book contains a highly useful section on how to spot the misuse of scaling in graphs and charts, and is well worth reading before you next look at visual summaries of research results.

In research, probabilities determine the odds of getting a particular result, based on some number of participants measured across some number of outcomes, due to random chance. Calculating these probabilities is the primary purpose of the statistical analysis performed in most quantitative health care research studies, and the resulting number at the end of the calculations is known as a statistic. If the probability, or *p* value, of obtaining those results for that number of participants is small enough, usually 5 out of a hundred, or even less, such as 1 out of a thousand, then we are willing to conclude that there is strong enough evidence that these results are not random. In fact, as we saw in the Ganmaa study example in the last chapter, no more than 5 out of 100 or 0.05 is the conventional level of acceptable statistical significance to rule out chance as a plausible alternate explanation for the results of the study.

Levels of Variables

Before we discuss the various types of statistics, it is helpful to understand that the variables used to format data can be characterized into four levels: nominal, ordinal, interval, and ratio. A **nominal variable** is expressed as a category, such as redhead, blonde, or brunette. An **ordinal variable** is one that is expressed as a ranked order, such as good, better, best, or never, seldom, often, always. **Interval** level **variables** can be expressed as numbers, and are the most familiar type of data – what we usually think of when we think of statistical data. **Ratio variables** are expressed as a numerical ratio of one thing to another thing, such as miles per gallon. These concepts are useful in understanding why we use different types of statistical analysis and under what circumstances one type is preferable, or more appropriate than another.

Types of Statistics

We will now look at how statistics are categorized. Stated briefly: **descriptive statistics** allow us to summarize and "crunch" a large number of observations into a condensed format. The calculation of descriptive statistics is usually straightforward. Most of us use descriptive statistics on a daily basis, for example, looking up the average temperature at a vacation destination during the month of January, or Googling the median price of a three-bedroom house in our neighborhood. **Inferential statistics** let us draw a conclusion about a population based on a randomly selected sample from that population, allow us to test hypotheses, and sometimes to make predictions as well. Most quantitative research studies contain reports using both descriptive and inferential analyses. The term **experimental statistics** refers to statistics used in experimental designs; most of the inferential methods described could be considered such.

• *Descriptive Statistics*

Descriptive statistics simply describe a data set, hence the name. They present the data generated in a study without generalizing them to a larger group. They contain the characteristics of the data, and most commonly include:

· the number of categories of responses for each variable

· the difference between the highest and lowest values for each variable, called the **range**

· the average values for each variable – the average of the numbers in a group is referred to as the **mean**

· the amount of variation or dispersal of the data around the average, meaning the degree to which individual results vary around the mean is the **standard deviation (SD)**

A **measure of central tendency** reflects where the middle of the data set is; there are three different ways in which the middle can be defined, depending on the level of variable. The mean, or average, is the measure of central tendency that is most familiar. The mean is equal to the sum of all the observations in the data set divided by the number of observations. It must be calculated using interval or ratio data – numerical values such as 3 or .67. The mean is often abbreviated as a capital X with a line over it: $\overline{X}$. Related to the mean, the standard deviation is a measure of the average variability around the mean – that is, how spread out the scores are. The more spread out from the average the individual scores are, the larger the standard deviation. It is sometimes abbreviated as the Greek letter sigma: σ.

Two other measures of central tendency are the **median** and the **mode**. The median is the midpoint at which half of the data set is above and half is below. It can be calculated with interval or ratio data, as in the example above of finding the median

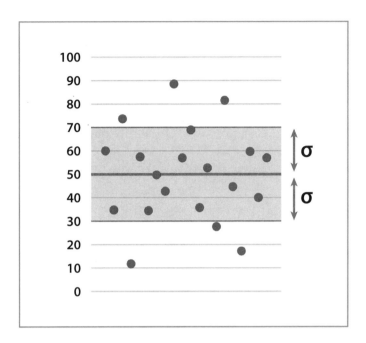

Figure 6.1 A data set with a mean of 50 and a standard deviation of 20.

Standard deviation [Online]. 2009 July 23 [cited 2009 July 24];
Available from: URL: http://www.wikipedia.org

home price, but also with ordinal data, data that can be expressed as a ranked order, such as letter grades: a B is lower than an A but higher than a C. If we say that the median grade for the course is a B, then we know that half of the students did better and half did worse.

The **mode** is the measure of the score value or category that has the highest frequency associated with it. In addition to describing interval, ratio, and ordinal data, it can also be used to describe the middle of a nominal data set, that is, categorical data such as eye color. It would be meaningless to say that the average eye color was 3.16, but we can say that in a particular group of kindergarteners, the eye color most frequently observed was brown.

Researchers typically do a preliminary analysis of the data by plotting each data point on a graph, to see how often each score is repeated. Such a graph provides what is called a **grouped frequency distribution** of a particular data set. Some authors may also include general information regarding the distribution of the data. Usually, most of the scores are bunched up in the middle, with very high or very low scores trailing off to either side, creating a bell-shaped curve on the line graph. This is called the **normal distribution**. Many real-life data sets, assuming they are large enough, have this bell shape and are said to be normally distributed. In the normal distribution, roughly 68% of the data points will be within one standard deviation of the mean. If we add another standard deviation, 95% of the data points will be contained, and three deviations will bring almost all our data points, 99.7%, under the curve. If the data are not normally distributed, researchers may run into problems later on when trying to apply inferential statistical testing.

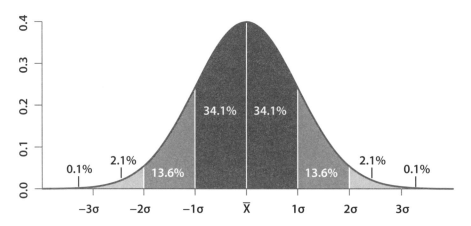

Figure 6.2 A plot of a normal distribution (bell curve). Each colored band has a width of one standard deviation.

Standard deviation [Online]. 2009 July 23 [cited 2009 July 24];
Available from: URL: http://www.wikipedia.org

• *Inferential Statistics*

Inferential statistics are used to make inferences about a population from measuring a sample of that population. Two of the most common applications of inferential statistics are **estimation** and **hypothesis testing**. When the Gallup organization conducts a voter survey, they select a sample that is representative of the population to which they want to apply the results. Based on the sample data, they can then estimate how the entire population as a whole will vote. If the sample is representative of the population, the estimate will be fairly accurate. The amount of error within that estimate can also be determined. Surveys frequently report results with a **margin of error**, usually two to three percentage points, that tells us the range of error that could be present in the estimate. You can probably find an example in any daily paper.

The amount of error in such an estimate gives us what is called a **confidence interval**, abbreviated as CI, and a probability is associated with it, usually 95%. This allows us to know that the true score lies within the specified range 95% of the time. For example, with a survey result stating that 69% of Outer Banks surfers reported that they were stung by jellyfish in August, with a margin of error of plus or minus 2.5 points, we can be 95% sure that the true percentage of stung surfers lies between 66.5% and 71.5%. And if this sample is representative, you might want to plan your beach vacation for July.

In hypothesis testing, statistics are used to determine whether any difference between the means of the groups compared is due to chance, or whether chance can be ruled out as an alternate explanation. Remember the concept of falsifiability – the idea that science works best by demonstrating a hypothesis to be false instead of true? In inferential statistics the mathematical equivalent is a concept called the **null hypothesis**. The null hypothesis proposes that there is no difference between the means of the groups compared in a study, for example, between the means of the outcomes measured in the treatment and control groups of an experimental study such as an RCT. In other words, the null hypothesis represents the idea that a study did not produce or observe a genuine effect, and the task of the researchers becomes to disprove the null hypothesis.

If an author can show that there is indeed a difference between the group means and that this is not a chance or random occurrence, the reader can feel confident in rejecting the null hypothesis, and the **alternate hypothesis**, that a true difference between the groups was observed, can be accepted.

The common abbreviation for the null hypothesis is H_0 and for the alternate hypothesis, H_1. Remember that the null hypothesis is that there is no difference between the groups, or in other words, that the groups' means are equal. This can be expressed as $H_0 = H_1$. The alternate hypothesis, that the groups' means are not equal, is expressed as $H_0 \neq H_1$. In nonparametric statistics, to which we will turn shortly, other measures of central tendency instead of the mean are compared.

Generally speaking, there are two kinds of inferential statistical testing: **tests of statistical significance** and **measures of association**. Tests of statistical significance tell us the probability that any observed differences between group means is due to chance. Measures of association do just that – they evaluate or measure the extent to which two variables are associated with each other, and the probability that the magnitude of this association is due to chance can be determined. Both kinds of tests have a stated assumption that the data set being tested is normally distributed. If this is not the case (if the distribution has a different shape than the usual bell-shaped curve), the test may not be accurate. A statistical test is said to be "robust" when its assumptions can be violated and yet still return a reasonably accurate estimate of the value for p.

P-Values and Effect Sizes

As we have stated previously, p stands for probability – in the reporting of research results, this refers to the probability that the results of any inferential statistical tests are due to chance. Because p values are closely related to sample size, any difference between group means will be statistically significant if the sample size is large enough. The p value tells us only that the results are not due to chance. While this is a necessary starting point, it says nothing about the magnitude of the observed effect or its clinical relevance.

A useful measure that is too rarely reported in health care research studies is the **effect size**, which is not dependent on sample size. We often use the concept of effect size in making everyday decisions. For example, a weight loss program may claim that it leads to an average weight loss of 25 pounds. In this case, 25 pounds is the purported effect size. Another example is a tutoring program that advertises that it raises school performance in math by one letter grade. This grade increase is the claimed effect size of the program. The larger the effect size, the easier it is to observe in a study's results.

Depending on the type of statistical test used, there are a number of different ways to calculate effect size. Most involve relatively simple equations based on the means and standard deviations of the two groups compared. The interested reader may visit web.uccs.edu/lbecker/Psy590/es.htm, University of Colorado professor Lee Becker's website, for a thorough discussion of the various ways to determine effect size based on the means and standard deviations for two groups. Try out the effect size calculator provided there.

The **odds ratio** is a kind of effect size, similar to the relative risk, that is often seen in epidemiological studies, particularly case-control studies. It is used when both the exposure and outcome variables are binary (also called dichotomous), that is, a yes or no situation. For example, consider a hypothetical study on whether smoking (exposure) affects the risk of having a myocardial infarction (outcome) in a sample of women. The data can be presented in a two-by-two table and would look like this:

Exposure	Outcome		Total
Smoker	*Myocardial Infarction*		
	Yes	*No*	
Yes	*a*	*b*	*a+b*
No	*c*	*d*	*c+d*
Total	*a+c*	*b+d*	*a+b+c+d*

Figure 6.3 A sample two-by-two table.

The odds ratio can be expressed simply as a times d, divided by b times c:

$$\text{Odds ratio} \; = \; \frac{ad}{bc}$$

This kind of table and calculation can be used for any dichotomous data, and is similar to one of the nonparametric tests of significance we will talk about a bit later, the *chi-square test*.

Statistical Power

Effect size has a direct relationship to **statistical power**. Power refers to the likelihood (probability) that a significance test of the difference between two means will be able to reject the null hypothesis, that is, to detect a genuine effect if one is present – the larger the effect, the smaller the sample size necessary to be able to detect it. Detection of small effects therefore requires large sample sizes, and many of the effects in health care research are small. This is why the relatively small sample sizes often seen in pilot studies are problematic, and why the savvy investigator will perform a **power analysis** at the beginning of such a study's design phase. With some idea of a study's potential effect size, or of the effect size the researchers want to be able to detect, the number of participants needed to achieve this can be calculated. Generally, the preference is for an 80% probability of rejecting the null hypothesis. In other words, if my research hypothesis is true, I want to have an 80% chance of demonstrating it. A 99% chance would be even better, but 80% is usually a more realistic goal in terms of the resources of time, money, and number of participants needed to conduct a study.

Another way to think of this idea is the concept frequently used in medical tests: the **false positive** and the **false negative**. Type 1 error, or **alpha**, where the null hypothesis is mistakenly rejected and the researchers prematurely break out the bubbly to celebrate their highly significant results, can be thought of as a false positive – the positive results are actually false. The probability level for alpha is traditionally set very low – the arbitrary *p* value of no more than .05. In the opposite situation of Type 2 error, or **beta**, the researchers fail to reject the null hypothesis and have a false negative – their negative results are actually false, and the value of their findings is lost to science because their sample was too small. Power is equal to 1 minus beta, and can be defined as being the probability of correctly rejecting H_0, the null hypothesis.

Type I and Type II errors were discussed in Chapter 3. As you have no doubt realized by now, these are both directly related to statistical power, and are inversely proportional to each other. Setting an appropriate alpha level guards to a reasonable degree against the possibility of committing Type I error, while having a reasonable degree of statistical power protects against Type 2 error. So, in the design phase of a study, the savvy researcher attempts to balance the risk of Type 1 and Type 2 error. The conventional levels of no higher than .05 for alpha and not lower than 80% for beta are the consensually accepted reasonable balance within scientific research generally. Occasionally pilot studies will set alpha at .10, which is considered a reasonable compromise in an exploratory situation.

One factor that affects the statistical power of a study is the total number of variables being measured, both exposure and outcome (or independent and dependent variables, depending on your field) – the more variables, the larger the *n*, or number of study participants that will be necessary. Variables measured also include those used as covariates. This is why unanticipated confounding variables present a dilemma: the researcher must decide whether to reduce the statistical power of the study or its internal validity. A handy book by Kraemer and Thieman titled *How Many Subjects?*[3] contains an excellent discussion of this topic, and has a complete list of tables that can be used to determine the number of participants necessary for a wide variety of study designs. No calculator needed; just look it up.

At this point, we have concluded a quick overview of basic statistical concepts, and hopefully some of mysteries faced when viewing study results tables will now be less obscure. Next we will consider some specific types of tests of statistical significance and measures of association, and learn how to tell if they are being misused.

Parametric and Nonparametric Statistics

Earlier in this chapter, we discussed descriptive statistics and measures of central tendency (where the middle of the data set is). Remember that the variables measured to create the data set can come in four different formats: nominal, ordinal, interval or ratio. To reiterate, a nominal variable is simply a named category, like eye color or sex. An ordinal variable produces data that is ranked in order, such as stages of cancer, or ratings of the depth of pressure used in applying a massage technique. Nominal and ordinal variables describe categories or qualities associated with the variable being measured. It wouldn't make any sense to say what the average sex of the participants in a study was. We can only count the number in each category – how many men and women participated in the study.

With interval and ratio variables, though, we can determine the average. Interval variables are things that can be measured with numbers, like age, cortisol levels or years of education. Ratio variables are also numbers and are expressed in terms of a ratio, like systolic over diastolic blood pressure, or the person-time units we saw in the Ganmaa study in Chapter 5. They are treated the same way for the purposes of statistical analysis.

It is important to distinguish among these different types of variables for two reasons. First, interval and ratio variables are usually assumed to be normally distributed (if the sample is large enough) and can be analyzed using **parametric** statistics. Nominal and ordinal variables require simply counting the number of things or people in each category or rank. These kinds of data must be analyzed using **nonparametric** statistics. Nonparametric tests are said to be "distribution-free" in that these analytical methods do not assume that the data set fits the normal distribution. There are also nonparametric tests for very small samples, another circumstance where the data cannot be assumed to be normally distributed. Second, it is certainly possible to express interval and ratio data in terms of categories; we could take blood pressure readings from people in a doctor's waiting room and group or categorize them according to high, normal, or low diastolic pressure. But we would lose a great deal of information and statistical power by doing so, because by compressing the actual readings into only three ranked levels we are losing detail and precision of measurement. In general this is a bad strategy for data analysis, and it is one that should raise a red flag if you see it employed in a study.

Types of Parametric Tests

The *t*-test was first developed by William S. Gossett [1876–1937], who published under the pseudonym of "Student." Gossett was a statistician employed by the Guinness Brewery in Dublin, Ireland, as a quality control supervisor, and could not publish under his own name because the company believed that secretly having a statistician on the payroll to test small batches of their stout gave them an edge over the competition. The *t*-test is the most basic test of statistical significance, and is still often used with small samples. If you can understand the logic that underlies the *t*-test, you will have a fundamental understanding of how many statistical tests work.

In the *t*-test, the means of two groups are being compared to each other. It is not enough to show that the means differ from each other – how much the variability in each group differs must also be considered. Within each group, then, the difference between each individual score and the mean is computed by subtracting the group mean from each score, and then averaging those for each group. This is the familiar standard deviation, the average amount of "spread-outedness" around the mean, in each group. The *t*-test compares the difference between the two means in relation to the average variability in each group. In simple terms, the formula for the *t*-test is:

$$\frac{\text{Difference between the Group Means}}{\text{Variability of the Groups}}$$

Almost all inferential statistical tests use some version of this basic formula, with greater or lesser degrees of complexity based on the study design. So, the next time you drink a pint of stout, raise your glass to "Student."

Independent and Paired *t*-tests

There are two types of *t*-tests: the **independent *t*-test**, used for two samples drawn from independent groups of subjects, and the **paired *t*-test** or **dependent *t*-test**, which is used for paired observations. What do we mean by independent samples? These are samples that are drawn from two different groups, for example, a randomly assigned treatment group and a control group. The two separate groups are not related and do not overlap.

The paired *t*-test is used when participants in two groups are matched on some characteristic, such as age or severity of illness, and then compared to each other, or when individuals are compared with themselves as in a before-and-after treatment situation. An example would be comparing range of motion in a group of gymnasts before and after massage. The gymnasts' range of motion at a particular joint would be measured before the massage intervention and then again afterward. The two measurements would then be paired with each other. Another example would be patients in a cancer unit paired based on medication use. This example can be seen in one of the studies we will examine in Chapter 7.

If a *t*-test is being used to compare one group to another, the informed reader will look to see which kind was used and consider whether the author has chosen wisely with regard to the type of *t*-test employed. If the author has used the independent *t*-test when the study design demands the paired *t*-test, a red flag should go up. The *t*-test is also directional, and the terms used are **one-tailed** and **two-tailed**. A one-tailed test predicts a difference in a single direction, positive or negative; a two-tailed test predicts a difference in either direction. The one-tailed test is appropriate only if the author predicted in advance which group would have the larger mean, based on prior observation or data. The two-tailed test is more commonly used.

In addition, a *t*-test should only be used for a single outcome variable. Remember that the more comparisons you make, the greater the chance of Type I error, which is the probability that one comparison will be significant by chance alone. In *PDQ Statistics*,[4] Norman and Streiner enjoy pointing out that this means that one out of every 20 published articles that report a statistically significant difference is wrong, and that we can only wonder which one it is!

Multiple comparisons are actually a serious problem in molecular genetics, where thousands of gene sequences may be compared at one time. According to stem cell scientist David Shaywitz, "A recent review of 85 published genetic mutations proposed to be associated with heart attacks demonstrated a validation rate of zero: there was insufficient evidence to suggest that any of the originally published associations reflected more than chance alone."[5]

Analysis of variance (ANOVA) is also a commonly used test of significance. It allows for comparisons among multiple groups that are assessed with the same outcome measure. A good example of a research study where ANOVA might be used would be comparing over-the-counter NSAIDs – is there any difference in how well the four major brands relieve headache pain? We could recruit a sample of tax accountants during the first two weeks of April and randomly sort them into four groups, one for each brand tested. Our null and alternate hypotheses would be:

No difference among the group means; they are all equal: $H_0 = H_1$
There is a difference; not all the group means are equal: $H_0 \neq H_1$

This is the most basic kind of ANOVA, and is called a **one-way analysis of variance**. In ANOVA, the variation both within the groups and between the groups is being partitioned and compared. This ratio can be simply expressed as:

$$\frac{\text{Variance between Groups}}{\text{Variance within Groups}}$$

The result is called the *F statistic*. The beauty of ANOVA is that it allows the researcher to make multiple comparisons among all the different groups without increasing the risk of committing a Type I error (and it takes much less time than doing a series of *t*-tests). There are more complex forms of ANOVA that involve two- and three-way comparisons, sometimes referred to as nested designs. For example, in our study of the four different pain relievers, we could perform a three-way ANOVA to compare medication brands by age groups and sex. Do some OTC medications work better for older people or younger people? Or for younger men or older women? **Repeated measures ANOVA** is often used for samples that are measured at various points over a period of time. This approach in effect multiplies the original number of participants by the number of occasions on which they are measured, and can help to compensate for a small sample size.

Multiple analysis of variance (MANOVA) is used for comparisons involving multiple outcome variables. Analysis of covariance, used to control for pre-existing differences between groups, has been introduced in previous chapters, and will be discussed in more detail in a moment. With all types of ANOVA, however, one should not be misled by a large F statistic, or lots of comparisons. Look at the means and standard deviations, and get some sense of the effect size.

Speaking of comparisons, sometimes in studies employing ANOVA you will see references to **post-hoc testing**. These are comparisons between two of the multiple groups in the study that are being tested for significance. The use of post-hoc tests ideally should be specified in advance, and they should be used only if the overall ANOVA reaches significance. A statistically significant F indicates that there is a difference somewhere among the multiple comparisons, but it doesn't specify which comparisons. The *Bonferonni procedure* controls for multiple comparisons and is used when planned contrasts between particular groups is anticipated by the investigator. There are two other acceptable post-hoc tests that also take multiple comparisons into account and do not require that specific comparisons be identified in advance; these are the *Tukey's test* and *Scheffe's test*. A positive *t*-test as a follow-up to an ANOVA that has failed to reach significance overall is a big red flag, and is most likely Type I error at work.

Correlation

Correlation refers to a group of statistical methods that are measures of association. A measure of association, as we have said before, looks at the extent to which two variables are associated with or related to each other. In mathematical terms, correlation indicates the strength and direction of a linear relationship between two variables. If there is no relationship, if the variables are completely independent of each other, the correlation will be 0. The correlation is 1 in the case of an increasing linear relationship and -1 in the case of a decreasing linear relationship. In other words, if the correlation is 1 or -1, as one variable increases or decreases, then so does the other, by the same amount. The closer the coefficient is to either -1 or 1, the stronger the relationship between the variables. Think of this concept as *co-relation*. The resulting statistic that shows the degree of correlation is called a **correlation coefficient** and is denoted as *r*.

There are several different coefficients that are used for different situations. The most frequently encountered is the **Pearson product-moment correlation coefficient**, which is used for two interval or ratio level variables. From the name, one would think it must have been developed by someone named Pearson, but it was actually introduced by the well-known statistician and psychologist Francis Galton. The simple formula for a Pearson product-moment correlation can be expressed as:

$$\frac{\text{Co-variance of the Two Variables}}{\text{Standard Deviation of First Variable x Standard Deviation of Second Variable}}$$

This is very similar to the way in which the *t*-test is calculated. Some measure of central tendency is being assessed in relation to the spread-outedness of the variables, and the resulting value for *r* shows how big the association between the two variables is, as well as its directionality. Just as with the *t* and F statistics, we can go to a table of critical values for *r*, look up the author's stated value for *r* and see for ourselves the probability of getting this result due to chance. Remember, however, that correlation does not equal causation, and that even if a cause-and-effect relationship is at work, correlation does not tell us which variable is the cause and which is the effect.

In most of the statistical situations encountered so far, there has been an interval or ratio level outcome variable and a nominal level exposure variable. **Regression analysis** is a measure of association that, like the Pearson correlation, assesses the association or relationship between two interval or ratio level variables, such as years of education and income. Regression predicts the value of one variable from our knowledge of the other. For example, we intuit that education and income are correlated with each other. Assuming that years of education is the exposure or independent variable, and income the outcome, so to speak, regression analysis allows us to measure the extent of the association between the two and determine how much of the variance of one variable can be explained by the other. Mathematically, the data points for income and years of education are plotted on an x-and-y graph and an equation is developed that has the best fit with the actual data. The strength of the relationship is expressed by the proportion of the variance explained by the exposure or independent variable. In this example, it would be the amount of variance in income explained by years of education.

Regression analysis is often used to make predictions based on the extent of the association between variables. An example is the predicted lifetime income for a high school graduate, which is often contrasted with the predicted lifetime income for a college graduate. When several exposure variables are used to predict a single outcome variable, it is called **multiple regression**. Multiple regression determines the relative proportion of variance explained by each of the variables used as predictors – the statistic reported is called an R^2. It is a quite powerful statistical technique that can be used in many of the same situations as ANOVA.

Analysis of covariance (**ANCOVA**) can be thought of as a combination of ANOVA and regression analysis. It compensates for preexisting differences between groups and works best when there is a relationship or correlation between the covariate and the outcome measure, for example with age (covariate) and blood pressure (outcome). However, if more than one covariate is used, they should not be correlated with each other. Using covariates makes the analysis more powerful in terms of detecting a difference in group means, but at the cost of requiring an increased sample size. ANCOVA is not a panacea for a poorly conceived study with serious preexisting imbalances between groups.

Nonparametric Tests

As stated previously, nonparametric tests involve comparisons based on nominal (categorical) and ordinal (rank-ordered) variables, and are considered to be distribution-free, that is, the data do not need to be normally distributed for the test to correctly estimate the probability that the null hypotheses is false. One class of nonparametric tests is based on the sign properties of the data; that is, all the observations above the median are given a + sign and all the observations below the median are given a − sign. Data may also be ranked in order. For example, patients might be asked whether they feel *extremely uncomfortable / uncomfortable / neutral / comfortable / very comfortable*. What scores should be assigned to the comfort categories and how is it determined whether the outcome would differ with a slight change in scoring? Some of these concerns are alleviated when the data are converted from categories to ranks. "Extremely uncomfortable" can be set to equal 1, "uncomfortable" can be set equal to 2, and so on. In this example, ranking provides more information than categories. More information is always better than less, at least in the statistical sense. In examining data there is no such thing as TMI (too much information).

There are many different nonparametric tests of significance and measures of association – there is a nonparametric equivalent for each of the parametric tests and measures discussed earlier. For example, the nonparametric equivalent of the Pearson product-moment correlation is known as *Spearman's rho*, which is used for ordinal level or ranked data. The odds ratio presented earlier could be considered a nonparametric test, since it uses two categorical exposure-and-outcome variables. Actually, these are binary or dichotomous yes/no conditions. The data consist of the number of people in each category who have the exposure or not, and the number who developed the outcome or not.

The **chi-square test** (χ^2) is the most commonly used nonparametric test. It can be employed both as a test of significance and as a measure of the association between two variables. Gregor Mendel's experiments with plant genetics were based on chi-square. It looks a bit like the odds ratio, and is often set up as a 2x2 table.

Chi-square is used when the data consist of frequency counts. Often in health care research there is a situation where researchers wish to compare observed frequencies with expected frequencies. For example, imagine that we have noticed what appears to be a cluster of leukemia cases in a town that has had a number of factories built in the last 10 years. We have access to statewide rates of leukemia in the population going back for a generation and can compare the number of observed cases of leukemia with the expected number of cases for the town based on this previous data. The null hypothesis is that there will be no difference between the observed and expected frequencies. The larger the value for chi-square, the greater the difference between the observed and expected frequencies. Chi-square can also be set up with individual data points, comparing observed results to the results we would expect based on probability.

Unlike most nonparametric tests, chi-square can also be used for interval data, keeping in mind that chi-square depends on a relatively large sample size. If the expected frequency in any cell of the chi-square table is less than 5, *Fisher's exact test* should be used instead.

Another commonly encountered nonparametric test is the *Mann-Whitney-U*, which is comparable to the *t*-test for independent samples. The *Wilcoxon rank sum* test is essentially the same as the Mann-Whitney-U. In both tests, the null hypothesis is that the samples come from the same distribution, whatever it may be and regardless of normality, and the data are in ranked order. The *Wilcoxon signed-ranks* test is a nonparametric equivalent to the paired *t*-test.

Summary

The goal of this chapter has been to demystify the statistical results commonly reported in published research. Understanding the basic statistical concepts presented here will give you greater confidence in deciphering the results section of an article. In general, look to see whether the study variables provide interval, ratio, ordinal, or nominal level data, and whether parametric or nonparametric tests have been used. Check that the appropriate statistical test has been selected based on the level of the data and the study design. Whenever possible, refuse to settle for p values alone. If two groups are being compared, use the means and standard deviations provided to calculate the effect size. And always use common sense when weighing the statistical evidence presented in an article.

References

1. McGervey J. *Probabilities in Everyday Life*. New York: Ballantine Books;1989.

2. Huff D. *How to Lie With Statistics*. New York: WW Norton; 1993.

3. Kraemer HC and Thiemann S. *How Many Subjects? Statistical Power Analysis in Research*. Newbury Park, CA: Sage Books; 1987.

4. Norman GR and Streiner DL. *PDQ Statistics*. BC Decker, Incorporated: Toronto; 1986, p 33.

5. Shaywitz, DA. Science is leading us to more answers, but it's also misleading us. *Washington Post* cited April 22, 2008. Available from: www.washingtonpost.com /wp-dyn/content/article/2008/04/18/AR2008041802868.html

Exercise

1. *With your newfound statistical knowledge, go to the BioMed Central website and choose an article of interest. Read the article, paying particular attention to the results section. Determine what level of data was provided from the study variables, and whether a parametric or nonparametric test was used. Is the statistical test performed appropriate to the study design? If possible, go to the Becker website and calculate the effect size.*

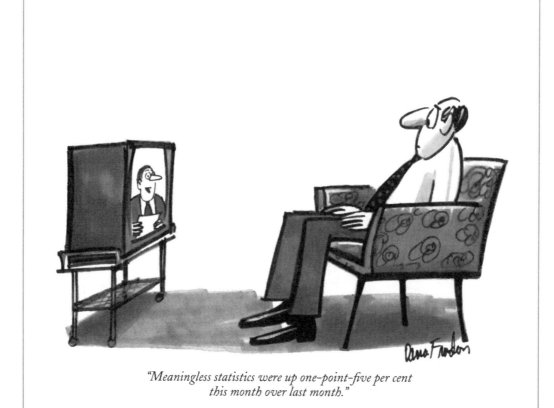

"*Meaningless statistics were up one-point-five per cent this month over last month.*"

Chapter 7:

How to Read a Quantitative Article

It is no kindness to a colleague – indeed, it might be the act of an enemy – to assure a scientist that his work is clear and convincing and that his opinions are really coherent when the experiments that profess to uphold them are slovenly in design and not well done. More generally, criticism is the most powerful weapon in any methodology of science; it is the scientist's only assurance that he need not persist in error.

P. B. Medawar

Learning Objectives

After completing this chapter,
the reader should be able to:

· *Use the questions in this chapter as a guide for critical evaluation of a quantitative journal article.*

· *Read the results section of an article with confidence.*

· *Differentiate between statistical and clinical significance.*

· *Identify the three alternative explanations that need to be ruled out in any study.*

· *Practice critical evaluation skills.*

Chapter 7: How to Read a Quantitative Article

In this chapter we get down to the specifics of how one critically reads a journal article. For each section of a typical clinical research article, questions to guide your evaluation are listed. These questions are presented as a general protocol. In this chapter the intention is to familiarize the reader with a systematic approach to the critique process. Concepts that have been previously introduced, especially statistical concepts, will be briefly reviewed as necessary. Later in the chapter we will model the practical application of the protocol through using it to analyze two quantitative journal articles. The questions used are oriented toward quantitative studies, which are still by far the most numerous in the health care literature to date. Critical evaluation of qualitative studies is discussed in the next chapter.

General Considerations

There are several general considerations to keep in mind as you read any article. First, remember the primary rule: *Be skeptical*. When an author is making assertions or claiming statements as facts, ask yourself on what basis these claims are being made, and whether some other plausible explanation is possible. It is the author's job to provide a convincing argument based on the evidence presented, rather than persuasion or emotional appeals. As you will remember from Chapter 3, plausible alternate explanations will generally fall into one of three categories: chance, bias, or confounding.

Another consideration is the general quality of the journal in which the article is published:

- *Is the journal peer reviewed?*

Being published in a prestigious journal does not automatically make an article better, but articles published in journals that lack a critical peer-review system have not been put through the same process of scrutiny and quality control. Look at the journal's guidelines for authors (likely available on its website) to determine whether submissions are subject to blind review, that is, where the reviewers do not know the authors' identities and therefore cannot be influenced by reputation or institutional affiliation. Despite the pleas of methodologists in every scientific discipline, poorly conceived and executed research projects are still undertaken, and articles describing their results are published somewhere every month.

Also check the fine print for author affiliations and funding sources of the study:

- *Who conducted and funded the research?*

The reader must consider whether or to what extent such relationships may have influenced the study findings.

The Abstract

In evaluating a research article's abstract, the key question to ask is:

- *What information, if any, is missing?*

The abstract should contain concise statements highlighting the context of the study, the research objective, the study design, information about the participants, the main outcome measures, the results, and the researchers' conclusions. Older articles are more likely to have unstructured abstracts that lack clarity or sufficient detail, are missing information, or use the first paragraph of the article as an abstract.

What is missing in the abstract is your first clue as to what to look for in the rest of the article. Basically, what piques your curiosity as you read the abstract? What details do you want to know more about?

The Introduction

The first question to ask after reading an article's introduction is this:

- *Is the study objective clearly stated?*

Although the abstract typically contains a statement of the study's objective, the introduction should clearly elaborate the specific hypothesis being tested or the research question being investigated. If the hypothesis is vague or too general, chances are that the study results will not provide useful information. An unclear or a poorly conceived hypothesis is a red flag.

The next question to ask is:

- *Are the study's relevance and context established?*

As was mentioned in Chapter 5, the purpose of the introduction is to set the stage for the rest of the article by providing a rationale for conducting this particular study and by placing the study in context through a concise but pertinent discussion of past studies related to the current research question. If you are reading critically and find that you are persuaded of the study's importance or necessity based on such discussion, the authors have likely done a good job of establishing relevance. As you become more familiar with the literature in your areas of interest, you will be able to judge for yourself how well the authors have succeeded in providing a balanced and accurate summary of previous studies.

Methods and Procedures

This is the section where we must get quite specific. There are a number of questions to ask and consider when evaluating the methods and procedures used in a study. If the authors have not already specified the study design in the abstract, it should be stated here. Generally speaking, all of the questions that follow should be answered by the authors with enough information so that a reader with the requisite time, money, and expertise could reproduce the study. The methods section is the part of the article where sources of bias and/or confounding are more likely to be discovered by the astute reader.

- *Is the sample well described, including inclusion/exclusion criteria and method of selection?*

Does the sample population, chosen to represent the larger population to which the results will be generalized, suit the study hypothesis? The study participants should also be described in sufficient demographic detail so that the reader can determine whether the results are likely to be applicable to his or her clinical practice. An explanation of the inclusion and exclusion criteria and the selection method used are necessary to help the reader judge whether the sample was chosen on the basis of convenience or whether each eligible participant had an equal chance of being selected. Without sufficient information about the researchers' sampling procedures it is difficult for the reader to evaluate the possibility or degree of sampling bias, and whether it is likely to over- or underestimate treatment effect.

Surveys are especially sensitive to sampling bias because the results are intended to be extrapolated to a much larger population, and a small error in the sample may be magnified many times over when projected onto the larger group. The results table will generally specify the estimated amount of possible error, or the margin of error, which should typically be less than 5%.

As an example, in the Ganmaa study cited in Chapter 5, the authors describe their sampling strategy for this particular study, but not for the Nurses' Health Study as a whole. Because it is well known in the health care research community, they refer readers to a previous study rather than repeat the information yet again. As you might imagine from the title, all participants in the Nurses' Health Study were recruited through the nursing registry of the state in which they were licensed. Do you think that this sample is randomly selected or representative of the US population as a whole?

The rationale for selecting the Nurses' Health Study sample is that because of their nursing education, respondents would be more likely to answer brief, technically worded questionnaires with a high degree of accuracy, and would also be highly motivated to participate in a very long term study. This is an example of the necessary trade-offs in research design – a sample that was truly selected randomly might not have provided data that was as accurate or might easily have a much higher rate of missing data, and of respondents dropping out, thus undermining the credibility of the results. The current rate of response for the Nurses' Health Study is 90%, which is considered excellent for a survey.

- *Were blinding procedures used, and if so, how well did they work?*

As has been previously discussed, blinding as a design feature helps to reduce or equalize the effect of expectation, and adds credibility to a study's results. Remember that with single blinding either participants or providers are blinded as to group assignment, while with double blinding both are unaware. It is important to be alert to the fact that investigators' efforts to blind study participants or treatment providers are not always adequate or successful. It is more impressive if the authors employ some method for gauging how well their blinding procedures worked, for example by going back and asking whether participants had realized which group they were in.

- *Is a comparison or placebo group part of the study design?*

The inclusion of these design features helps reduce potential bias and adds credibility. When evaluating the use of a comparison or placebo group in a quantitative study, the important consideration is whether the study's groups are alike in every respect that may influence the outcome except the treatment or intervention being tested. This is the reason that random assignment to group is such a powerful design feature for increasing the internal validity of a study – it ensures that the groups will be similar even in terms of unanticipated characteristics that could influence outcomes to be measured.

- *For an intervention (treatment) study, is the treatment procedure well described?*

Clearly, with any intervention a sufficient description of the treatment protocol is crucial for the reader to be able to determine whether it seems appropriate to the study hypothesis. For complementary therapies, this issue is particularly important as it relates to ecological validity. As discussed in Chapter 3, ecological validity refers to the idea that if a study proposes to evaluate the overall usefulness or safety of a therapy, such as massage or acupuncture, the treatment protocol employed in the study should reflect the way such treatment is used and practiced in the real world. Otherwise the study may be assessing the safety or effectiveness of a narrowly defined protocol that is not representative of the therapy being investigated. If a sham treatment was used for the comparison group, the same issues of validity and appropriateness arise. In other words, for the sham to appear to be valid and maintain blinding, it must closely resemble the treatment under evaluation, yet not produce the intended treatment effect.

- *Was treatment randomly assigned, and is the method of randomization described?*

Just as random selection of participants is necessary to avoid introducing bias, so is random assignment to group. As described previously, the best method of randomization is based on the use of a computer-generated table of random numbers or one that has previously been published in a statistical textbook. If the method is not specified or is somehow assumed, the reader should be wary.

- *Are the outcome measures well described and appropriate given the hypothesis?*

Apply common sense again – do the measures used make sense in relation to the study's hypothesis? Can you understand them from the description given to the reader? If a measurement tool is relatively new or unfamiliar, such as a newly developed personality inventory, for example, the authors should provide information on its reliability and validity, and on how these were determined.

The reliability of a new measurement tool is often determined based on administering the instrument two or more times and comparing the results to see if they are reasonably similar, or correlated. This method is called **test-retest reliability**, and the higher the correlation, which is expressed as a value such as 0.87 (87%), the better.

Validity is also commonly estimated by administering the new instrument along with a more established one that measures the same concept or attribute, and again comparing the results to see how much they are alike. For example, two instruments that measure anxiety should produce similar scores that are highly correlated with each other. If the correlation is less than 50%, the two instruments do not appear to be measuring the same construct. The procedures used to determine a measurement tool's reliability and validity, and their statistical results, should be described in sufficient detail for the reader to decide whether these are reasonable.

- *Are the methods used in calculating both descriptive and inferential statistical analysis described?*

As was outlined in the previous chapter, descriptive statistics present a study's results (or data set) without generalizing them to a larger group. They simply present the characteristics of the data – such as the age range of participants, average years of education, or means and standard deviations of outcomes measured before and after treatment. Inferential statistics are used to draw conclusions about observed differences between groups, and whether these differences can be extrapolated to a larger population. Most inferential statistical tests, such as the *t*-test, are designed to determine statistical significance – whether the results represent a meaningful result or are due to chance alone. Measures such as ANOVA also estimate the strength of an association between two variables or among a group of variables. Analyses that perform this function are useful because they provide an estimated measure of just how much of an outcome is due to the treatment(s) being tested.*

The choice of which type of test to use is partly dependent on the level of data involved. For example, as was discussed in the preceding chapter, the *t*-test is an example of a test that requires interval level data, whereas the chi-square test (χ^2) can be used with categorical data.

The methods used in any inferential statistical analysis should make sense in relation to the study hypothesis and the number of outcome measures (dependent variables). A commonly used measure of both significance and the strength of an association is analysis of variance (ANOVA), because a great deal of information about relationships among the exposures (independent variables) and how these affect the

---

* In technical language, what percentage of the variance can be attributed to the independent variable – remember that ANOVA stands for "analysis of variance."

outcome measure can be examined. A related technique, called analysis of covariance (ANCOVA), is sometimes used to factor out the influence of demographic variables when these are unequally distributed between groups prior to treatment, to make the groups comparable. For example, imagine a study where two groups were used to assess the effect of exercise on blood pressure, and through attrition one group's mean age was younger than the other by the end of the study. To make the two groups comparable again, age might be used as a factor (covariant) in an analysis to remove its confounding effect on blood pressure.

More sophisticated tests using multivariate analysis should be employed when multiple outcomes, which are usually correlated to one another to some extent, are being measured. Multivariate analysis controls for the problem of multiple comparisons among the same group of variables. The most common method is multiple analysis of variance (MANOVA), used when there are more than two groups being compared across multiple outcome measures. Another method is *Hotelling's T^2*, used for only two groups.

The key issue is that the particular statistical procedures chosen should be described in understandable detail, and should make sense in relation to the study design and variables. A complete description of the numerous statistical tests in existence and their proper use is beyond the scope of this book; indeed it would be a textbook in itself. A terrific resource, called *PDQ Statistics*[1] and written by Geoffrey Norman and David Streiner, is a concise yet thorough and often humorous guide to statistical tests, with clear explanations of their proper uses and how to spot their misuse.

Authors may also present the results of a power analysis, which is used to determine how many participants were needed to have at least an 80% chance of finding statistical significance. While this calculation is normally part of the planning stage of a study, some authors choose to report it as a way to justify the sample size chosen. As a rough guideline regarding sample size, there should be at least 10 participants per outcome measure to have adequate power.[1] Planned comparisons between groups, that is, specified in advance of the data collection, may also be presented here, as well as the level of statistical significance that will be accepted. The conventional level is .05, or five out of a hundred, although pilot or exploratory studies may set a less stringent alpha level of .10.

Finally, because computers are almost invariably used now to actually crunch the raw numbers, it is common practice to mention not only the statistical tests used but also the specific software package, including the version, used to compute them.

Results

Reading the results table in a journal article for the first time can be an intimidating experience for anyone who is not already comfortable with grasping quantitative information presented in visual form. One way to demystify tables and graphs is to think of them as a type of executive summary presented in a specific kind of shorthand. Breaking down the process into pieces and knowing what questions to ask helps.

As you look at any table of results, the first question to ask is:

• *Are the tables and graphs clearly labeled?*

Identify the demographic results and the inferential results; these will typically be presented in separate tables. Look carefully at the demographic data to determine whether any groups that are being compared to each other are sufficiently matched in terms of factors that could influence the dependent variables or outcomes. In looking at the inferential results, distinguish the treatment or independent variables from the outcome or dependent variables. What level of variable are these – nominal, ordinal, interval, or ratio? Were parametric or nonparametric tests used?

• *Are all the participants accounted for?*

Look back to the abstract or methods section for the total number of participants who were enrolled in the study. Check to see if that number matches the sample size listed in the results table, usually abbreviated as *n*, signifying the number of participants included in the statistical analysis. If the numbers do not match, are the participants who dropped out of the study taken into account in some way? People may choose to leave a study for many different reasons – they leave the area, their life circumstances change, the treatment is unpleasant, or the record-keeping is too time consuming. Regardless of the reasons for drop-out, the risk is that the results may be skewed such that the study may over- or underestimate the effect of treatment.

• *Are means and standard deviations provided?*

This information, as part of the descriptive statistical analysis, is usually presented at the beginning of this section's table, or in a separate table if there is more extensive information to warrant it. Because the descriptive analysis is the summary of the raw data before the authors manipulate it, you should view with suspicion any article that fails to list means and standard deviations. Means are usually expressed as a number next to the standard deviations (SD), which are in parentheses with a plus or minus sign. It typically looks something like this: 45.1 (± 3.46). In this example, 45.1 is the mean, plus or minus a standard deviation of 3.46. It is useful to look at these at the study baseline and then compare them to post-treatment outcomes. Large standard deviations mean that there is a great deal of individual variation around the mean. When standard deviations are small, it means the individual scores are more tightly grouped around the mean. If the size of the standard deviation is larger for the baseline measures and then gets smaller for the same outcomes post-treatment, it may indicate a stronger or more consistent treatment effect.

- *What results of statistical analyses are provided?*

The methods section should describe the plan for the statistical analysis, made during the design phase of the study, in advance of the actual collection of the data. Depending on the method of analysis, some final statistic such as a t or χ^2 value is arrived at, and the value of this number determines whether or not statistical significance has been reached. You will often see an additional column labeled DF, which stands for **degrees of freedom**. The DF is used to calculate the final statistic, and is related to the sample size or n. Usually DF = $n - 1$. Most statistics texts have appendices with tables of the critical values necessary for statistical significance with the t-test, F-test, or chi-square, and you can look up the value of the study statistic and the degrees of freedom to verify that the authors' results are reported correctly.

Next to these numbers you will generally see a column labeled p. The value of p indicates the probability that the statistic is due to chance. The smaller the number, the better the odds that the results are not due to chance. The generally accepted standard for p is .05 or less, meaning that the likelihood of these results occurring from chance alone is smaller than or equal to 5 in 100, or 5%. A p value of .001 means the probability is no more than 1 in 1000. The .05 limit is an arbitrary convention that has become entrenched in most health care literature,* although researchers are free to specify in advance what limit of p will be accepted.

As has already been mentioned, in a pilot study with a small sample size, the investigators may decide that a p value of .10 will be adequate. In a study with

---

* *This number was not handed down on a stone tablet, as one of my professors liked to point out, saying, "Surely, God loves the .06 just as much as the .05."*

multiple outcomes, investigators may choose to set the p value at .01 to take into account the multiple comparisons among the outcome variables. Although using a multivariate analysis such as MANOVA would be more appropriate, this technique is still considered permissible.

The value of p is often the first thing readers look at in a results table. However, p indicates only whether or not results are due to chance, and is highly sensitive to sample size. With a sufficiently large sample, it is easy to reach statistical significance. For small samples with p values that are close but do not reach the .05 level, the possibility of Type II error should be kept in mind. A more useful measure of clinical relevance is the effect size, discussed in more detail in the previous chapter, which is the magnitude of an effect and gives a direct indication of how effective a particular treatment is. While methodologists have been stressing the importance of reporting effect sizes for many years, it is still relatively rare for researchers to report them, with the exception of systematic reviews.

The final question to ask in this section is:

- *Are all the research outcomes reported?*

If the authors include a number of outcome measures but show data only for outcomes that favor or support their hypothesis, the results are suspect. Most peer-reviewed journals would refuse to publish an article with selective reporting of results.

Now that you have a stronger foundation from which to read a quantitative study's results section, take a second look at this section of the Ganmaa article in Chapter 5. It is an interesting example of a sophisticated epidemiological analysis. Notice that the relative risks computed for each category of caffeine consumption include confidence intervals (CI), which you will remember are an estimate of how much measurement error is present in the result – in this case the relative risk of developing breast cancer given the amount of caffeine consumption – and are similar to the margin of error typically reported for opinion polls and surveys. A 95% CI means that we can be confident 95% of the time that the true mean for the outcome reported will fall within the specified range. And certainly in this study, small sample size is not a problem! There is more than enough statistical power to detect quite small effects, even though multiple comparisons were made and several covariates entered into the analysis.

Discussion or Conclusions

Having sorted through the tables, graphs, and charts in the results section, you are ready to read the authors' interpretation of what the numbers mean. The first question to ask in this section is:

- *Are the authors' comments justified based on the results, and do they follow logically from the results?*

Are the conclusions consistent with the data presented, or do the authors go out on a limb making statements that are only tenuously or not at all supported by the data? Do the conclusions make sense in light of the data that has been presented?

Another question is:

- *Do the authors identify weaknesses or limitations in the study design and statistical analysis?*

As discussed in Chapter 3, flaws can be found in any study, no matter how well designed and executed it is. A trustworthy and thoughtful discussion will openly admit the potential biases and limits of the study so that readers can make up their own minds about how much weight to give these. Authors may even suggest ways that future studies might improve upon theirs. Looking back at the Ganmaa study, the authors offer several possible explanations for their findings of a lack of an association between caffeine consumption and breast cancer, and mention the possibility – slight but still possible – that their cohort design contained an unmeasured confounding variable even though they took many known breast cancer risk factors into account. They also present the results of other animal studies that support their conclusion. This is a competent example of such a discussion.

The next question is related to the previous issue of statistical significance:

- *Is the clinical significance of the study discussed?*

As previously mentioned, a large sample size practically guarantees that statistical significance will be reached. However, this does not mean that the results are clinically useful or meaningful. For example, imagine a new drug that is demonstrated to reduce the amount of time that patients are deprived of oxygen to the brain following a stroke by an average of five seconds. With a large enough sample size, the p value could be less than .001. Certainly, such results are not due to chance. But will a five-second reduction make a clinically significant difference in the survival rate or the prognosis for long-term recovery of most stroke patients?

- *Are the conclusions consistent with the study objectives?*

How do the authors relate their results to the study objectives and hypotheses? Have they done what they set out to do in terms of answering their research question? What degree of uncertainty has been reduced by the current study?

Related to all of the above is this question:

- *Would this study influence the way I practice?*

A primary goal of clinical research is to improve the quality and delivery of health care. The major measure of a study is its impact on clinical practice. In most cases, study results pertain directly to treatment decisions, but not always. In the example of the Ganmaa study, the question might become: Would I stop drinking my morning coffee to reduce my risk of developing breast cancer? Probably not, based on the evidence presented, and definitely not if I were a postmenopausal woman.

References

In looking over the reference list, ask yourself:

- *How up-to-date and appropriate is the reference list?*

Check the publication dates. It is generally better to have more recent references, although in some cases older references are useful because of historical significance or relevance to a particular phase of study or time frame in research processes on a subject. Also, check whether the titles of the references cited seem relevant to the study.

- *Did the authors examine other articles focusing on similar designs, population, and outcomes?*

The titles of the citations are again a good clue. As you become familiar with the literature in your areas of interest, you will also have a better sense of how well the authors have accomplished both these tasks.

Some General Comments

The goal of this chapter thus far has been to introduce a way of thinking about the quality of an article, and to provide some tools to begin breaking down the process of critical thinking into manageable steps. The questions listed here are generally useful, but each one may not always apply to every type of article you may encounter. For example, a case study should not be measured with the same yardstick as a clinical trial. Use your judgment, experience, and common sense.

Critically evaluating a journal article is also a skill that develops with practice. Having come this far, you hopefully have developed a better understanding of the scientific method and how it is applied in the clinical research setting, as well as some specific guidelines for critiquing an article. The primary objective is to be reasonably skeptical as you read, and to always ask yourself whether some other explanation is possible. The bottom line for any study is this:

- *How credible is it? Do chance, bias, or confounding provide a plausible alternate explanation for the results?*

If the answer is yes, the study may be flawed and the results should be interpreted very cautiously.

The approach presented in this chapter is suited to the evaluation of experimental or intervention studies, especially clinical trials. Other types of designs such as case studies or meta-analyses will have other concerns, as discussed previously in Chapter 4. As you evaluate quantitative studies generally, keep in mind that any flaws in a study may be due to challenges faced by the researcher(s), who may have encountered ethical considerations, logistical problems, or technical difficulties that could not have been anticipated or reasonably avoided. Try to take a balanced perspective. Almost every study contains flaws when examined closely; the crucial questions are whether these allow chance, bias, or confounding to be plausible alternate explanations for the study findings, and whether the authors are aware of and discuss any limitations.

We will now apply our guidelines to two pilot intervention studies to gain more concrete experience in critical evaluation. The subject of the first article is the use of massage to reduce pain among hospitalized patients who have cancer. The second is a report of the effects of reflexology on anxiety, cortisol levels, and melatonin secretion. It is advisable to do a quick read of each article first, just to get an overall sense of it, and then to go back and read each section in detail, answering the critique questions by yourself or in a small group. It is better to avoid reading author comments until after you have completed your own critique. You may find it helpful to make a copy of the article so you can read it through with a pen or highlighter and make notes regarding questions or comments as you read.

Study Example #1: Massage and Cancer Pain

The Effect of Massage on Pain in Cancer Patients

Sally P. Weinrich, PhD, RN: Associate Professor, College of Nursing, University of South Carolina; Martin C. Weinrich, PhD: Associate Professor, Department of Epidemiology and Biostatistics, School of Public Health, University of South Carolina, Columbia, SC.

From the College of Nursing and the Department of Epidemiology and Biostatistics, School of Public Health, University of South Carolina, Columbia, SC.

Address reprint requests to Sally P. Weinrich, PhD, RN. College of Nursing, University of South Carolina, Columbia, SC 29208.

Applied Nursing Research, Vol. 3, No. 4 (November), 1990: pp.140-145.
©1990 by W.B. Saunders Company.

Abstract: *Evaluating the effectiveness of nursing interventions in decreasing pain is a top priority for clinical research. Unfortunately, most of the research on cancer pain relief has been limited to treatment studies involving the administration of analgesics. Research is needed to determine which nonanalgesic methods of pain control are effective and under what conditions. Consequently, an experimental study was designed to test the effectiveness of massage as an intervention for cancer pain. Twenty-eight patients were randomly assigned to a massage or control group. The patients in the massage group were given a 10 minute massage to the back; the patients in the control group were visited for 10 minutes. For males, there was a significant decrease in pain level immediately after the massage. For females, there was not a significant decrease in pain level immediately after the massage.*

There were no significant differences between pain 1 hour and 2 hours after the massage in comparison with the initial pain for males or females. Massage was shown to be an effective short-term nursing intervention for pain in males in this sample.

Introduction: *Cancer pain remains a frequent and neglected health problem. Thus, proper control of cancer pain is one of the most important issues in the field of oncology (Benedetti & Bonica, 1984; Pritchard, 1988). Dennis, Howes, and Zelanska (1989) found that 715 nurses identified evaluating the effectiveness of nursing interventions in decreasing pain as one of the top priorities for clinical research. Likewise, 85% of an international sample of 669 nurses believed that more emphasis should be given to the management of cancer pain (Pritchard, 1988).*

Every year, approximately 780,000 Americans experience moderate to severe pain due to cancer or cancer therapy (Benedetti & Bonica, 1984). Bonica (1985) estimates that 20% to 40% of cancer pain is inadequately managed. Of Pritchard's (1988) international sample of 669 nurses, 15% believed that cancer patients in their units were given no relief from cancer pain. In a study by Donovan and Dillon (1987) involving 96 patients, only 43% of the patients recalled a nurse discussing anything about their pain with them. Most of the research on cancer pain relief has been limited to treatment studies involving the administration of analgesics (Dalton, Toomey, & Workman, 1988). There is a gap in the literature concerning methods of treatment other than medication for cancer pain.

Current nursing practice needs to consider nonanalgesic methods of pain control as useful adjuncts to pharmacologic therapy of individual patients (Barbour, McGuire, & Kirchhoff, 1986; Daake & Gueldner, 1989; Dalton et al., 1988; Donovan & Dillon, 1987). Pain intensity has been reported to be reduced by a wide range of behaviors including massage, verbalizations, heat and cold application, position changes, distraction, strenuous activity, movement restriction, breathing exercises, hypnosis, relaxation, biofeedback, and guided imagery (Barbour et al., 1986; Wilke, Lovejoy, Dodd, & Tesler, 1988).

Research is needed to determine if and under what specific conditions massage is therapeutic. Massage is thought to be very relaxing and to greatly increase a feeling of well-being (Glaus, 1988). In addition to these benefits, massage is believed to be effective for the relief of pain through the stimulation of the production of endorphins (Tappan, 1988). It is assumed that physiological, mechanical, and reflex effects are accomplished with a 10-minute massage (Tappan, 1988). Dalton et al. (1988) found in their study that the use of massage brought "moderate" and "quite a lot of relief" for 3 of the 5 subjects. Similarly, Barbour et al. (1986) found that massage was reported to decrease pain by 75% in 58 outpatient cancer patients. This pilot study was conducted to confirm the reported effect of massage on pain for cancer patients.

The conceptual framework for this research was the gate control theory of pain (Melzack & Wall, 1982), which includes both sensory and emotional components for pain perception (McGuire, 1987). According to this theory, pain that arises as a result of noxious stimulation (such as cancer pain) may be decreased or increased in its passage from peripheral nerve fibers to those in the spinal cord by the action of a specialized gating mechanism situated in the region of the dorsal horns of the cord (Daake & Gueldner, 1989). The gating mechanism's impact is in modulating sensory input before pain perception and response occur (Barbour et al., 1986). Techniques such as massage, manipulation, relaxation, heat, and ice packs close the gate to the central nervous system (Barbour et al., 1986), resulting in a decrease in pain. Conversely, central activities such as anxiety, excitement, and anticipation may open the gate, resulting in an increase in pain (Daake & Gueldner, 1989).

Method

Research Question: *The purpose of this pilot study was to measure the effect of massage on pain for cancer patients. It was hypothesized that cancer patients who received a 10-minute massage would experience significantly less pain than cancer patients who did not receive a massage.*

Subjects: *Patients were randomly selected from a 30-bed oncology floor of a private hospital in the southeastern United States. Patients were paired based on previous frequency of medication for pain, tranquilizer, or antiemetic effect. Frequencies used for* *pairing were as follows: within 4 hours (n = 2) within the last 4 to 8 hours (n = 0), within the last 9 hours or more (n = 16), or no medication (n = 10). Each pair of patients was randomly assigned to a treatment or control group.*

A total of 28 cancer patients (14 in each group) participated in the research project. No patients dropped out of the study after they consented to participate. The sample consisted of 18 males and 10 females, 22 whites and 6 blacks. The age range was 36 to 78 years with an average age of 61.5 years old. Of the sample, 21% (n = 6) were receiving radiation; 21% (n = 6), chemotherapy; and 11% (n = 3), a combination of radiation and chemotherapy. Eighteen of the subjects had received medication within the 3-day time period before initiation of the study. Seven of the subjects received medication within 4 hours before the intervention, and 7 of the subjects received medication within the 2-hour time period after the intervention.

Instrument: *A Visual Analogue Scale (VAS) (Figure 1) was used to measure the self-report of pain intensity (McGuire, l988). The scale consists of a 10-mm line with end points of* no pain *and* pain as bad as it could possibly be.

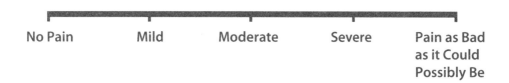

No Pain   Mild   Moderate   Severe   Pain as Bad as it Could Possibly Be

Figure 1 Visual Analogue Scale.

Each patient was asked to place a mark through the line at the point that best described how much pain he or she was experiencing at that particular moment. The point on the line is measured and used as the score. The VAS assumes equal intervals for scoring. The VAS has been shown to be a reliable and sensitive measure of the patient's subjective experience of pain (Chapman et al., 1985; Ohnhaus & Adler, 1975; Syrjala & Chapman,

1984). Price, McGrath, & Rafii (1983) have validated the use of the VAS in chronic and experimental pain. Revill, Robinson, & Rosen (1976) demonstrated that the VAS was reliable on repeated measurements ($r = 0.95$, $p < .001$). Cronbach alpha reliability for this study was 97.*

Procedure: *A 1-hour training session on massage technique, interviewing procedure, and the use of the VAS was provided to the data collectors before the research project began. Seven senior nursing students conducted the intervention activities for the paired groups. All of the interviews and interventions (massage or control) were carried out between 9 a.m. and 12 noon. The massage and interviewing procedures of each student were validated at the completion of both days of the study.*

Initially, each patient was asked to indicate the current level of pain on the VAS. For the treatment group, the patient was given a 10-minute Swedish massage to the back by the data collector. The back was massaged in a slow, continuous, upward manner with the use of lotion. The muscles of the back provided the direction for the massage. For the control group, no physical contact was initiated, and the data collector sat and visited with the patient for 10 minutes. The control was intended to account for the possible non-specific effects of the data collector's time and effort with patients. For both the control and treatment groups, data collectors were instructed to respond as they usually would to verbal comments of patients. Immediately after the procedure, patients in both the control and treatment groups were asked to indicate their level of pain. Self-reported levels of pain were collected again 1 and 2 hours after the intervention. Data on medication taken during the time of the study was retrieved from patient charts after the last self-reported pain level was obtained.

---

*r, called the correlation coefficient, is a measure of how closely one measure corresponds to another measure, like weighing yourself several times on the same scale on the same day, and seeing how close the scores are. The higher the value of r, the more closely correlated the measures are to one another. Correlation is often used to show the degree of relationship between variables.

Findings

On a VAS scale of 0 to 10, self-reported pain levels before the procedure ranged from 0 to 9, with a mean of 2.6. Subjects in the treatment group had higher levels of initial pain (M = 3.1) than subjects in the control group (M = 2.2). Gender difference existed in the level of pain, with males in the treatment group having the highest levels of pain (M = 4.19) (Table 1). Mean pain levels immediately after the procedure, 1 hour after the procedure, and 2 hours after the procedure are shown in Figure 2.

Analysis of covariance and repeated measures were performed to detect group differences in perceived pain over time. The VAS level of pain before the procedure was the covariate in the analysis of covariance. Repeated measures were used to measure changes in the VAS level of pain immediately after the procedure, 1 hour, and 2 hours after the procedure. Medication taken before the study and medication taken during the study were included in the analyses. Significant differences between gender and massage intervention led to separate analyses for males and females. For males, there was a significant decrease in pain levels immediately after the massages ($F(5,13) = 8.24$, $p = .01$). For females, no

Table I – Mean (Standard Deviations) Pain Levels on the Visual Analogue Scale

Time of Measurement	Treatment Group			Control Group			
	Males	Females	Both	Males	Females	Both	Total
Initial	4.19 (2.6)	1.65 (2.7)	3.1 (2.8)	1.93 (2.7)	2.73 (4.2)	2.2 (3.0)	2.6 (2.9)
Immediately after the Procedure	2.93 (2.3)	1.43 (2.3)	2.3 (2.3)	2.06 (2.7)	2.63 (4.3)	2.2 (3.1)	2.3 (2.7)
1 Hour after the Procedure	3.03 (2.1)	1.40 (2.2)	2.3 (2.2)	1.87 (2.6)	2.63 (4.3)	2.1 (3.0)	2.2 (2.6)
2 Hours after the Procedure	2.38 (2.1)	1.40 (2.2)	2.0 (2.1)	1.09 (1.2)	2.35 (4.4)	1.5 (2.4)	1.7 (2.3)

Making Sense of Research

significant difference was found after the massage (F(4,6) = 2.52, p = .17) In the repeated measures analyses, there were no significant differences between pain 1 hour and 2 hours after the massages in comparison with the initial pain for males or females. Age had no significant effect on pain at any of the four VAS measures. For both males and females, there was no significant difference in the control groups.

Evaluating the effect of medicines yielded interesting and surprising results. Medication given 1 and/or 2 hours after the procedure was not significantly associated with a decrease in self-reported pain levels for the sample as a whole (F(5,23) = 0.36, p = .56), for the pain level at 1 hour after the procedure (F(5,23) = 1.25, p = .28). and for the pain level 2 hours after the procedure. Medication given 1 to 4 hours before the procedure was not significantly associated with a decrease in pain at the measure of pain taken immediately after the intervention (F(4,24) = 1.44, p = .24) or 1 hour after the intervention (F(5,23) = 3.09, p = .09). However, this medication was associated with a decrease in pain 2 hours after the intervention (F(5,23) = 9.03, p = .006). When the analyses were performed separately

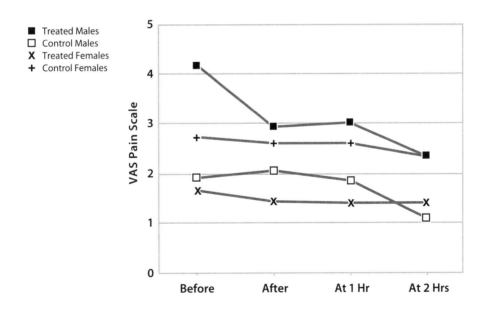

Figure 2 Mean Level of Pain by Gender and Procedure Group

for males and females, medications given before the intervention were significant for the females (F(3,7) = 29.37, p = .002), but not for the males (F(3,15) = .03, p = .87). In summary, medication was not effective in reducing pain levels for any of the subjects until more than 2 hours after administration of the medication.

Discussion

In this pilot study, pain relief was significantly decreased immediately after a massage for males, but not for females. Although there was a decrease in pain for the males 1 and 2 hours after the massage, it was not significantly different from the decrease in pain for the females or for the control group (males or females). According to this study's conceptual framework, the gate control theory of pain, the massage could have temporarily closed the gate for the males, decreasing the pain.

The low intensity of pain in the control group (males and females) and the females in the experimental group is a limitation of the study. Significance was obtained for the subjects who had high levels of pain (males in the experimental group). Additional research on subjects in high levels of pain is needed to determine whether the benefit of a massage extends to all persons with high levels of pain or applies only to males. Subjects were paired and divided into control or experimental groups based on the variable of frequency of medication before the study. It was assumed that frequency of medication would be related to pain levels with patients who had more pain taking more medication. In this study, the patients who had more pain did not take more medicine. Consequently, the treatment group had higher pain levels than the control group. We recommend that future studies on pain intervention use a self-reported measure of pain as the variable for pairing rather than the frequency of medication, as was done in this study.

Similarly, this study did not use gender as a basis for division into control or treatment group. In this study, males had higher self-reported levels of pain than females. Gender difference in the effect of a massage as well as the effectiveness of medication are apparent in this study and require further research. Also, gender differences in methods of coping with pain need to be explored. Could the males use fewer coping behaviors for pain than the females, resulting in increased effectiveness of the massage? Or perhaps, there is greater social acceptability of massage in the males than in the females.

This pilot study provides support for use of alternative methods of pain alleviation, such as massage in males, simultaneously with medication. The males in this study obtained an immediate decrease in pain levels after the massage. Medication was not effective in reducing pain levels until more than 2 hours after administration of the medication for any of the subjects. Based on the males in this pilot study, massage could be used for immediate pain relief, and medication could be used for long-term (2 hours) pain relief in males. Future research needs to focus on the complementary effect of medication and massage.

The Donovan and Dillon (1987) study showed that nurses usually do not discuss pain with patients. The impact of discussing pain with patients needs to be evaluated. Donovan (1989) has also discovered that the environment in which care is given is important to a patient's pain relief. The effect of the environment needs to be studied, as well as the effect of the provider. For example, would pain alleviation be different for a back rub given by a family member, a primary nurse, a staff nurse, or a student nurse?

References

1. *Barbour, L., McGuire, D., & Kirchhoff, K. (1986). Nonanalgesic methods of pain control used by cancer outpatients. Oncology Nursing Forum, 136: 56-60.*

2. *Benedetti, C., & Bonica. J. (1984). Cancer pain: Basic considerations. In C. Benedetti, C.R., Chapman, G.M. Moricca (Eds.). Recent Advances in the Management of Pain (pp. 71-101). New York, NY: Raven.*

3. *Bonica, J. (1985). Treatment of cancer pain: Current status and future needs. In H.L. Fields, R. Dubner, & F. Cervero (Eds.), Advances in Pain Research and Therapy, 9: 589-616. New York. NY: Raven.*

4. *Chapman, C., Casev. K., Dubner. R., Foley, K., Gracely, R., & Reading, A. (1985). Pain measurement: An overview. Pain, 22: 1-31.*

5. Daake. D.R., & Gueldner, S.H. (1989). Imagery instruction and the control of postsurgical pain. Applied Nursing Research, 2: 114-120.

6. Dalton, J., Toomey, T., & Workman, M. (1988). Pain relief for cancer patients. Cancer Nursing, 11: 322-328.

7. Dennis, K., Howes, D., & Zelauskas, B. (1989). Identifying nursing research priorities: A first step in program development. Applied Nursing Research, 2: 108-113.

8. Donovan, M., & Dillon, P. (1987). Incidence and characteristics of pain in a sample of hospitalized cancer patients. Cancer Nursing, 10: 85-92.

9. Donovan, M.I. (1989). An historical view of pain management: How we got to where we are! Cancer Nursing, 12: 257-261.

10. Glaus. A. (1988). The position of nursing. Cancer Nursing, 11: 250-253.

11. McGuire, D. (1987). The multidimensional phenomenon of cancer pain. In D.B. McGuire & C.H. Yarbro (Eds.), Cancer Pain Management (pp. 1-20). Orlando, FL: Grune & Stratton.

12. McGuire, D. (1988). Measuring pain. In M. Frank-Stromborg (Ed.), Instruments for Clinical Nursing Research (pp. 333-356). Norwalk, CT: Appleton & Lange.

13. Melzack, R., & Wall, P. (1982). The Challenge of Pain. New York, NY: Basic Books.

14. Ohnhaus, E., & Adler, R. (1975). Methodological problems in the measurement of pain: A comparison between the verbal rating scale and the visual analogue scale. Pain, 1: 379-384.

15. Price. D., McGrath, D., & Rafii, A. (1983). The validation of visual analogue scales as ratio scale measures for chronic and experimental pain. Pain, 17: 45-46.

16. Pritchard, A.P. (1988). Management of pain and nursing attitudes. Cancer Nursing, 11: 203-209.

17. Revill, S., Robinson, J., & Rosen, M. (1976). The reliability of a linear analogue for evaluating pain. Anaesthesia, 31: 1191-1198.

18. Svrjala, K., & Chapman, C. (1984). Measurement of clinical pain: A review and integration of research findings. In C. Benedetti, C.R. Chapman, G.M. Moricca (Eds.), Recent Advances in the Management of Pain (pp. 251-264). New York. NY: Raven.

19. Tappan. F. (1988). Healing Massage Techniques. Norwalk, CT: Appleton & Lange.

20. Wilke, D., Lovejoy, N., Dodd, M., & Tesler, M. (1988). Cancer pain control behaviors: Description and correlation with pain intensity. Oncology Nursing Forum, 15: 723-731.

Critical Evaluation Questions

1. What information, if any, is missing from the abstract?

2. Is the study objective clearly stated in the introduction?

3. Are the study's context and relevance clearly established?

4. In the methods section, is the sample well described, including inclusion /exclusion criteria and method of selection?

5. Were blinding procedures used, and if so, how well did they work?

6. Is a comparison or placebo group part of the design?

7. Is the treatment procedure well described and appropriate given the hypothesis?

8. Was treatment randomly assigned, and is the method of randomization described?

9. Are the outcome measures well described and appropriate given the hypothesis?

10. Are the methods used in calculating both descriptive and inferential statistical analysis described?

11. In the results section, are the tables and graphs clearly labeled?

12. Are all the participants accounted for?

13. Are means and standard deviations provided?

14. What results of statistical analyses are provided?

15. Are all the previously specified research outcomes reported?

16. In the discussion section, are the authors' comments justified, based on the results?

17. Do the conclusions follow logically from the results?

18. Do the authors identify weaknesses or limitations in the study design or analysis?

19. Is the clinical significance of the study discussed?

20. Are the conclusions consistent with the study objectives?

21. How up-to-date and appropriate is the reference list?

22. Did the authors examine other articles focusing on similar designs, populations, and outcomes?

23. The last question to consider about an article: Based on the results of this study, would it influence the way you practice?

Critical Evaluation

Now that you have read through the article once, go back and read each section again, this time attempting to answer the critical evaluation questions. Remember to be somewhat skeptical as you read. If you can locate the journal's website, or a hard copy of the journal, check the guidelines for authors to determine whether the journal sends out its submissions for blind review by other experts in the field, that is, without author information, so that editorial readers are not influenced by author identity or affiliation. If editors or reviewers and their credentials are listed, determine if you can the extent of their expertise about the complementary therapy being studied and other areas of expertise relevant to the study.

Comments on this Study's Abstract

- *What information, if any, is missing?*

This abstract uses a narrative format rather than the standardized one, so the reader has to work a little harder to pull out the relevant information. The research question is introduced, and the design is described in general terms. The methods are not described in detail, but you can identify the number of subjects, and that the subjects were randomly assigned to either a treatment group who received a 10-minute massage or a control group who were visited for 10 minutes. The results are described in general terms and a conclusion reached. Based on the information in this abstract, the research hypothesis sounds very broad and the methods used to answer it raise questions because they seem inadequate to such a large task. A knowledgeable reader will plan to scrutinize the methods section carefully.

Comments on the Introduction

- *Is the study objective clearly stated?*

Yes. The authors cite two other studies where massage was used to reduce cancer pain and state that they conducted a pilot study to confirm the reported effects of massage on pain for cancer patients. Note that one of the other studies (Barbour, 1986) was a survey of cancer outpatients – even without familiarity with the Barbour study, you can get a sense of this from the title of the article as listed in the references. However, the specific research question is not stated until the methods section of the article.

- *Are the study's context and relevance clearly established?*

The authors provide a compelling case for the importance of conducting the study in light of the problem of pain related to cancer, and the role that other interventions (in addition to medication) can play. Because massage is reported by cancer patients to be a frequently used method of pain reduction, the authors give a clear rationale that justifies the need for a study evaluating the effects of massage on cancer pain. They also provide the gate control theory of pain as a conceptual framework for their argument.

The authors provide a reference (Tappan, 1988) as the basis for their assumption that physiological, mechanical, and reflex effects are accomplished with a 10-minute massage. There is no mention of studies or clinical anecdote to support this assertion in the Tappan edition cited, in either the sections on effects of massage or on massage and pain. The Barbour survey is used twice to support a statement describing the proposed neurological mechanism of the gating response. From the context, a reader might think the survey was instead a laboratory-based study. A less knowledgeable reader, unfamiliar with the literature, might give more credibility to these statements than is warranted. A surprising omission in this section is a failure to cite a 1986 study by Sims on the use of slow-stroke back massage, which used a very similar protocol in a hospital setting.

Another problem with this article's review of the literature is that an important area of previous research is missing altogether. There is a large body of studies investigating differences between how men and women report their pain and respond to treatments for pain. No mention of these studies or the general issue of gender differences in regard to pain is made in the introduction, and this is a serious omission.

Comments on the Methods Section

- *Is the sample well described, including inclusion/exclusion criteria and method of selection?*

The description of the subjects is sketchy at best, and the method of randomization is not mentioned. Although some demographic data are given for the sample as a whole, no table that describes the demographics of each group for comparison purposes is provided. From the information given it is impossible to determine the male to female ratio, age, and ethnicity in each group. No inclusion/exclusion criteria are given. In terms of selection, subjects were recruited from a 30-bed unit, and 28 of 30 possible patients agreed to participate. In essence, this appears to be a convenience sample drawn from a small, private, community-based hospital.

Although subjects from each group were matched according to medication for pain, anxiety, and nausea, no information is given regarding the type of cancer, stage of disease, or type of chemotherapy. Therapists who have worked with people with cancer know that different cancers cause varying degrees of discomfort, that the later stages of cancer are more likely to have metastasized to other locations such as the spinal vertebrae, which can cause severe pain, and that some chemotherapy drugs are harder to tolerate than others. It seems likely that the patients in this relatively small sample may not have been truly comparable to one another, in other words, that there was a great deal of individual variation that could have influenced the results. While such a varied sample would theoretically have greater generalizability, remember that this trade-off also equals less internal validity.

- *Were blinding procedures used, and if so, how well did they work?*

No blinding procedures are described.

- *Is a comparison or placebo group part of the design?*

Yes. Subjects in the treatment group were compared to those who received a 10-minute conversational visit, in an attempt to control for the nonspecific effects of attention. Little is said about the parameters for the visit, such as whether a script was followed, or whether patients were encouraged to respond to open-ended questions. In addition, the 10-minute visit does not control for the nonspecific effects of touch.

- *Is the treatment procedure well described and appropriate given the hypothesis?*

Yes and no. The authors state that the massage was performed by senior nursing students who received an hour-long training in massage, interviewing procedure, and how to administer the Visual Analogue Scale. Thus, the reader can conclude that the people providing massage received less than an hour of training specifically in how to perform the massage. In addition, the gender of the students is not specified.

From the description, it appears that the massage consisted of 10 minutes of effleurage to the back, following the direction of the back muscles. This standardized protocol is problematic in relation to the research question. An experienced therapist familiar with the needs of people with cancer would tailor the treatment to the individual patient's need, which would likely increase the effectiveness of the intervention. It also seems possible that more than 10 minutes of massage could be needed to produce effective pain reduction in this population. Finally, the study looks at the effect of a single massage on only one occasion – perhaps a larger "dose" of massage over a longer period of time, with multiple sessions, would yield different results.

- *Was treatment randomly assigned, and is the method of randomization described?*

Treatment is stated to have been randomly assigned, but the method of randomization is not described. Subjects were paired, however, based on their use of medication, in an attempt to control for the influence of this variable.

- *Are the outcome measures well described and appropriate given the hypothesis?*

Yes. A clear description, along with background information justifying the use of the Visual Analogue Scale, is included. Data on medication use was taken directly from each patient's chart. Both seem appropriate to the research question.

- *Are the methods used in calculating both descriptive and inferential statistical analysis described?*

Not in the methods section. These are included in the results section instead. The authors used analysis of covariance to control for the higher level of initial pain reported by males in the treatment group. From the authors' description, it is difficult to tell whether plans for statistical analysis were specified in advance, or were selected afterwards based on what the data showed.

Comments on the Results Section

- *Are the tables and graphs clearly labeled?*

Yes, the tables and graphs are straightforward and fairly easy to read. The graph of the Visual Analogue Scale pain data is easier to grasp visually compared to the explanation in the text. The VAS pain is an interval level variable, and patient gender is a nominal level variable. The repeated measures ANOVA and ANCOVA are parametric tests, and seem appropriate to the study design. Unfortunately there is no table of participant demographic data.

- *Are all the participants accounted for?*

Yes. No patients dropped out of the study after agreeing to participate.

- *Are means and standard deviations provided?*

Yes. Means are given for the demographic data in the text; means and standard deviations are provided for the VAS data in Table 1. Standard deviations are given in parentheses. Notice the relative size of the means and the standard deviations – the SDs are fairly large. This tells the reader that there is a large amount of individual variation in the pain scores. A graph showing the change in pain scores over time by group is also given in Figure 2. Values for *p*, the level of statistical significance, are given in the text.

- *What results of statistical analyses are provided?*

The results of analysis of the VAS data are presented in Table 1 and Figure 2. Some demographic data and the results of an analysis of the medication use, along with their *p* values, and more of the VAS data are all included in the text. The analysis of the medication data is difficult to read – a third table or graph might have made this information easier for readers to grasp. It appears that because of unanticipated differences between males and females in the sample, a separate and additional analysis was performed, in an attempt to rule out medication use as an explanation for the observed results.

Although values for *p* are given, the effect size is not reported, nor is a power analysis included to determine whether the sample size was adequate to detect a true difference between groups. Notice too that there is a fairly large initial difference between the treatment and the control group. A possible alternative explanation for the reduction in pain following the treatment could be regression to the mean, a concept explained in Chapter 1.

- *Are all the previously specified research outcomes reported?*

Yes. The primary outcome specified is the patient's level of pain, as measured using the VAS. Data on medication use was also collected from the patients' charts.

Comments on the Discussion Section

- *Are the authors' comments justified, based on the results?*

This is often a difficult question to answer. In this case, the authors speculate that the gate control theory worked only for the males. Does this seem likely to you? It does appear that there are some gender differences in terms of how males and females responded to the massage; however, because the sample was not more homogeneous it is difficult to say whether the differences were due to gender or some other factor. Remember that each group consisted of fourteen patients, and that the number of males relative to females per group is not specified. While we do not know precisely how many males are being compared to how many females in the treatment group, it seems probable that the numbers are quite small. How willing should we be to make a clinical generalization based on such a small sample size?

- *Do the conclusions follow logically from the results?*

Given the problems already discussed in the design of the study, arguably they do not. The ambiguous results seen in this study could be due to flaws in the design that introduced a large amount of individual variation. The methods used are clearly not a good fit for answering such a broad research question. It certainly seems possible that there are plausible alternate explanations for the results. For example, perhaps the males in the study were responding to being massaged by a female nursing student. In addition, 10 minutes of effleurage on the back performed by an untrained student is probably not the most effective or even valid method to assess whether massage therapy is helpful in reducing pain for people with various types and stages of cancer.

- *Do the authors identify weaknesses or limitations in the study design or analysis?*

The authors do identify one limitation – the relatively high baseline pain intensity among males in the treatment group, compared to the females in the treatment group and the entire control group. The authors also discuss their assumptions regarding the spurious relationship between pain levels and medication use, and make some recommendations for future research.

One limitation previously identified in our discussion is the lack of any mention on the subject of pain and gender differences. Another major limitation not discussed by the authors is the absence of understanding of massage therapy as it is clinically practiced. A major weakness of this study is the operational definition of massage, which was ill suited to provide reliable or optimal pain relief for the participants.

Finally, the sample size is small for the number of statistical analyses that were performed. A careful reader would wonder whether there was sufficient power to detect a true treatment effect. The large reduction in pain seen among males in the study may have been the result of statistical error – too many tests performed on too little data, with a large amount of individual variation mixed in. This is another reason why unusual findings often require replication in order to be considered credible.

- *Is the clinical significance of the study discussed?*

Some recommendations for the use of massage in addition to medication are made. However, based on these results, would you as a hospital administrator decide to immediately implement a massage therapy program? It would appear that the results support providing massage for male patients with cancer but not females, a type of decision making that requires stronger evidence than this study presents.

Because the study measures pain, the question also arises: what degree of pain reduction is clinically meaningful? There must be a standard defined by the authors or that makes sense to the reader, and this is not provided. For example, the authors could give the percentage of patients who experienced a reduction in pain, or the extent of pain reduction, as demonstrated by visual analogue scale scores.

- *Are the conclusions consistent with the study objectives?*

This is difficult to say – on the surface, yes, but the logic of the conclusion seems tortuous, and the analysis of the medication data appears to be an afterthought. In general, this study raises more questions than it answers, as do the authors in the discussion section. Based on the small sample size, lack of fit between the overly broad research question and the methods used to answer it, and other possible explanations for the statistical results, the informed consumer of research would not place a high degree of confidence in the findings.

Making Sense of Research

Comments on the Reference List

- *How up-to-date and appropriate is the reference list?*

The reference list seems adequate and current given the publication date of the article.

- *Did the authors examine other articles focusing on similar designs, populations, and outcomes?*

The authors considered other studies on pain in cancer patients. Given the paucity of research on massage at the time when this study was planned, conducted, and published, it is not surprising that other contemporary studies on massage are not cited – not many existed.

- *Based on the results of this study, would it influence the way you practice?*

Probably not. As stated before, the flaws in this study and the ambiguous nature of the results make it difficult to place a high degree of confidence in it. It seems as likely that chance, bias and confounding could explain these findings as much as the conclusion put forward by the authors. A hospital administrator considering whether to implement an oncology massage program for male patients but not for female patients would have difficulty justifying that decision to a board of directors based on this study alone. At the same time, the authors do state clearly that this is a pilot study, meant to test the pragmatic aspects of the study design, methods, and procedures, and that they did not anticipate their findings. An investigator planning a future study in this area would find some useful information; this is one reason that some journals have begun to publish negative results.

Surprisingly, even though this is a small pilot study with several design flaws, it is still frequently cited in the massage therapy literature, largely because of its use of random assignment to group. If you look at the references for any of the early meta-analyses or later systematic reviews of massage therapy, or for other kinds of studies focusing on pain or on symptom relief from cancer and its treatment, you will see this study cited again and again. We can only hope that future investigators will read the study in its entirety, not just the abstract.

Study Example #2: Massage and Acupuncture for Postoperative Symptom Management

Symptom Management with Massage and Acupuncture in Postoperative Cancer Patients: A Randomized Controlled Trial

Wolf E. Mehling, MD, Bradly Jacobs, MD, MPH, Michael Acree, PhD,
Leslie Wilson, PhD, Alan Bostrom, PhD, Jeremy West, BA, Joseph Acquah, OMD,
Beverly Burns, OMD, Jnani Chapman, RN, CMP, and Frederick M. Hecht, MD
Osher Center for Integrative Medicine (W.E.M., B.J., M.A., L.W., J.W., J.A., B.B., J.C., F.M.H.),
and Department of Epidemiology and Biostatistics (A.B.), University of California,
San Francisco, California, USA

Journal of Pain and Symptom Management Vol. 33 No. 3 March 2007

Abstract

The level of evidence for the use of acupuncture and massage for the management of perioperative symptoms in cancer patients is encouraging but inconclusive. We conducted a randomized, controlled trial assessing the effect of massage and acupuncture added to usual care vs. usual care alone in postoperative cancer patients. Cancer patients undergoing surgery were randomly assigned to receive either massage and acupuncture on postoperative Days 1 and 2 in addition to usual care, or usual care alone, and were followed over three days. Patients' pain, nausea, vomiting, and mood were assessed at four time points. Data on health care utilization were collected. Analyses were done by mixed-effects regression analyses for repeated measures. One hundred fifty of 180 consecutively approached cancer patients were eligible and consented before surgery. Twelve patients rescheduled or declined after surgery, and 138 patients were randomly assigned in a 2:1 scheme to receive massage and acupuncture (n = 93) or to receive usual care only (n = 45). Participants in the intervention group experienced a decrease of 1.4 points on a 0-10 pain scale, compared to 0.6 in the control group (P = 0.038), and a decrease in depressive mood of 0.4 (on a scale of 1-5) compared to ± 0 in the control group (P = 0.003). Providing massage and acupuncture in addition to usual care resulted in decreased pain and depressive mood among postoperative cancer patients when compared with usual care alone. These findings merit independent confirmation using larger sample sizes and attention control. J Pain Symptom Manage 2007;33:258-266.

Funding for this study was provided by the Mount Zion Health Fund, San Francisco, California. The authors confirm that this material is original research and has not been published otherwise, with the exception of a presentation at the 2005 Bay Area Research Symposium, San Francisco, October 2005 and a poster presentation at the North American Research Conference on Complementary and Integrative Medicine, May 2006, Edmonton, Alberta, Canada.

Address reprint requests to: Wolf E. Mehling, MD, Osher Center for Integrative Medicine, University of California, San Francisco, 1701 Divisadero St., Suite 150, San Francisco, CA 94115, USA. E-mail:mehlingw@ocim.ucsf.edu

Accepted for publication: September 4, 2006.

Keywords

Cancer, surgery, symptom management, cancer pain, acupuncture, massage

Introduction

More than 40% of people with cancer report using complementary and alternative medicine (CAM) therapies.[1] Leading cancer centers in the United States offer massage and acupuncture to inpatients and outpatients. A recent review concluded that the judicious integration of these therapies into cancer patient care is warranted, although strong evidence of measurable benefits is often missing.[2] A National Institutes of Health consensus panel and numerous clinical trials support the efficacy and safety of acupuncture for postoperative pain, postoperative nausea and vomiting, and perioperative anxiety[3], and the National Comprehensive Cancer Network guidelines[4] recommend consideration of massage and acupuncture for symptom management.

A systematic review on the effects of massage in cancer patients concluded that massage confers short-term benefit on psychological well-being, including anxiety, and that it may confer benefits on physical symptoms; more trials are needed.[5] We found only one small study published on the effect of massage in the postoperative setting that suggested it might reduce postoperative pain.[6]

Reviews of acupuncture for perioperative or chemotherapy-induced nausea and vomiting have concluded that acupuncture is efficacious.[7-10] Acupuncture reduced cancer pain in three uncontrolled single-arm studies[11-13] and in one randomized placebo-controlled trial.[14] Systematic reviews of acupuncture for various noncancer pain conditions[15] and three clinical trials of acupuncture for noncancer perioperative pain[16-18] reported improvement. Although these data on acupuncture and perioperative pain are promising, limitations include variance in the timing of the intervention and noncancer-related diagnoses.

In summary, the literature suggests that the level of evidence for the use of acupuncture and massage in the management of perioperative symptoms in cancer patients is relatively strong for the use of massage for anxiety and acupuncture for nausea, and is encouraging but nonconclusive for the use of acupuncture or massage for pain. The combination of massage and acupuncture for symptom management in perioperative cancer patients has never been studied. Massage and acupuncture are components of traditional Chinese medicine (TCM) and, as such, often are used in combination. Although mechanisms of action are still unclear for both modalities, they are viewed as complementary and additive within the frame of TCM. Recently, the Institute of Medicine report on "Complementary and Alternative Medicine in the United States" strongly recommended innovative study designs, including studies of combinations of therapies.[19]

We conducted a randomized, controlled clinical trial exploring the effect of a combination of massage and acupuncture added to usual care vs. usual care alone on postoperative symptoms (pain, nausea, and mood) and costs for symptom-related medications in hospitalized cancer patients in the first three days after cancer-related surgery.

Methods

Participants: *Patients who were at least 18 years of age and scheduled to undergo cancer-related surgery requiring hospitalization for at least 48 hours were eligible to participate in the study. Patients were recruited during their preoperative anesthesia screening clinic visit. Cancer surgery was defined as any surgery related to a diagnosis of malignancy but including one of the following five groups: breast cancer surgery, either mastectomy or reconstructive surgery; abdominal surgery for intestinal or hepatic malignancies; pelvic surgery for ovarian, uterine, or cervical malignancies; urological surgery for testicular, prostate, bladder, or renal malignancies; and head and neck cancer surgery. Patients were excluded if they were not fluent in English, were diagnosed with deep vein thrombosis, or were receiving blood-thinning medication.*

Recruitment: *The study was approved by both the Committee of Human Research at the University of California, San Francisco (UCSF) and the Protocol Review Committee of the UCSF Cancer Center. Participants were recruited during their preoperative clinic visit scheduled for the medical and anesthesia clearance for the surgery planned for the following days. As part of the standard preoperative information package, all patients received a flyer describing the study. After reviewing data obtained from the clinic schedule, the research assistant approached consecutive patients potentially eligible for the study and, when they were eligible and interested, obtained informed consent.*

Randomization: *Following the baseline symptom assessment on postoperative Day 1 (POD1), the research assistant opened, at the bedside, a consecutively numbered, opaque envelope containing the random assignment to the intervention or control group. Using a computerized random number generator, these envelopes were prepared by the study statistician, who had no contact with the participants. To make participation as attractive as possible, we chose a 2:1 randomization scheme favoring the intervention.*

Interventions: *Massage and acupuncture were each provided on POD1 and POD2 at the bedside by one of two certified massage therapists and by one of two licensed acupuncturists. Practitioners had over 10 years of clinical experience treating cancer* patients and had been credentialed and privileged by UCSF. The timing and sequence of massage and acupuncture was variable due to the providers' schedules and the patients' postoperative procedures scheduled for the same days.

Massage comprised standard ("Swedish") massage (applying kneading and strokes to soft tissue and muscles), and acupressure-type foot massage. Duration varied from 10 to 30 minutes depending on the participant's clinical needs and condition; the intended duration of 30 minutes could not always be achieved due to nursing care requirements (mean duration 20 minutes, SD ±3).

Acupuncture treatment was based on symptom report and physical exam and was semistandardized according to leading symptom (e.g., pain or nausea): a standardized core set of acupuncture points according to TCM was used for each presenting symptom and additional points were added (and documented) depending on history and examination at the discretion of the practitioner. We used 34-gauge needles (manufacturer: Seirin, Japan) at the following standardized points: for pain, large intestine-4, spleen-6, and auricular points corresponding to the area of pain; for nausea, pericardium-6 and stomach-36; for anxiety, liver-3, large intestine-4, and Yin Tang. An average of 10 acupuncture needles (range 4-14) were placed bilaterally in symmetrical points and unilaterally for auricular points to a depth of 1 fen to 3 tsun until de qi was obtained and were retained for 20 minutes. Patients in the control group received usual care and were offered a 30-minute massage after completion of the questionnaire on POD3.

Measurements: Baseline demographic and medical history data were collected by questionnaire during the preoperative anesthesia clinic visit. Baseline clinical data were collected at the bedside before randomization on POD1. We collected further clinical data at three time points: on POD1 and POD2 within 3 hours after interventions (or equivalent time points) and on POD3 (no intervention). When the patient was discharged from the hospital prior to the final POD3 assessment, we contacted the patient over the phone. Data on costs of pain-, nausea-, and anxiety-related medications, on procedures, anesthesia, pathology, and length of hospital stay were obtained after the patient's discharge from the hospital from chart review and electronic databases. Costs were assessed for the entire postoperative hospital stay for all variables except medications, which were compared for the first three postoperative days only.

The primary outcome was the between group difference in pain scores on an 11-point (0-10) pain numeric rating scale (NRS) for severity of current pain and for pain during the previous 24 hours. Secondary outcome measures included the following: 1) nausea on an 11-point (0-10 nausea NRS for current nausea intensity and nausea during the previous 24 hours, similar to a measure used previously;[20] 2) vomiting as the self-reported number of vomiting episodes during the previous 24 hours; 3) mood by tension (six items) and depressive mood (eight items) subscales of the Profile of Mood States Short Form (POMS-SF)[21] (reported as unweighted average score across all individual items, range 1-5); and 4) costs of health care, as assessed by type of care for the postoperative stay, except for medications, which were compared for the three-day study period only.

Statistical Analyses: Estimating that 150 patients would agree to participate in this study during a three-month recruitment period and a 20% drop-out rate, we expected to obtain complete data from 120 patients. With a 2:1-randomization scheme, this would suffice to show a change score difference of 1.1 points on the pain NRS between treatment and control groups (estimated SD of 2.0^{20}), with alpha of 0.05 and beta of 0.2, using a two-sided t-test.

Repeated measures for pain, nausea, mood scales, and number of vomiting episodes were compared by mixed-effects regression analyses. We controlled for significant (P < 0.1) differences in baseline characteristics and for baseline values of the outcome variables. t-Tests were used to compare the sameday prepost intervention changes in symptom scores and health care costs. For analysis of medication cost data by categories, which included many zeros, we used a randomization test (SAS PROC MULTTEST)[22] with 100,000 resamples.

We conducted prespecified exploratory subgroup analyses for trends in the four different surgery groups to see if there were particular types of surgery in which the intervention *appeared to be particularly useful or ineffective, without expecting to obtain statistical significant differences for between-group comparisons. Intention-to-treat analyses included all patients as randomized irrespective of whether they actually received the intervention, no intervention, or only part of it. We used SAS and Stata software[22,23] to perform statistical analyses.*

Results

From the preoperative clinic schedule, we identified 180 consecutive, potentially eligible cancer patients, of whom 150 were eligible and consented before surgery to enroll in the study. Of these 150 patients, 12 ultimately did not participate because the surgery was rescheduled or they declined participation after surgery. The remaining 138 patients were randomly assigned to the intervention (93) or control (45) groups (Figure 1).

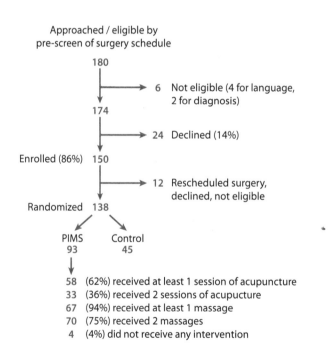

Figure 1 Recruitment and randomization
(PIMS = Perioperative Integrative Medicine Service)

Patient characteristics at baseline are summarized in Table 1. They were similar in both groups with the exception that the intervention group was more educated and more depressed (45% of standard deviation).

TABLE I – Patient Characteristics (n=138)

	PIMS	Control
Demographics		
Sex (female)	48 (52%)	20 (44%)
Age	55.9 (±1.9)	59.2 (±1.7)
Ethnicity (white)	63 (69%)	35 (78%)
Education (college +)	61%	53%
Medical history		
Type of cancer		
Abdominal/pelvic (GI, gyn)	23 (25%)	7 (16%)
Prostate/testicular	16 (18%)	14 (31%)
Bladder/kidney	19 (21%)	11 (24%)
Breast	18 (20%)	7 (16%)
Presurgery narcotic use[a]	15%	14%
Characteristics of surgery		
General anesthesia only	64%	68%
Epidural	31%	25%
Hours of anesthesia	5.4 (±1.7)	4.5 (±2.2)
Hours of procedure	3.8 (±1.8)	4.1 (±2.4)
Symptoms postoperative – Day 1 (baseline)		
Depressive mood[b]	1.7 (±0.8)	1.4 (±0.4)
Tension/anxiety[b]	2.1 (±0.9)	1.8 (±0.9)
Painc	3.5 (±2.2)	3.1 (±2.4)
Nausea[c]	0.7 (±2.0)	0.6 (±1.7)
Episodes of vomiting[d]	0.6 (±2.0)	0.3 (±1.6)

Data presented as n (%), mean (±SD), or %.

PIMS=Perioperative Integrative Medicine Service; GI=gastrointestinal; gyn=gynecologic.
[a] Current use of narcotic medication in preoperative week.
[b] POMS Likert scale 1–5.
[c] NRS, 0–10.
[d] Number of episodes of vomiting per last 24 hours.

The average baseline pain score (range 0-10; mean 3.4 ±2.3) improved by 1.1 in the intervention group compared with 0.1 in the control group after the first intervention on POD1 (P = 0.01). Thirty-four of 90 (38%) patients in the intervention group improved their pain score by at least two points, compared with eight of 44 (18%) in the control group (P = 0.02). The average time interval between the intervention and the following assessment was 3 hours (SD 4.2 hours; range 0.08-12.4). Average pain scores improved from POD1 baseline (prior to first treatment) to POD3 in the intervention group by 1.6 vs.0.6 in the control group (P = 0.04; Table 2, top rows). Thirty-eight of 88 (43%) patients in the intervention group improved their pain score by at least two points, compared with 11 of 43 (26%) in the control group (P = 0.05). Since 31% of participants reported mild (less than 3/10) or no pain at baseline, we performed a post hoc subgroup analysis to mitigate floor effects. Among patients reporting moderate-to-severe (at least 3/10) pain at baseline on POD1, average pain scores improved during the study period by 1.8 points in the intervention group (P < 0.0001) and by 0.3 points in the control group (P = 0.34; Table 2, bottom rows; Fig. 2). Repeated measures analyses in all 138 patients for all time points from POD1 to POD3 showed a statistically significant improvement in pain for the intervention group, whereas the control group remained essentially unchanged. Mixed-effects regression analyses over all four time points showed a significant (unadjusted: P = 0.036) between

TABLE II – Mean Pain Scores (±SD) in All 138 Patients and in 90 Patients with at Least 3/10 Pain After Surgery

	n	POD1 Pre	POD1 Post	POD2 Post	POD3	Change POD1-3	P[a]
All 138 patients	PIMS (93)	3.5 (±2.2)	2.5 (±2.1)	2.2 (±1.9)	2.1 (±1.8)	−1.4 (±2.2)	0.038
	Control (45)	3.1 (±2.4)	3.1 (±2.3)	2.9 (±2.4)	2.7 (±2.0)	−0.6 (±2.3)	
Symptomatic patients (n=90)	PIMS (62)	4.3 (±2.0)	3.0 (±2.2)	2.2 (±1.8)	2.5 (±1.9)	−1.8 (±2.3)	0.001
	Control (28)	3.6 (±2.1)	3.6 (±2.3)	3.8 (±2.2)	3.3 (±1.9)	−0.3 (±2.3)	

PIMS=Perioperative Integrative Medicine Service.
[a]Mixed-effects regression analyses for repeated measures from baseline POD1 to POD3 controlled for education, baseline pain, and depression.

group difference for the average pain curves, which was not altered by controlling for level of education, baseline depression, and baseline pain (adjusted: P = 0.038).

When compared to the control group and using all enrolled patients irrespective of the presence of the respective symptom, we found a standardized effect size (ES) for the change in pain from before to after the first intervention on POD1 of 0.68, and from baseline to POD3 of 0.36. In the symptomatic patients with pain of at least 3/10, ES was 0.65 with a mean reduction in pain by 25.5%.

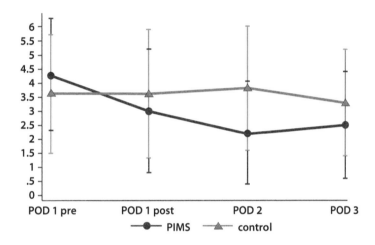

Figure 2 Pain scores at all time points in patients with pain of at least 3/10 at baseline (90 Patients, 62 PIMS, 28 control). (POD = postoperative day; PIMS = Perioperative Integrative Medicine Service)

Prespecified subgroup analysis by type of cancer showed significant improvement for pain among patients undergoing prostate and testicular surgery (n = 30, P = 0.04). Exploratory analysis among those reporting pain demonstrated the greatest ES for patients undergoing abdominal (gastrointestinal and gynecologic) surgery and prostate/testicular surgery (ES 0.98 and 0.97, n = 21 and n = 14, respectively; Table 3).

In an exploratory analysis of actual treatment received, we found patients receiving massage only (n = 33) reported greater improvement in pain after their first massage on POD1 than patients in usual care (P = 0.03).

TABLE III – Mean Change (±SD) Scores for Pain from Baseline to Postoperative Day 3 by Diagnostic Subgroups for Patients with at Least 3/10 Pain at Baseline (n=86)

Subgroup of Cancer (n)	PIMS (n)	Control (n)	P^a	ES
Prostate/testes (14)	−1.9 (±1.5) (9)	−0.2 (±2.2) (5)	0.03	0.97
Abdominal (GI, gyn) (21)	−2.3 (±2.2) (16)	+0.2 (±3.6) (5)	0.13	0.98
Breast (17)	−1.9 (±2.6) (14)	−0.3 (±0.6) (3)	0.14	0.66
Kidney/bladder (19)	−2.1 (±1.8) (11)	−2.3 (±2.0) (8)	0.86	−0.10
Others (15)	−2.6 (±1.8) (10)	−2.4 (±3.0) (5)	0.30	0.09

PIMS=Perioperative Integrative Medicine Service; GI=gastrointestinal; gyn=gynecologic.
[a]Mixed-effects regression analyses for repeated measures from baseline POD1 to POD3 controlled for education, baseline pain, and depression for complete subgroups irrespective of baseline

Secondary outcomes, such as nausea, vomiting, and mood, were different between groups only for depression (P = 0.003), after adjustment for baseline differences (Table 4). In patients with at least mild depression at baseline (n = 56), ES was 0.67 favoring the intervention. After controlling for education and depression, as well as for baseline nausea or anxiety, both nausea and tension/anxiety improved in the intervention group on POD1 more than in the control group (P = 0.043 and 0.048, respectively), but these improvements

TABLE IV – Secondary Outcomes Mean Change (±SD) Scores for Nausea, Vomiting, Anxiety/Tension, and Depression from Baseline to Postoperative Day 3

	PIMS	Control	P^a	n
Nausea[b]	−0.3 (±2.3)	−0.1 (±2.1)	0.26	88+43=131
Vomiting[c]	−0.6 (±2.0)	−0.1 (±1.9)	0.20	88+43=131
Anxiety/tension[d]	−0.3 (±0.9)	−0.02 (±1.0)	0.15	88+43=131
Depression[d]	−0.4 (±0.7)	+0.01 (±0.5)	0.003	88+43=131

PIMS=Perioperative Integrative Medicine Service; GI=gastrointestinal; gyn=gynecologic.
[a]Mixed-effects regression analyses for repeated measures from baseline POD1 to POD3 controlled for education, baseline pain, and depression for complete subgroups irrespective of baseline
[b]NRS, 0–10.
[c]Number of episodes of vomiting per last 24 hours.
[d]Likert scale 1–5; unweighted average score across all individual items.

were not maintained on POD2 and POD3. Although the ESs for the treatment of vomiting were relatively high (ES 0.36), the small sample size with this symptom (n = 30) limited the ability to find a statistically significant difference between groups (P = 0.20; Table 4).

Only 25 (18% of all) patients (18 intervention, 7 control) reported any degree of nausea, of whom 12 received both acupuncture and massage on POD1. Pre-postintervention (same day), the patients reporting nausea improved by 4.5 (SD ±3.1) on an 11-point scale with the intervention and by 2.1 points (SD ±3.1) without (between-group difference P = 0.13). Health care utilization and costs were not different between intervention and control groups with regard to the average length of the hospital stay (5.2 vs. 5.0 days; P = 0.66), total hospital costs ($14,556 vs. $14,819; P = 0.87), total direct hospital costs (defined as excluding overhead costs: $8,378 vs. $8,559; P = 0.84), or medication costs (during POD1-3: $184 vs. $169; P = 0.71). Subgroup analyses by therapeutic categories of medication demonstrated differences in the costs for average sleep and antianxiety medications ($5 vs. $16 in 22 intervention vs. 6 control patients, who used these medications; P = 0.02), amounting to an average of $1 vs. $2 over all 136 patients (P = 0.42). No differences were identified for pain, antiemetics, or laxative drug classes.

Discussion

We found that a bedside service of massage and acupuncture in addition to usual care resulted in decreased pain and depressive mood among postoperative cancer patients when compared with usual care alone. Massage and acupuncture could add to symptom management in cancer care if confirmed by a larger clinical trial.

These results confirm in part findings from the largest, although uncontrolled, published study to date of massage among over 1200 cancer patients[20] unrelated to any surgery. In that study, for symptom measures obtained at baseline and within 3 hours after massage, the investigators reported an ES of 0.85 for pain and of 1.12 for anxiety. Mean improvements (SD) for pain and anxiety were 40.2% (±40.9) and 52.2% (±39.5), respectively. Tension/anxiety, rather than depression, was the predominant mood symptom and was the overall symptom with the largest treatment ES. However, ESs in uncontrolled studies are not compared to the effects of usual care or natural course of symptoms. Using identical assessment instruments, the findings in our controlled study in a postoperative setting were more modest: When compared to the control group and using all enrolled patients irrespective of the presence of the respective symptom, we found a smaller ES pre-postintervention (same day) of 0.68. When taking the improvement with usual care in the control group into account, the mean pain reduction from baseline in symptomatic patients was 25.5%.

We could not replicate the benefits for anxiety, however. Several factors might explain the discrepancy. First, our control group used more sleep/antianxiety medications than the experimental group, perhaps masking any difference in the anxiety/tension score. Also, the time interval between the intervention and the following assessment averaged 3 hours, with a range up to 12 hours. In exploratory analyses for POD1, we found no correlations between 1) length of time interval from massage to assessment, and 2) change in pain scores, but a strong correlation for the interval following acupuncture.

The "natural" course of acute symptoms in the hospital care setting immediately after surgery is quite different from the setting of chronic disease management. In the surgery setting, the interval between the study intervention and the following assessment is subject to wide fluctuations in pain and anxiety, depending on variables such as getting out of bed, having an epidural catheter removed, or receiving intravenous or epidural medications. Consequently, there is greater variability in reporting symptoms among postoperative patients than other settings. Median time of day for the assessment of outcome measures was around 2 PM and similar in both groups on all days.

Overall, we were unable to demonstrate any differences in health care costs over the entire hospital stay or for the three-day postoperative study period, except for a reduction in antianxiety/sleep medication costs. The small difference we saw for antianxiety/sleep medications might be an effect of the intervention, as it has been previously found that massage decreases anxiety.[5] Unfortunately, there were too few subjects and infrequent reporting of symptoms to more clearly determine whether these medications were masking a treatment effect. Both the short postoperative time period for following these costs and our lack of data on the exact analgesic amounts used with as needed orders were limitations in our ability to detect differences in cost that might exist between groups. We are not surprised by the lack of a difference in length of stay (LOS). When LOS is short, it is a relatively insensitive measure of change for many treatments, especially when patients are discharged to intermediate care centers and home care. Further study should conduct a cost-benefit analysis taking into account both the economic costs and the noneconomic costs and benefits in a more complete economic model of the value of a new intervention. Until such analyses are available, hospital administrators will have to decide whether the added value from patient satisfaction and reduced pain warrants adoption.

Our resources were limited and did not permit the inclusion of an attention control group to isolate nonspecific treatment effects. Thus, it is possible that expectation or attention may have contributed to observed effects. However, the inclusion of a control group in this study, even without attention control, is an advance over similar prior uncontrolled studies.

Our analyses were potentially limited by a floor effect caused by numerous patients with no or minimal postoperative symptoms due to excellent postoperative pain management by usual care. Patients were enrolled into the study before surgery, which made it impossible to predict which patients would report significant symptoms after the surgery. Effects were stronger in subgroup analyses of those patients with significant symptoms at baseline, although particular care must be exercised in the interpretation of post hoc subgroup findings. However, results remained robust for improvement in pain when we included the entire study sample.

The patients in our sample were predominantly Caucasian-American and relatively well educated. Education has shown to be a factor in patients' expectations toward CAM. We cannot rule out that patients' expectations are a mediator for the observed effects, and our results might not be generalizable to a different population. Nonetheless, controlling for level of education did not change the results of our analyses.

Our results need confirmation by a larger trial that includes an attention control. A high acceptance rate, short recruitment time, minimal patient burden, and high patient satisfaction (data published elsewhere[24]) support the feasibility of such a trial. Several lessons for future efficacy studies can be learned from our study, which could be seen as a pilot study in regard to its limited scope. Postsurgery symptoms could guide stratified randomization, and subgroup analyses defined by baseline symptoms can be planned before recruitment. Due to our study design and our budget limitations, we were not able to separate the contributions of massage or acupuncture alone from the effects of the combination of these treatments; future multiarm studies would benefit from comparing these combined treatments to individual modalities. Effort should be made in standardizing the time interval between intervention and follow-up assessment. Patients from more diverse populations may allow more generalizable results. Measurement of patient expectations would permit assessment of the influence of expectation on treatment outcomes. Inclusion of more patients with anxiety and more frequent data collection on this symptom would allow a more refined assessment of relationships between drug use and anxiety scores. Despite these limitations, our results indicate that massage and acupuncture are likely to be a valuable addition to postoperative symptom management in cancer patients.

Acknowledgments

The authors thank John Hillman and Matthew Gitlin for their invaluable support with electronic data collection and data organization, the team at the UCSF PREPARE clinic staff for their support with patient recruitment, the nurses at Mount Zion Hospital wards for support with the intervention, Jeffrey Pearl for support from the hospital administration, Susan Folkman and Sylver Quevedo for support from the Osher Center for Integrative Medicine, Donald Abrams and Susan Folkman for manuscript review, and, in particular, the patients for their participation.

References

1. Lee MM, Lin SS, Wrensch MR, Adler SR, Eisenberg D. Alternative therapies used by women with breast cancer in four ethnic populations. J Natl Cancer Inst 2000;92(1):42-47.

2. Deng G, Cassileth BR. Integrative oncology: complementary therapies for pain, anxiety, and mood disturbance. *CA Cancer J Clin* 2005;55(2):109-116.

3. NIH-Consensus Conference. Acupuncture. *JAMA* 1998;280(17):1518-1524.

4. Benedetti C, Brock C, Cleeland C, et al. NCCN practice guidelines for cancer pain. *Oncology (Huntingt)* 2000;14(11A):135-150.

5. Fellowes D, Barnes K, Wilkinson S. Aromatherapy and massage for symptom relief in patients with cancer. *Cochrane Database Syst Rev* 2004;(2). CD002287.

6. Nixon M, Teschendorff J, Finney J, Karnilowicz W. Expanding the nursing repertoire: the effect of massage on post-operative pain. *Aust J Adv Nurs* 1997;14(3):21-26.

7. Mayer DJ. Acupuncture: an evidence-based review of the clinical literature. *Ann Rev Med* 2000; 51:49-63.

8. Vickers AJ. Can acupuncture have specific effects on health? A systematic review of acupuncture antiemesis trials. *J R Soc Med* 1996;89(6):303-311.

9. Ezzo J, Vickers A, Richardson MA, et al. Acupuncture-point stimulation for chemotherapy induced nausea and vomiting. *J Clin Oncol* 2005;23(28):7188-7198.

10. Lee A, Done ML. The use of nonpharmacologic techniques to prevent postoperative nausea and vomiting: a meta-analysis. *Anesth Analg* 1999;88(6):1362-1369.

11. Filshie J, Redman D. Acupuncture and malignant pain problems. *Eur J Surg Oncol* 1985;11(4): 389-394.

12. Leng G. A year of acupuncture in palliative care. *Palliat Med* 1999;13(2):163-164.

13. Alimi D, Rubino C, Leandri EP, Brule SF. Analgesic effects of auricular acupuncture for cancer pain. *J Pain Symptom Manage* 2000;19(2):81-82.

14. Alimi D, Rubino C, Pichard-Leandri E, et al. Analgesic effect of auricular acupuncture for cancer pain: a randomized, blinded, controlled trial. *J Clin Oncol* 2003;21(22): 4120-4126.

15. Ezzo J, Berman B, Hadhazy VA, et al. Is acupuncture effective for the treatment of chronic pain? A systematic review. *Pain* 2000;86(3):217-225.

16. Wang B, Tang J, White PF, et al. Effect of the intensity of transcutaneous acupoint electrical stimulation on the postoperative analgesic requirement. *Anesth Analg* 1997;85(2):406-413.

17. Wang RR, Tronnier V. Effect of acupuncture on pain management in patients before and after lumbar disc protrusion surgery-a randomized control study. *Am J Chin Med* 2000;28(1):25-33.

18. Lin JG, Lo MW, Wen YR, et al. The effect of high and low frequency electroacupuncture in pain after lower abdominal surgery. *Pain* 2002;99(3):509-514.

19. Institute of Medicine, Committee on the Use of Complementary and Alternative Medicine by the American Public. *Complementary and alternative medicine (CAM) in the United States. Prepublication copy. 2005:109-129.*

20. Cassileth BR, Vickers AJ. *Massage therapy for symptom control: outcome study at a major cancer center. J Pain Symptom Manage 2004;28(3):244-249.*

21. Baker F, Denniston M, Zabora J, Polland A, Dudley WN. *A POMS short form for cancer patients: psychometric and structural evaluation. Psychooncology 2002;11(4):273-281.*

22. SASv9. *Cary, NC: SAS Institute Inc., 2001.*

23. Stata9.1. *Statistics/data analysis. College Station, TX: Stata Corporation, 2005.*

24. Mehling W, Jacobs BP, Acree M, et al. *Acupuncture and massage improve patient satisfaction in post-operative cancer patients. Feasibility data from a randomized controlled pilot trial. Poster presentation/abstract at North American Research Conference on Complementary and Integrative Medicine, May 2006, Edmonton, Canada. 2006. 266 Vol. 33 No. 3 March 2007 Mehling et al.*

Critical Evaluation

Comments on the Abstract

- *What information, if any, is missing?*

This article also uses a narrative abstract. Most of the information is clearly laid out – the research question as well as a brief description of the study rationale, design, and methods used. A description of the patients and how they were selected is given, along with some attrition data and a brief summary of the results. Subject areas that we will want to read more closely include the descriptions of participant recruitment and selection, of the outcome measures used, and of the massage and acupuncture protocols. We will also want to pay close attention to the statistical methods employed and their results.

Comments on the Introduction

- *Is the study objective clearly stated?*

Yes, very clearly. The goal of the study is to evaluate the effect of a novel combination of massage therapy and acupuncture in addition to usual care, to relieve postoperative symptoms compared to usual care alone.

- *Are the study's context and relevance clearly established?*

Yes. The authors provide a reasonable rationale for investigating the combination of acupuncture and massage as an intervention to reduce postoperative symptoms of pain, nausea and mood for cancer patients in particular. They cite previous research to support their choice of outcome measures related to each intervention. In general, their case is that a large percentage of people with cancer use these therapies, and while previous research demonstrates some beneficial effects for each therapy, no prior study has used the interventions in combination. Thus, this study will add new information to the existing knowledge base. We also learn that costs associated with the hospital stay will be assessed.

Comments on the Methods Section

- *Is the sample well described, including inclusion/exclusion criteria and method of selection?*

Yes, the inclusion and exclusion criteria are clearly defined and make sense. The method of selection allows for a cross-section of surgical patients as potential participants, and the various types of cancer are described. The method of recruitment and selection should not bias the results since all the patients who were eligible for the study were approached. Given the stressful nature of the recruitment environment – patients were approached during their preoperative anesthesia workup, where blood draws, X-rays, and other tests are given along with a great deal of paperwork to complete – the relatively large number of willing participants is impressive.

- *Were blinding procedures used, and if so, how well did they work?*

Although neither the participants nor the practitioners were blinded, one could argue that some blinding was used, since the study statistician who prepared the random assignment to the intervention or the control group had no contact with the participants.

- *Is a comparison or placebo group part of the design?*

Yes. The comparison group in this study is one that received standard care alone. In many clinical trials, it makes sense to compare a novel intervention to the usual treatment. In this study, the design of standard care plus the massage/acupuncture intervention compared to standard care alone allows the researchers to see whether the intervention offers any additional benefits above and beyond the usual postoperative care. To promote participation in the study and avoid resentment on the part of those assigned to the control group, a greater number of participants were assigned to the intervention group and the control group members were offered a massage at the end of their hospital stay after all the data had been collected.

- *Is the treatment procedure well described and appropriate given the hypothesis?*

Yes. If a reader were planning to replicate this intervention study, or to design one similar to it, there is enough information here to do so. The description of the massage intervention is fairly thorough, and of the acupuncture intervention, quite thorough. Experienced practitioners were used to provide both of the interventions and were allowed to exercise clinical judgment within the confines of the study.

- *Was treatment randomly assigned, and is the method of randomization described?*

Yes, treatment was randomly assigned using a table of random numbers and sealed consecutively numbered envelopes.

- *Are the outcome measures well described and appropriate given the hypothesis?*

Yes, they appear to be, based on the literature cited. The inclusion of both physiological and psychological symptoms is a plus. The Profile of Mood States is a well-known, reliable and valid measure for assessing depressive mood and tension, and a reference is cited describing the measurement properties of the shorter version of this instrument used in the study. Shorter versions of existing instruments, with reasonably similar ratings of reliability and validity, are often developed to reduce the burden of research participation among patients who are hospitalized or otherwise medically fragile.

- *Are the methods used in calculating both descriptive and inferential statistical analysis described?*

Yes. The authors present the results of their power analysis, to show that they had planned to recruit a sufficiently large sample to have an 80% probability of detecting a difference in pain scores of 1.1, with the threshold for statistical significance set at $p = .05$. The particular statistical test used to determine significance was a regression analysis, which also controlled for the effects of education, depression and baseline pain. For changes in pre-post symptom scores and health care costs, the frequently used two-tailed *t*-test was performed. "Two-tailed" refers to the fact that the test will detect a difference between the groups in either direction; it is a more stringent test. As was mentioned previously, stating the plan for statistical analysis in advance of data collection enhances the credibility of a study's results by avoiding "fishing expeditions" where multiple tests are performed on the data in an effort to find meaningful patterns. In this case the authors planned ahead of time to explore possible differences based on type of surgery. Another example of using a more stringent analytic approach is the use of intention-to-treat analysis – there will be more about that in the next section.

Comments on the Results Section

- *Are the tables and graphs clearly labeled?*

Yes, these are straightforward and easy to read. The patient characteristics in Table I contain means and standard deviations for the categorical and interval level variables. Subsequent tables contain interval level data for pain and secondary outcomes of anxiety/tension, depression, nausea, and vomiting. The regression analysis and *t*-tests performed are parametric tests and seem appropriate to the study design. One table that is not included, however, is a summary of the health care utilization and costs data, which was not statistically significant. Figure 1, which provides a summary of the recruitment and randomization sequences, with numbers of patients at each stage and in each group, is especially helpful in answering the next question.

- *Are all the participants accounted for?*

Yes. Notice that the rate of attrition – 12 participants out of the original 150 who were enrolled in the study – is relatively small at a little over 1%. The reasons participants stated for dropping out are also given. The authors note that the analysis is based on intention-to-treat, meaning that once the remaining 138 participants were randomized to the control or the intervention group they were included in the analysis, regardless of the number of massage or acupuncture sessions completed – 4% received no intervention. This is consistent with the principle, "Once randomized, always analyzed." Using intention-to-treat is a conservative approach that makes it more difficult to reach statistical significance, that is, a *p* value of .05 or less. Many methodologists believe that data from clinical trials should always be analyzed using this approach; if statistical significance is reached using an inherently more conservative method, one can have a higher degree of confidence that the results are not due to chance.

- *Are means and standard deviations provided?*

Yes, means and standard deviations are provided for both the demographic and outcome data. Notice that the standard deviations are relatively small, making it more likely that the reduction in postoperative symptoms is really a consequence of the massage/acupuncture treatment. Compare these means and standard deviations to those reported in the previous study example.

- *What results of statistical analyses are provided?*

The results of the descriptive analysis of the demographic data and the inferential analysis of the outcomes measured are included. Table I provides background data about the participants so that the reader can see how comparable the two groups were. Notice that the pain analysis took into account preexisting levels of baseline postoperative pain, education level, and depressed mood, in effect ruling them out as plausible alternate explanations for the observed results. The analysis of the change score data, which uses the degree of change between postop pain on Day 1 to Day 3 pain as the outcome, is impressive. Notice how the standard deviations in the intervention group are smaller compared to those in the control group. Results for change scores among the secondary outcomes of nausea, vomiting, and anxiety/tension were smaller and did not reach significance, with the exception of depression.

In addition, the authors get points for including not only the usual p values, but also the effect size of the intervention. Effect size is a measure of the strength of the relationship between two variables. In health care research we often want to know not only whether a treatment has a statistically significant effect, but also the size or magnitude of any observed effects. As was mentioned earlier, the fact that a result is statistically significant does not mean that it is clinically meaningful.

- *Are all the research outcomes previously specified reported?*

Yes, although it would have been helpful to see the descriptive results of the secondary outcomes, i.e., the means and standard deviations, and not just the change scores. Health care utilization and costs data are reported as part of the results section narrative.

Comments on the Discussion Section

- *Are the authors' comments justified, based on the results?*

Yes. The discussion of the observational study by Cassileth and Vickers is both accurate and useful, as are the recommendations or "lessons learned" for future studies in this area.

- *Do the conclusions follow logically from the results?*

Yes, it appears that the combined acupuncture/massage intervention did reduce the postoperative symptoms of pain and depression compared to standard care alone, based on the strength of the randomized controlled design and the strength of the statistical results.

- *Do the authors identify weaknesses or limitations in the study design or analysis?*

Yes, they do this in the discussion of the reasons why they may have failed to observe an effect in the rest of the other outcome variables. The authors also discuss the limits of how widely the study can be generalized based on the participants' ethnicity and higher-than-average levels of education – the results may not be applicable to patients with different ethnic backgrounds or educational levels. The discussion of effect sizes, and comparison of this study with the Cassileth and Vickers study, is helpful in explaining the difference made to the effect size reported in the prior study by adding the standard care control group. It is interesting to speculate what adding an attention-only group to control for nonspecific effects would do to the results of a future study in this area.

- *Is the clinical significance of the study discussed?*

Yes. The study results support the use of massage and acupuncture for postoperative symptom management, particularly for pain. However, notice that how the degree of improvement in pain is reported can affect your opinion. Which sounds larger and more impressive, a decrease in pain of 1 point on a 0 to 10 scale, or a decrease of 25.5%? When results are reported in percentages, make sure to look at what numbers are used to compute these percentages.

- *Are the conclusions consistent with the study objectives?*

Yes, overall. The study hypothesis and objectives are clearly stated, and the design and the methods used are congruent with these. Contrast the strength of the design and the appropriateness of the methods used here, especially the intervention protocols, with those in the previous study on massage and cancer pain. This is clearly a much stronger study, and a good contrast to the previous one since it was also based in a hospital setting and utilized some of the same outcome measures, such as pain and medication use. Obviously, after a close examination of both studies, it is clear that much more care and planning went into the design and conduct of this study. The authors also undoubtedly benefited from the knowledge gained through other studies on this topic during the intervening years between the first and second examples.

Comments on the Reference List

- *How up-to-date and appropriate is the reference list?*

It is both up-to-date and competent – the citations seem pertinent and succinct.

- *Did the authors examine other articles focusing on similar designs, populations, and outcomes?*

Yes. The references also include several systematic reviews.

- *Based on the results of this study, would it influence the way you practice?*

Without question. A massage therapist or acupuncturist familiar with the hospital setting could certainly consider working with postoperative clients during their hospital stay, and use this study to support a client's request for their services. Although it is not perfect, this is a well-designed and thoughtfully conducted study. A careful reader can have a fairly high degree of confidence that the observed results are an effect of the treatment.

Summary

Evaluating health care research critically takes knowledge and pragmatic skills. In this chapter we have developed a protocol for systematically reading and critiquing quantitative studies. Putting into practice what you have learned, you are developing the ability to improve the quality of the care you provide to your clients through integrating new information. Be reasonably skeptical, and remember that no study is perfect and that researchers often face a number of practical challenges that can limit their findings. The issue is always whether the flaws in a given study provide a plausible alternate explanation for the observed results, to the extent that the validity of the study is undermined. In the next chapter, we will apply critical evaluation to qualitative studies.

Reference

1.   Norman GR, Streiner DL. *PDQ Statistics*. Toronto: B.C. Decker Inc; 1986.

Exercise

1.   *Go to a reference in the second study. Find the article and read it critically in its own right, and then consider it in relation to its role in informing the authors of the Mehling et al study.*

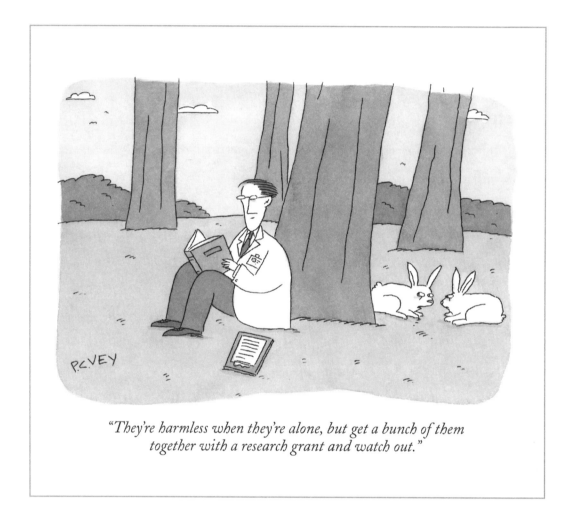

"They're harmless when they're alone, but get a bunch of them together with a research grant and watch out."

Chapter 8:

How to Read
a Qualitative Article

*We cannot know a priori which observations are relevant
and which are not.*

P. B. Medawar

Learning Objectives

After completing this chapter,
the reader should be able to:

- *Describe the major differences between qualitative and quantitative research paradigms.*

- *Name three types of qualitative approaches and their theoretical basis.*

- *List three design strategies that enhance the trustworthiness of qualitative research.*

- *Feel more confidence in critiquing qualitative studies.*

- *Discuss the advantages of a mixed methods approach.*

Chapter 8: How to Read a Qualitative Article

Qualitative Inquiry

As we discussed in Chapter 1, qualitative methods were developed largely out of the need for a different approach to answering questions of interest in the social sciences. Many important and useful questions cannot be answered using quantitative methods. For example, "What proportion and demographic segments of the public use complementary therapies?" clearly requires a quantitative approach, but, "How do people decide to seek a complementary practitioner?" is a different kind of question that necessitates a qualitative strategy.

Although qualitative research has historically been the domain of social scientists like anthropologists and sociologists, qualitative methods are now being used more often by biomedical researchers to give depth and understanding to their quantitative work. While developing a written survey to assess smoking behavior, for example, a researcher* conducted focus group interviews with smokers to pilot test a written questionnaire. In it, the researcher used the terms "quit" and "stop" interchangeably. For the smokers in the group, the two terms had opposite meanings – "stop" meant to become a nonsmoker, while "quit" was only temporary. Had the researcher not incorporated qualitative methodology into the design of her study through the use of these interviews, the survey instrument would have been fatally flawed, and she would have unknowingly reached an erroneous conclusion.

Qualitative methods are especially useful when exploring uncharted territory because variables of interest may be poorly understood, ill-defined, or uncontrollable. The qualitative approach has a great deal to offer in the exploration of complementary therapies, where so much is still unknown, and much of the territory is still being mapped out.

Qualitative methods are based on a divergent set of assumptions from quantitative methods. These include the following:

- that there is no single "objective" reality and that there may be multiple equally valid realities
- that the observer affects the phenomena observed

* *Paige Hornsby, personal communication, April 1995.*

· that what is true in one situation or context may not necessarily be applicable to other situations or contexts in the way that quantitative research is usually generalized

According to Michael Quinn Patton[1] qualitative inquiry is also distinguished by its use of several themes. These include:

· an emphasis on studying situations as they occur naturally, without manipulation by the researcher, and on studying them as unobtrusively as possible

· an openness to emergent design, where outcomes are not predetermined but are instead allowed to develop from immersion in the collected material – design strategies may change as the researcher's understanding of a process deepens, or in response as a situation changes

· an emphasis on detailed description (referred to as "thick" or "rich" description) that includes direct quotations portraying participants' views and experiences

Qualitative research also values the personal insights and experiences of the researcher as part of the inquiry process, recognizing, however, that while complete objectivity is impossible, a neutral attitude toward whatever content that may emerge is essential. The researcher should have no personal axe to grind. While the qualitative researcher's experience is inevitably colored by culture, education, and personal beliefs, he or she recognizes that the challenge is to suspend these as much as possible when observing and reporting. Just as with quantitative methods, analysis and interpretation of the data must always be grounded in and supported by the data.

Types of Qualitative Approaches

There is no single qualitative method. Qualitative methods have been developed based on diverse approaches to knowledge used in fields such as anthropology, sociology, psychology, education, and even philosophy. There are many different theoretical bases that provide a methodological foundation for qualitative approaches; we will mention only three of the more commonly used ones here. Many of the references listed at the end of this chapter offer excellent introductions to the subject, and the interested reader can learn more about designing qualitative inquiry from these sources.

• *Grounded Theory*

Grounded theory is rooted in sociology. It was developed to help better understand human behavior through generating explanatory models[2] based on empirical data. Imagine that we wish to investigate a chosen phenomenon, for example, the internal processes and stages that massage therapy students go through as they develop their professional identity. Using grounded theory, a researcher would identify and select knowledgeable participants who could provide a range of experiences and perspectives. The researcher would then systematically sample, collect, and analyze data throughout the course of the study, primarily through observing and interviewing the participants. As a picture of the phenomenon begins to develop, the researcher continues to purposively sample, collect, and analyze the data, based on the emergent theory, with each phase informing the next round of data collection and analysis, until a comprehensive theory integrating all the available information is fully formed.

Emergent is a key word here – the research design cannot always be specified in advance since the researcher does not know what will be discovered. One informant may identify other key informants, or identify new issues to be investigated. Grounded theory is an ongoing and highly responsive process. Its strength is that the generated theories and models are strongly rooted in the data, and that they continue to be revised as more data become available. This type of continuous revision is called an **iterative process**.

A feature of grounded theory that is sometimes incorporated into other approaches is the use of **negative cases**. Negative cases are examples that are contrary to the prevailing data and that are purposefully sought out by the researcher to provide a different and more complete perspective. These can sometimes be the exception that proves the rule, and their presence increases the credibility of a study's findings. Including negative cases reflects an attempt to build a theory or model that accounts for all the data generated, rather than ignoring information that does not fit the theory.

• *Ethnography*

Ethnography developed from anthropology and relies on that field's traditional use of participant observation and fieldwork methods, that is, immersion in a culture as both an observer of and participant in that culture, combined with copious note-taking. It is based on the assumption that any group of people will, over time, develop a culture. Ethnography answers the question: "What is the culture of this group?" Culture is a particular shared way of defining the world, the relationship of the group to it and to each other, and accepted standards of behavior, such as the proper way to make a request between members compared to non-members of the group. Simply, culture is the means by which we separate "us" from "them." By this definition, the idea of culture is not limited to geographic location or ethnic heritage but can refer to any group of people, for example, organizations, religious groups, or people in schools or workplaces. Ethnographic techniques could be used to study the culture of a particular complementary therapy training program, of a hospital ward, or of a software corporation.

The researcher's challenge in this approach is to maintain the dynamic tension between the perspectives of the neutral observer and the engaged participant. Each informs the other. Participating in the culture even as an outsider helps the qualitative investigator understand it from the insider's perspective. Think of movies such as *Witness* or *The Last Samurai*, where the protagonist goes to live for a time in a radically different culture and whose understanding of that culture (and often himself) is changed or deepened as a result. A risk of the ethnographic approach is that the investigator may emotionally overidentify with the study's participants and lose the ability to remain a neutral observer. An important aspect of the ethnographic method is that the researchers keep detailed journals; one reason for this is to help separate observation, experience, and interpretation, as part of an **audit trail**. Potential biases are identified and noted, and an attempt is made to take these into account. The audit trail provides a written record to document both the data and the researchers' analytic process, so that anyone could follow and understand how they reached their conclusions.

• *Phenomenology*

Phenomenology is based within the field of philosophy, and is sometimes seen as synonymous with qualitative methods. Its focus is on understanding the essence and structure of the experience of a phenomenon for a group of people, from their perspective. The phenomenological approach attempts to uncover the lived experience of an event and distill it down to its essential features. For example, what is the fundamental nature of the experience of becoming a first-time mother? Or the experience of receiving and living with a terminal diagnosis? What does it mean to be an acupuncturist? Phenomenology attempts to truly get inside another person's skin, to see and experience the world through his or her eyes.

From a phenomenological perspective there is no objective reality – the subjective details of the individual's experience and the interpretation of its meaning are necessary to understand its essence. Women may have very different individual experiences of becoming a mother for the first time, yet there are likely to be common threads or themes that identify regular features of a universal experience, such as the impact of sleep deprivation. In a sense, phenomenology attempts to generate a more general and comprehensive model from specific and individual cases. An issue that can arise especially with this approach is how to determine when enough individuals have been sampled. The only way that the investigator can know is when no new features or information are discovered through participant interviews, sometimes termed "saturation" or "redundancy." As in other qualitative approaches, participants are selected purposefully, based on their knowledge or experience, rather than at random.

Data Analysis in Qualitative Research

The units of data in qualitative research are words rather than numbers, so the way in which such data are analyzed is necessarily different than for quantitative data. Most often, the words that participants provide in qualitative data collection are recorded in written or oral format – orally collected data is typically transcribed to ensure fidelity of the content. The collected words are then usually analyzed using a method called **content analysis**, which is exactly what it sounds like – an analysis of the content of all the study data.

Content analysis is commonly employed in phenomenological and ethnographic studies. In addition to health care research, content analysis is used in many diverse fields, including marketing, literature, cultural studies in areas such as gender issues, sociology, psychology, and many other areas of inquiry. The basic method of content analysis is simple: the data coder determines the presence of certain words or concepts within the transcript of an interview. Software especially designed for this purpose is often used. These words or concepts may be quantified and analyzed for their meanings and relationships. To conduct a content analysis on interview data, the interview must be transcribed into a written text and then broken down and coded into meaningful and manageable categories, possibly on a number of levels – word, phrase, theme, for example – and then examined in terms of the concepts expressed. The researcher can use one of the two basic methods of content analysis: **conceptual analysis** or **relational analysis**.

In conceptual content analysis, the existence and frequency of concepts is established, usually through counting the number of repetitions of words or phrases. For instance, imagine that you are conducting a study on the experience of being a first-time mother. Using conceptual analysis you could determine how many times words such as "amazing," "overwhelmed," "exhausted," or "blissful" appear in the interview transcripts. Relational content analysis goes a step further by examining the relationships among the concepts identified. Additional words or phrases such as "excited," "sleep deprived," or "with love" might appear in conjunction to previously identified concepts. The different meanings that emerge as a result of these new groupings are then explored.

Trustworthiness in Qualitative Research

Lincoln and Guba[3] have identified four aspects of trustworthiness in qualitative research, which they believe can be applied equally to all types of qualitative studies (and to quantitative studies as well). These are: truth value, or **credibility**; **transferability**; **consistency**; and **neutrality** or *confirmability*. The rigor of qualitative research depends on attention to these factors.

- *Credibility*

Analogous to internal validity, credibility in qualitative research is based on describing and reporting the perspectives of study participants as clearly and as accurately as possible. The methods used to select participants, to collect data, and to analyze the data should be appropriate to the study question and clearly described. As in quantitative research, the conclusions of the study should be supported by the data presented. In qualitative studies, the results are usually the actual quotes of participants that exemplify the conclusions of the researcher. It is up to the reader to decide whether the research procedures and data presented provide a plausible alternate interpretation of the study findings.

- *Transferability*

Similar to generalizability, this criterion refers to the capacity of a study's findings to be applied to other contexts, settings, or groups. Although it can add to the utility of any study, transferability is not required for a qualitative study to be credible. Because qualitative research often emphasizes the unique nature of a situation, what is true in one setting or among one set of group members may not necessarily be true in other similar circumstances. In terms of applying results to clinical practice, a qualitative study may provide insight into the nature of client experience or give a practitioner a different or broader perspective on a particular issue. In this way, a study without high levels of transferability can still have clinical relevance.

- *Consistency*

This is the qualitative equivalent of reliability, that is, consistency over a period of time or across groups or settings such that the study data are internally congruent. As with transferability, the emphasis on unique experience in much qualitative research means that this type of consistency may not always be relevant, depending upon the research question or the nature of the particular study.

However, another type of consistency can be seen in qualitative studies where researchers employ **triangulation**. Triangulation refers to the use of multiple methods of data collection, or methods of analysis, or analysts. For example, a study might employ participant observation by the researcher together with interviews with knowledgeable informants conducted by other members of the research team. When there is internal consistency among the study results using multiple methods of data collection or analysis, confidence that the study findings are an accurate reflection of the phenomenon being studied is greatly increased.

- *Neutrality*

This criterion relates to freedom from bias in the research process and in the reporting of results. Neutrality can be increased by studying participants over a longer period of time or through prolonged contact with them, and by including diverse perspectives. The researcher attempts to gain a broader perspective and to collect as much information from as many differing points of view as possible. As was mentioned earlier, the researcher also attempts to identify his or her own biases by keeping a written journal where possible biases are noted, and through consultation with other researchers. The use of negative cases is a design feature that increases neutrality.

Evaluating Qualitative Research

Patton[1] succinctly identifies the following three areas of evaluation for readers of qualitative research:

1. The use of rigorous and appropriate methods for collecting high-quality data, and for analyzing the data, that address issues related to validity and reliability from the viewpoint of verification. For example, interviews should be audio- or videotape recorded, rather than using written notes that only summarize participants' words. The use of videotape additionally allows the inclusion of nonverbal behavior in the analysis of the data. For a fascinating illustration of this approach in the field of interpersonal psychology, read any of John Gottman's books on couples therapy. Triangulation, for example through the use of multiple of data coders, also increases both validity of the themes uncovered and the reliability of the method of data analysis performed.

2. The qualifications of the researcher – clearly training and experience are important, as well as track record, status in the field, and methods of self-presentation in the research situation. The qualifications of the researcher are especially important in qualitative research because the researcher is both the instrument of data collection and the core of the process of data analysis.

3. An appreciation, familiarity, and degree of comfort with the assumptions of the qualitative paradigm, including naturalistic inquiry, holistic thinking, and the use of qualitative approaches.

Based on these criteria, there are several basic questions to consider when reading any qualitative study and evaluating its trustworthiness. Most will sound familiar because their underlying concepts are often inherently the same as those used in evaluating quantitative research.

Critical Evaluation Questions for Qualitative Studies

1. Is the research question clearly articulated?

2. What assumptions underlie the study; what qualitative approach forms its theoretical basis?

3. What are the qualifications, experience, and perspective of the researcher(s)?

4. What techniques and methods were used to ensure the integrity of the results as well as their accuracy?

5. Are the methods used in data collection and analysis described in sufficient detail?

6. Given the theoretical approach and the purpose of the study, are the methods used appropriate?

7. Are the results credible?

8. Do the results justify the conclusions?

9. Are the results applicable to other settings?

10. Are the results clinically meaningful?

While the methods used in qualitative research are quite different from those used in quantitative studies, they can be applied as rigorously. It is just as important in a qualitative study that the research question be clearly formulated as it is in a quantitative study. The methods and procedures used in the study, such as the strategy and rationale for participant selection, should make sense and be appropriate in regard to the research question or study objective. In particular, the care with which data is collected and analyzed is equally if not more crucial in a qualitative study. Because qualitative data is often not "measurable" in the same way that numerical data is, documentation of data collection and analysis strategies allows readers to understand the researcher's approach and to see whether they reach substantially similar conclusions.

In collecting interview data, it is standard practice to audiotape interviews for later transcription while the researcher also makes written notes about nonverbal behavior or nuances that cannot always be captured aurally. Videotaping of interviews is becoming more common with the advent of relatively inexpensive digital video cameras. Content analysis of interview data is often assisted by the use of software programs that sort responses based on criteria such as key words or phrases, and may perform frequency counts and analysis. Methods used in the data collection and analysis of a study, including the use of any software packages, should be spelled out in sufficient detail for the reader to understand exactly what was done, and why.[4]

Other considerations in evaluating quantitative research, such as the clarity and thoroughness of a review of the literature, or the appropriateness of the references cited, may also be relevant depending on the individual study. Some qualitative researchers may choose to avoid an extensive literature review in an effort to remain unbiased on a given topic, and the reader will have to decide if this is a reasonable strategy or not.

The examples used in this chapter are concerned with difficult issues such as breast cancer, mastectomy and chemotherapy, and childhood abuse. The qualitative approach is well suited to investigating questions related to the sensitive nature of these topics, and puts a human face on what can be an abstract concept. Students often find that reading high-quality qualitative research is both intellectually and emotionally engaging. As you read the following study, think specifically about the questions listed in the preceding box.

Study Example #1: Mastectomy, Body Image, and Massage

Mastectomy, Body Image and Therapeutic Massage: *A Qualitative Study of Women's Experience*

Bredin, Mary MA RGN

Macmillan Research Practitioner, Macmillan Practice Development Unit, Centre for Cancer and Palliative Care Studies, Institute of Cancer Research at the Royal Marsden Hospital NHS Trust, London, UK

Accepted for publication 24 June 1998.

Correspondence: Mary Bredin MA, RGN, Macmillan Research Practitioner, Macmillan Practice Development Unit, Centre for Cancer and Palliative Care Studies, Institute of Cancer Research at the Royal Marsden Hospital, Fulham Road, London SW3 6JJ, UK.
E-mail: maryb@ICR.ac.uk

Full Text of: Bredin: J Adv Nurs, Volume 29(5). May 1999. 1113-1120
Journal of Advanced Nursing © 1999 Blackwell Science Ltd.

Abstract

Despite the wealth of literature concerning the impact of breast loss on a woman's body image, sexual and psychological adjustment, there have been few studies within the medical and nursing literature directly quoting a woman's private perspective; how in her words she experiences her changed body. Furthermore, there is a lack of evidence-based interventions for addressing the problem of altered body image (ABI); healthcare professionals often feel at a loss in knowing how to help women cope (Hopwood & Maguire 1998).[11] In this study in-depth interviews were undertaken to explore three women's experiences of breast loss with particular focus on body image issues; a second phase piloted a massage intervention as a means of helping them adjust to living with their changed body image. Listening to their experience, in combination with the therapeutic massage, allowed deep access and insight into the nature of the women's trauma. The experiences of the three women in this study suggest there may be a group of women whose needs are overlooked and who, despite their prosthesis and reassurances that they are disease-free, opt to conceal the problems they have in living with a changed image. The availability of a body-centred therapy might help with certain aspects of adjustment as revealed by this study.

Introduction

A great deal has been written and researched on the psychological and social effects of mastectomy. This research has shown that whereas all cancer causes anxiety about the disease and its progression, mastectomy threatens some women with a distressing disturbance of body image, partly because of the breast's symbolic and physical association with being a woman.

This paper reports on a qualitative study which explored three women's experiences of breast cancer with a particular focus on body image issues. The study incorporated two phases; the first phase was to interview three women about their experiences of mastectomy, and a second phase offered each woman a body-centred intervention involving massage and listening, as a means of helping them adjust to their changed body image. While the study shows that the women's distress was clearly multi-dimensional, it also revealed that their bodily loss remained a potent focus for their distress and a reminder of a wider sense of disruption. According to the women's accounts the intervention in some ways met their need to reveal (implicitly and explicitly) their secret loss and sense of being different.

Background: The Issue of Body Image Within Breast Cancer Research

In the light of the breast's emotional and symbolic significance much has been written about the impact of its loss through breast cancer. The literature on breast cancer which includes assessment of altered body image (ABI) is generally concerned with the psychological and psycho-social effects of mastectomy compared with breast conservation, adjuvant treatment and breast reconstruction (Fallowfield et al. 1986, Kemeny et al.

1988).[5,14] *These studies found that women have a more satisfactory body image following breast conservation; a fairly consistent finding despite the researchers offering no clear definition of body image nor standardized inventories to measure it (Schover et al. 1995). While it appears that women receiving conservative breast surgery report improved body image ratings, studies assessing the effects of surgery on psychological morbidity show similar levels of anxiety and depression regardless of the treatment given (Fallowfield & Hall 1991).[6] Furthermore, the advantage women may gain in terms of greater body image satisfaction following breast conservation may be offset by an increased fear of cancer and its possible recurrence (Fallowfield et al. 1986).[5]*

The supposition that fear about breast loss may take precedence over the fear of having a diagnosis of cancer may be erroneous, according to Fallowfield & Hall (1991).[6] They explored this issue with a sample of 269 women in a prospective multi-centre study designed to evaluate the psychological outcome of different treatment policies in women with early breast cancer (Fallowfield et al. 1990).[7] At the first post-operative interview the majority (159/244) gave 'fear of cancer' as their primary fear rather than the fear of losing a breast; only 12% of the sample (18 women who received mastectomy and 14 who received lumpectomy) felt that losing a breast was worse. This finding is similar to that of an earlier study by Peters-Golden (1982)[19] who examined perceptions of social support among 100 breast cancer patients and 100 disease-free individuals. Within the breast cancer group recurrence and spread of cancer and the consequences of treatment regimes took precedence over fears of losing a breast. Peters-Golden commented that researchers' assumptions that breast loss is the primary concern for women facing breast cancer may only serve to detract from the gravity of facing a life-threatening illness. Undoubtedly, these issues are blurred and for each woman reactions will vary considerably, depending on the emotional significance a woman attributes to her breast and her ability to adjust to having a life-threatening disease. Priorities at diagnosis and following treatment can change in significance over time; healthcare professionals need to be aware of this so that they can respond appropriately regardless of the nature of problems encountered.

Some of the earliest studies of mastectomy and body image explored whether mastectomy resulted in a negative body image (Polivy 1977, Jamison et al. 1978).[20,12] For example,

Polivy (1977)[20] examined the impact of mastectomy on feminine self-concept and body image. An important finding from this study was that immediately following surgery, mastectomy patients showed no body image alteration whereas patients undergoing breast biopsy showed a decline in body image and self-image. She suggested that both these groups used denial as a defense mechanism. However, for those women who learned their results were negative denial was no longer needed, therefore their self-image scores worsened postoperatively, while scores of those who had mastectomy showed little change. In contrast, 6-11 months after mastectomy significantly worse scores for body image and total self-image were evident. Polivy concluded that breast cancer and its treatment by total breast amputation are intrinsically both more anxiety-provoking and likely to leave a woman feeling worse about her body. However, she also commented that denial was an important part of the defense process whereby a woman who has undergone a mastectomy integrates her changed body into her new self-image.

In contrast to Polivy's (1977)[20] findings, it has been argued that many women will not always suffer irreparably as a consequence of mastectomy (Price 1990).[21] Price (1990)[21] cites Anderson (1988)[1] who reported that women who had undergone mastectomy apparently recovered remarkably well, despite a lack of structured support. Some felt positively about the experience because it had removed the threat of the cancer. Confirming Anderson's (1988)[1] finding, Krouse & Krouse (1982)[15] examined a small sample of women: breast cancer patients (n = 9); gynaecological cancer patients (n = 5); and a non-cancer comparison group (n = 5). Assessments of depression and body image in the mastectomy group at 1, 2 and 20 months showed that after a brief initial crisis there was a total adaptation by the end of the study. In contrast, patients with gynaecological cancer had increased feelings of depression and worsening body image scores even at 20 months following surgery. However, it is not clear from the study what the authors mean by 'adaptation' and the small sample size makes it difficult to generalize the findings. More recently, Schover et al. (1995) conducted a retrospective study comparing psycho-social adjustment, body image and sexual function in women who had either breast conservation (n = 72) or reconstruction (n = 146) for early stage disease. Overall, fewer than 20% of women reported poor adjustment on the domains measured which included psycho-social distress, body image and sexual satisfaction. The two groups did not differ greatly in their results; however, women who had undergone chemotherapy had more sexual dysfunction, poorer body image and psychological distress. The authors conclude that it is important to identify women at high risk for psycho-social distress and they suggest that screening should be routine for women undergoing chemotherapy or reporting having a troubled marital relationship, feeling unattractive, dissatisfaction with sexual relationships or poor social support.

To summarize, it seems that not all women will find living with a mastectomy problematic. None the less, when a body image problem does exist it may not be apparent to health professionals initially; patients are often afraid of admitting they have a problem. For their part, doctors and nurses may be reluctant to enquire, perhaps because they feel they lack the time or skills needed to cope with the distress that inquiry might reveal (Hopwood & Maguire 1988).[11] The present study suggests that there may be a group of women who, following breast cancer treatment, fail to reveal ABI distress, possibly because it may become apparent months later, when 'life' is meant to be returning to some sense of normality.

Body Image: Theoretical Considerations

The concept 'body image' is a construct deriving from different dimensions of body experience. Many authors have attempted to define the 'body image' phenomenon, the earliest and most frequently quoted definition was formulated by the German neurologist Paul Schilder who wrote:

> "The image of the human body means the picture of our own body which we form in our mind, that is to say the way in which our body appears to ourselves."
> (Schilder 1950, p. 11)[25]

Schilder's definition implies the highly subjective nature of the body image: as an inner representation of how one thinks and feels about one's body it may bear no relationship to how one's body appears to others. This subjectivity is also shaped by cultural and social influences and incorporates both unconscious and conscious subjective experience (Cash & Pruzinsky 1990).[2] These are important considerations when attempting to capture and assess a woman's experience of her changed body image. Such perceptions and feelings may not always be easily translated into language. They can be difficult to articulate when they remain embedded in the realm of 'body experience' and a 'body language' beyond conscious thoughts, words and concepts.

The Study and its Methods

The first phase of the study explored three women's experience of breast loss following mastectomy. In the second phase of the inquiry a body-orientated intervention (therapeutic massage) was offered to each woman. The sample size was limited to three participants because of the time required to undertake the massage intervention. Each woman who entered the study had been identified as having a body image problem by their consultant oncologist or breast care nurses. Because of the difficulties in defining what constitutes a 'body image problem,' it was agreed that there would be no specific selection criteria; practitioners invited women to take part who:

1. showed signs of having significant problems in adapting to the loss of their breast
2. revealed that they were particularly distressed about their changed appearance

Ethical permission was granted, and three women were invited to join the study. The women had to be currently cancer-free following mastectomy, aged between 25 and 65 years, and referred not later than 1 year after their original diagnosis.

Each woman participated in two 1-hour semistructured interviews and six sessions of therapeutic massage. The initial interview and subsequent massage sessions were conducted by the author. The follow-up interview was conducted by an independent researcher who focused on the effects of the massage intervention. Field notes were kept throughout and all interviews were taped and transcribed. Data analysis was undertaken following Guba & Lincoln's research methods (Guba & Lincoln 1985).[10]

The Massage Intervention

Each session began with talking for a short time, to gauge how the participant was feeling and to discuss concerns about the massage. Participants were offered a choice of where to be massaged: foot, arm, face or back, depending on preference. Sessions started with a short relaxation where the participant was invited to become aware of her breathing, notice how her body was feeling and to consciously let her limbs relax. The massage consisted of light gentle effleurage strokes only, and once completed the participant was encouraged to lie quietly. She would then be invited to talk for a short while if she so chose.

A Rationale for the Intervention

A rationale for the intervention was developed out of the author's prior experience of working with breast cancer patients. There were two components to the intervention:

1. Body Concept

An important aspect of adjusting to a changed body image may be the manner in which an individual describes or creates an account of her body in relation to self. This has been described by Price (1994)[22] as the 'conceptual element' of the body image construct which may feature in patients' accounts of their symptoms and coping style. When addressing ABI distress it may be important to help a woman articulate or express her body's story; the image of and feelings she has about her body and the meaning her breasts have held for her. If, as part of her story for instance, a woman conceptualizes her breast as being 'mutilated' or 'grotesque' it is likely that she will experience increased distress about her changed image. Because of her embarrassment and fear of being stigmatized, she may not want to draw attention to such feelings even though they may colour her whole experience. In such circumstances, it may be helpful for a person telling her story simply to have her experience heard and acknowledged by an empathic listener (Mitchell 1995).[16]

2. Body Perception

A second aspect of the body image relates to how we sense our bodies physically through sensations and feelings. If a mastectomy results in distorting surgical scars, pain, skin numbness and muscular tension for instance, this will colour a woman's experience of her body. There are a number of ways in which massage might affect body perception. For example, offering a woman structured touch within a safe therapeutic context might enable her to address the bodily dimension of her distress. By having another person 'touch the untouchable', i.e. her damaged body, a woman might begin to re-experience her traumatized body in a more positive way (Peters et al. 1996).[18] Emotional suffering may itself be felt as physical pain and muscular tension (Pruzinsky 1990);[23] massage can influence this (Ferrell-Torry & Glick 1992).[8] Illness and disfigurement can lead to feelings of being different and unacceptable (Murphy 1987);[17] touch is a type of communication that transcends the usual boundaries between people. It can enable a person to feel 'held', to feel safe and accepted (Corner et al. 1995).[3] It can be a very immediate expression of another person's ability to tolerate the unacceptable.

Findings

Four key categories emerged from the data, as follows:

1. *the women's experience of their changed bodies*
2. *the effects of breast loss on self*
3. *effects of breast loss on social identity*
4. *experiences of the massage*

The findings from the first three categories reflected the multi-dimensional nature of the women's experience; they expressed loss and difference at every level of their being. These categories are not distinct; they tend to overlap with each other, indicating the complexity of the subject matter. The fourth category, 'experiences of the massage,' directly reflected questions asked in the second interview about the women's experience of the intervention.

Women's Experiences of Their Changed Bodies

Each woman spoke of how she perceived and experienced her body—changes not only in sensations to the breast area but also within her whole body. For example, they all mentioned a variety of physical perceptions: numbness, coldness, skin sensitivity, stiffness, soreness, pain and lymphoedema in the arms. These were all unpleasant sensations which served as a constant reminder of their mastectomy experience. For example, 'Jane' was troubled by the sensitivity of her skin around her scar site. She was also affected by the change in the shape of her chest. The sense of the whole of her body feeling different made her self-conscious about her shape:

> *"You feel lopsided, there is no doubt about that and it's very strange when you haven't got the prosthesis on after a bath or moving in bed ... it's flat, it's noticeable..."*

'Sarah' initially could not look at herself, preferring to take her baths in the dark:

> *"Well, for three months I didn't even look at myself, I just put a lot of bubbles in the bath, I didn't look at all."*

Four months after her mastectomy Sarah had managed to look at her breast but still did not like what she saw:

> *"I don't like looking at it, if the towel falls down I just wrap it round it because I don't like looking at it."*

'Vicky' had undergone a double mastectomy. Physically she experienced pain locally around her scar sites and was troubled by lymphoedema in both arms:

> *"They [the arms] ache all the time and I'm in pain all the way down there all the time, and that rubs against your body so when I go down the road I have to hold my arms out."*

Her body image had altered, but when Vicky was dressed she was less disturbed by this:

> *"I think my scars are ugly. They are more grotesque than I thought they would be, I thought they would be a lot neater than they are ... and therefore my whole body shape is out of proportion. When you look in the mirror you look grotesque, but when I put my clothes on I don't give it a lot of thought."*

For Sarah and Jane, difficulty in adapting may have been hindered by interpretations of their experience being like an 'amputation' or 'mutilation':

> *"I suppose to an extent I feel deformed. That's probably the best way to describe it ... and your appearance has changed quite radically ... I think it's possibly one of the most mutilating things that a male or female can have done." [Jane]*

Effects of Breast Loss on Self

It has been suggested that, as a consequence of western medicine's tendency to objectify the body and 'fix' the part that has gone wrong, a woman's breast has often been considered as detachable and replaceable (Young 1992)[28]. However, whether or not she likes her breasts, they are a part of her self-identity; the loss of one (or both) may feel as if she has lost a part of her self. The statements made in this category indicate that the women had experienced more than just a bodily change; something felt different at a deeper level of the self:

> *"I know I don't look any different from the outside world but it's difficult to put into words; it's just there. You are different and there's no getting away from it." [Jane]*

For Sarah, her breasts were deeply bound up with her womanly image. Speaking of her reflection in the mirror she commented:

> *"I don't like it. That's not me any more."*

Vicky acknowledged her sense of incompleteness and difference:

> *"I am different. I had the most rounded boobs and I was proud of them. Although they were big, they were an important part of my life and now they are gone and yes there is this loss there—I feel diminished in some way but I couldn't tell you in what way; incomplete I suppose you would say."*

Effects of Breast Loss on Social Identity

As an inner representation, the body image may bear no relationship to how a person's body appears to others. A person might feel, for example, that her body is ugly, beautiful, large or small at different times when in fact her external physical appearance has not changed. This subjectivity can be influenced by social interactions which in turn determine the body image and influence self-worth (Schain 1986, Foltz 1987).[24,9] The women's statements suggested that their experience of breast loss had affected their social identity. All mentioned concealment, withdrawal, concern about others noticing, self-consciousness and changed behaviour with family/partners. Their statements indicated that they could cope as long as they kept up an appearance of looking normal by wearing their prosthesis and concealing their 'difference':

"…. when I'm dressed I can cope with it. When I'm dressed nobody needs to know." [Sarah]

Jane felt different not only to herself but also in relation to other women:

"I found it quite easy with my female friends on a one to one basis. But on a more than one to one basis I felt they are a woman and I am not, sort of thing. I don't know why, it's just the way you react I suppose."

Sarah felt uncomfortable with her partner:

"I get sort of panicky if he goes to walk in the bathroom. I don't want him to touch me at the top at all … because you are worried that he might touch the one that is not there …"

Vicky did not have a partner but the idea of having another relationship was out of the question for her:

"I think if there had been a thought at the back of mind of finding a mate prior to the operation there would be no thought now."

For each of the women there was an indication that they needed to hide the distress they felt from those around them; for example:

"When my mum was here … I couldn't wait for her to go so I could cry because I wasn't going to cry while she was here. When she went I just sat on the stairs and sobbed and sobbed." [Sarah]

Jane experienced conflict in not wanting to express how she felt:

"I mean you sort of feel grateful in one way and guilty for feeling upset and different."

Experiences of the Massage

The findings within the fourth category showed that each woman had felt positive about the intervention. Despite precautions to avoid bias by using an outside researcher to conduct the second interviews, it is possible that the women may have felt less comfortable reporting negative experiences because of their relationship with the researcher/practitioner. However, there was no indication within the interview material or in their unrecorded communications that they had found the intervention unhelpful. In contrast, there were

clear examples of how each woman had benefited from the sessions. Initially there was
some apprehension about the intervention:

> *"The first time I was very apprehensive because I wasn't sure ... and I always found it hard*
> *to relax ..." [Sarah]*

Both Sarah and Vicky had suffered with numbness and pain in their arms as a consequence
of their mastectomies. Sarah reported that the massage had helped her arm 'to feel part of
her body' once more and Vicky had found it helpful in reducing discomfort in her arms:

> *"You know there were days when I didn't know where to put my arms and yes the massage*
> *certainly helped my arms then ..."*

All three women reported that the massage had helped them relax. For example, Sarah
was surprised that she could let herself relax as she 'had always been one of those people
who couldn't', Vicky reported that she always 'had a lovely nap after the massage' and
then she felt 'great'; Jane, too, was surprised at how it made her feel:

> *"I just like the feeling of the massage and it did make me feel more relaxed. You know it sort*
> *of sends you off into another world almost. It's superb, I never would have imagined it*
> *would have that sort of effect..." [Jane]*

Sarah and Vicky reported that they were sleeping better:

> *"I wasn't sleeping at all, I mean every hour looking at the clock, but since my massage the*
> *last few weeks I've had good nights' sleep which I hadn't had for 8 months..." [Sarah]*

Vicky was feeling more comfortable with touching her breast scars, and Sarah was able to
look at herself once more:

> *"When M. came I found touching my scars terrible, you know I didn't even touch them ...*
> *but now it does not bother me, I cream them and massage them and no problem." [Vicky]*

> *"A few months back I'd covered myself up because I didn't like looking but I don't avoid the*
> *mirror as much as I would have before." [Sarah]*

At times even gentle body-work such as therapeutic massage can 'open up' and bring to
the surface previously suppressed emotions. This may be helpful, but practitioners also

need to be aware that such a reaction may be potentially harmful. During the 6 weeks that Jane came for massage she had a period of feeling low, and it could be argued that the massage opened up feelings which previously she had suppressed:

> "I had these couple of weeks of feeling pretty grim ... it was unfortunate that it happened while I was coming to see her but I think it was purely coincidental. On the other hand it might not have been ... I think it had to come out and I think it was important to do it really. I've certainly felt better since..."

Jane was given the choice to stop the sessions if she felt they were too disturbing because of feelings aroused. She chose to continue and talked about her grief of having cancer; in this way she was held physically and emotionally while she confronted feelings that had previously been too private and painful to reveal.

Sarah's dissatisfaction with her body and her fear of her partner's reaction to the sight of her breast had led her to conceal her wound totally. During the 6 weeks she came for the massage she resumed sexual relations with her partner, and she managed to show her breast to a friend:

> "I didn't look at it for the couple of months myself anyway, now I look at it ... I mean I can cope now, I mean at one time a while back if a towel dropped off me I'd have been ... but now if it drops I don't ... And actually my friend, I actually showed her the other week."

Vicky's story suggests that the intervention was an opportunity to be touched at a time when her body felt 'repulsive':

> "I haven't got a partner so I am not touched ... I think I felt my body was a bit repulsive and therefore people would not want to touch me and I think the massage helped me ..."

She also had found it helpful to talk:

> "I can't talk to the family and I haven't got a close personal relationship with somebody I could actually share so yes I shared it with M. and therefore she has helped me through quite a lot of feelings."

As well as talking about their massage experience, a strong theme to emerge from the second round of interviews was the women's ability to accept and cope with their changed self-images:

"You just learn to live with it in the same way you learn to live with other things, you know people with amputations and things like that I suppose. The same with bereavement, you don't get over it but you learn to cope with it and I think this is much the same." [Jane]

"Yes I've got used to my scars, I didn't like them at first I thought they were ugly. Well they are still not pretty but I've got used to them and I've accepted that they are there and it's the body I've got to live with now." [Vicky]

"Oh yes I'm feeling better because I suppose I'm coping with it better, accepting it I suppose that's all you can do." [Sarah]

Discussion

It is widely acknowledged that a small percentage of women will develop significant problems adjusting to their body image as a result of mastectomy. Body image distress can be experienced not just in terms of an impaired sense of femininity or sexuality; it can have a profound impact on the 'whole' of one's being (Coyler 1996).[4] Revelation of distress may be hindered by a fear of stigma, as a consequence of living in a culture where womanhood is bound up with having a perfect body and blemish-free appearance. It is not easy for health-care professionals to become aware of the problem of ABI distress post-treatment since, as this study revealed, some women will try to conceal their loss, physically and emotionally, under an outward desire to be seen as 'normal.'

The current management of breast cancer aims to rid the body of the disease, and as yet there is no consistent approach to identifying women at risk of ABI. The issue may be compounded by the difficulty in defining what the term a 'body image problem' means. An implication from this study is the need for a working definition. Practitioners must to be able to differentiate 'normal' and 'abnormal' reactions to breast loss—practical assessment tools are also needed.

When distress is encountered, how can body image problems be treated? While there is evidence to suggest that specialist nurses can and do provide invaluable counselling and support for women identified with ABI (Watson et al. 1988, Wilkinson et al. 1988)[26,27] such resources are often stretched; practitioners may feel they are limited in what they can offer.

It appears, moreover, from the private experiences of the three women in this study that subjective body experience and 'shocking' emotions can be too shameful to voice and (in some cases) literally beyond words. Can healthcare professionals help women find a language to express bodily distress and discomfort? Perhaps the multi-dimensional nature of the experience needs to be taken into account so that nursing care can attend to the three dimensions of experience: body, self and interpersonal self. While it may simply be enough for a woman to disclose her story and have her feelings acknowledged, the availability of a body-centred approach such as therapeutic massage could be valuable for woman with ABI problems post-mastectomy. The findings from this study suggest this would be worth exploring in more depth.

The three cases presented in this study are not necessarily typical of how women respond to or cope with the loss of a breast. The findings cannot be generalized. The women took part in the study because they were having difficulty in coming to terms with their changed body images. Statements made in the second interview about 'coping better' cannot be attributed entirely to the intervention, since it is possible they might have adjusted in their own time without such support.

However, it appears from their statements that the intervention helped them in important ways to cope at a time when the body had become an 'unacceptable' object. It may, for example, have provided some containment for what was previously uncontainable (Judd 1993)[13]; the untouchable and unspeakable perceptions of a changed body. It provided an opportunity for the women (literally and figuratively) to reveal themselves, and talk at a time when they felt isolated in their distress. Finally, it may have helped reduce bodily tension and discomfort, enabling relaxation and promoting sleep.

This tentative exploration of a body-orientated intervention suggests there may be potential scope for introducing it into clinical practice, but it must be acknowledged that there would be several difficulties in doing so. The notion of introducing a complementary therapy such as massage into an area where there is a gap in conventional health care has implications. Like any intervention massage may be harmful. Few research studies exist demonstrating its efficacy and many professionals understandably consider it unsafe to refer a patient to an unknown and unproven resource. There are no clear guidelines for appropriate referral or contraindications. For instance, the women in this study clearly had differing needs. According to their comments Sarah and Vicky found the massage helpful; Jane found the relaxation aspect useful too, but the massage itself may have been too physically and psychologically invasive, given her previous ways of coping. Undoubtedly, this type of intervention invites disclosure at a time when a woman's coping mechanisms might actually require her to deny her loss. Nursing research into this area is required and must be evaluated as part of an integrated approach to managing body image problems in breast cancer patients, about whose incidence we still know so little.

Conclusion

The experiences of the three women in this study are unique. Although not generalizable, the findings raise some important concerns and questions which challenge the approach currently adopted by healthcare practitioners. They imply that the current approach to managing women post-mastectomy may at times compound the experience of difference that leads some women to conceal their sense of loss inappropriately, with disturbing physical and emotional consequences. The immediate response to helping women adjust to their breast loss is to replace the irreplaceable: the prosthesis is fitted along with the reassurances that they are disease-free. Conventional management colludes with women's sense that their feelings of loss and disfigurement should be kept secret—the implicit imperative is to conform to being normal. It may be that this collusion between patients and professionals makes them pretend that adjustment is happening when in fact it is not.

As Jane's conflicting feelings implied, it was because she felt grateful to be rid of her cancer that she felt she should not express her anger and distress.

We should consider whether a body-centred intervention involving massage could be valuable in a multidisciplinary approach to preventing and treating distress after mastectomy. The findings from this study indicate that it introduced a clinically useful extra dimension which allowed significant disturbing experiences and feelings to be talked about, touched on, and met in a way that went beyond words.

Acknowledgements

With thanks to Dr. Tim Sheard and Dr. David Peters for their support and advice.

References

1. Anderson J. (1988) *Coming to terms with mastectomy. Nursing Times* 84, 41-44. Reprinted in *Body Image Nursing Concepts and Care* (Price B. ed.), Prentice Hall International Ltd, Herts (1990), pp. 235-239.

2. Cash T. & Pruzinsky T. (1990) *Integrative themes in body-image development deviance and change.* In: *Body Images Development, Deviance, and Change* (Cash T. & Pruzinsky T., eds), Guilford Press, London, Chapter 16, pp. 337-338.

3. Corner J., Cawley N. & Hildebrand S. (1995) *An evaluation of the use of massage and massage with the addition of essential oils on the well-being of cancer patients.* The Centre for Cancer and Palliative Care Studies, The Institute of Cancer Research, The Royal Marsden NHS Trust, London.

4. Coyler H. (1996) *Women's experience of living with breast cancer. Journal of Advanced Nursing* 23, 496-501.

5. Fallowfield L.J., Baum M. & Maguire P. (1986) *Effects of breast conservation on psychological morbidity associated with diagnosis of early breast cancer. British Medical Journal* 293, 1331-1334.

6. Fallowfield L.J. & Hall A. (1991) *Psychosocial and sexual impact of diagnosis and treatment of breast cancer. British Medical Bulletin* 47, 388-399.

7. Fallowfield L.J., Hall A., Maguire G.P. & Baum M. (1990) *Psychological outcomes of different treatment policies in women with early breast cancer outside a clinical trial. British Medical Journal* 301, 575-580.

8. Ferrell-Torry A. & Glick O. (1992) *The use of therapeutic massage as a nursing intervention to modify anxiety and the perception of pain. Cancer Nursing* 16, 93-101.

9. Foltz A. (1987) *The influence of cancer on self concept and life quality. Seminars in Oncology Nursing* 3, 303-312.

10. Guba E.G. & Lincoln Y.S. (1985) *Naturalistic Inquiry.* Sage, London.

11. Hopwood P. & Maguire G.P. (1988) *Body image problems in cancer patients. British Journal of Psychiatry* 153, 47-50.

12. Jamison K.R., Wellisch D.K. & Pasnau R.O. (1978) *Psychosocial aspects of mastectomy: I. The women's perspective. American Journal of Psychiatry* 135, 432-436.

13. Judd D. (1993) *Life-threatening illness a psychic trauma: psychotherapy with adolescent*

patients. In: *The Imaginative Body—Psychodynamic Therapy in Health Care* (Erskine A. & Judd D., eds), Whurr Publishers, London, pp. 87-112.

14. Kemeny M.M., Wellisch D. & Schain W. (1988) Psychosocial outcome in randomised surgical trial for treatment of primary breast cancer. *Cancer* 62, 1231-1237.

15. Krouse H. & Krouse J. (1982) Cancer as crisis: the critical elements of adjustment. *Nursing Research* 31, 96-101.

16. Mitchell A. (1995) Therapeutic relationship in health care: towards a model of the process of treatment. *Journal of Interprofessional Care* 9, 15-20.

17. Murphy R.F. (1987) The damaged self. In: *The Body Silent* (Murphy R.F. ed.), Dent and Sons Ltd, London, pp. 73-95.

18. Peters D., Bredin M., Daniel R. & Clover A. (1996) Clinical forum: breast cancer. *Complementary Therapies in Medicine* 4, 178-184.

19. Peters-Golden H. (1982) Breast cancer: varied perceptions of social support in the illness experience. *Social Science in Medicine* 16, 483-491.

20. Polivy J. (1977) Psychological effects of mastectomy on a woman's feminine self concept. *Journal of Nervous and Mental Disease* 164, 77-87.

21. Price B. (1990) Body Image Nursing Concepts and Care. Prentice Hall International Ltd, Herts, pp. 235-239.

22. Price B. (1994) The asthma experience: altered body image and non-compliance. *Journal of Clinical Nursing* 3, 139-145.

23. Pruzinsky T. (1990) Somatopsychic approaches to psychotherapy and personal growth. In: *Body Images Development, Deviance, and Change* (Cash T. & Pruzinsky T., eds), Guilford Press, London, pp. 296-315.

24. Schain W. (1986) Sexual functioning, self-esteem and cancer care. In: *Body-Image, Self-Esteem, and Sexuality in Cancer Patients* (Vaeth J.M., ed.), 2nd edn. Karger, Basel, pp. 15-23.

25. Schilder P. (1950) The Image and Appearance of the Human Body. International Universities Press, New York, p. 11.

26. Watson M., Denton S., Baum M. & Greer S. (1988) Counselling breast cancer patients: a specialist nurse service. *Counselling Psychology Quarterly* 1, 25-33.

27. Wilkinson S., Maguire P. & Tait A. (1988) Life after breast cancer. *Nursing Times* 84, 34-37.

28. Young M.I. (1992) The breasted experience: the look and the feeling. In: *The Body in Medical Thought and Practice* (Leder, D. ed.), Kluwer Academic Publishers, The Netherlands, pp. 215-230.

Critical Evaluation

- *Is the research question clearly articulated?*

Yes and no. The author primarily intends to explore the nature of three women's experience of breast cancer with a focus on body image issues. As part of this question, she also wants to explore whether massage, as a body-centered intervention, might be helpful as a means of helping the women adjust to a changed body image. These are two separate research questions and foci. The author has combined what could have been two separate yet related studies into a single one. We will want to read closely to see how successfully she manages to combine the two different questions.

- *What assumptions underlie the study; what qualitative approach forms its theoretical basis?*

This study is clearly relying upon assumptions common to the qualitative paradigm; the title tells us so. In terms of its theoretical basis, the study is based on phenomenology in that it explores the nature of the participants' experience of their changed bodies following the loss of a breast, and of the massage intervention. The term "experience" in the title of any study is often an indication that the study is qualitative and that a phenomenological approach is being used. This study cannot be considered a phenomenological study in the strict definition of that term, however, because it does not seek to understand and communicate to the reader the essence of the experience of altered body image in relation to mastectomy and massage therapy. We can say that it is a descriptive study, and that the author uses the technique of "thick description." Although the author's conclusions are certainly grounded in the data presented, no theory is developed.

- *What are the researcher's qualifications, experience, and perspective?*

Little information about the author's qualifications is presented. From the author information paragraph, the reader can determine that she is a nurse who works in a cancer research unit, and from the text, that she has some experience giving massage. It is not clear whether she has published other articles on this or on similar topics; no citations from previous studies authored by her are listed in the references. She does not appear to be endorsing any strong position about the use of massage for women struggling with an altered body image following mastectomy, presenting both the observed benefits and potential cautions based on the participants' statements.

- *What techniques and methods were used to ensure the integrity of the results as well as their accuracy?*

The author attempted to avoid bias by having an associate conduct the post intervention interviews so that participants would not feel the need to please her. Although interviews were taped and transcribed to ensure accuracy, the reader who is unfamiliar with the work of Lincoln & Guba is at a loss to understand exactly how the researcher proceeded in terms of the data analysis process. Triangulation of the data analysis, such as having more than one person reading, sorting, and coding the interviews to identify common themes in the women's experiences, would increase the accuracy and verifiability of the results. Jane's experience could be considered a lucky negative case – the study design did not allow the author to deliberately seek out someone who might have had a poor or unpleasant experience with massage.

- *Are the methods used in data collection and analysis described in sufficient detail?*

The description of the study methodology is somewhat vague. Lincoln and Guba are well-known qualitative methodologists, and the reference to their work in the text is to a popular textbook, a handbook of general qualitative research methods. More detailed information is necessary for us to determine just how the data were analyzed. Purposeful sampling was employed, by asking oncologists and nurses to identify patients who appeared to be having difficulty adjusting to the loss of a breast and who could acknowledge this verbally. Other inclusion/exclusion criteria were set as well, although no rationale for their use is given.

- *Given the theoretical model and the purpose of the study, are the methods used appropriate?*

This is a difficult question to answer. Certainly, this can be considered a small sample even for a qualitative study. A somewhat larger sample size with more features such as triangulation in the data analysis and a more highly defined theoretical approach such as grounded theory might have increased the applicability of the findings. Sampling to the point of redundancy, that is, continuing to identify and interview participants until no new information is forthcoming, would also have increased the study's credibility.

One way to view this study is to look at it as a pilot study, with its stated purpose of exploring the participants' experience and the usefulness of massage therapy as an intervention. The author justifies her sample size in terms of the limited resource of time, since she is providing the massage intervention. We can infer that money is also a limited resource, or else the sample size could have been increased by hiring another therapist to provide massage. Another question is raised by the massage intervention itself; it is described in very general terms, and given that there were only three participants, it is surprising that more detailed information about the sessions for each participant is not provided. Nor is the duration of the individual sessions. The two different research questions addressed require different approaches, and a mixed methods study with a slightly larger sample size might have provided more useful results.

- *Are the results credible?*

Within the previously stated limitations (and there are several), yes. The author has explored the research question, not quite as fully as we might have liked, but as well as possible under the practical limitations she faced. Certainly, the topic of body image in breast cancer is quite clinically relevant and the results of this study are meaningful, if only to raise awareness and sensitivity to these issues among other care providers. Not every woman who has undergone a mastectomy will have difficulty with adjusting to a changed body image, but most do, for some period of time and to varying degrees. Older women have often experienced particularly difficult surgeries and treatment protocols without the benefit of the public awareness and support systems available to breast cancer survivors now. The study also provides some suggestions for additional ways to help patients dealing with these concerns. A practitioner unfamiliar with the potential body image issues faced by many women with breast cancer would likely find this study helpful as background information.

- *Do the results justify the conclusions?*

Yes, again within the stated limitations of the study. This study could be a good source of pilot data for the development of a larger scale study exploring the same issue, or for a study evaluating the usefulness of massage in addressing body image distress. In general, the author's interpretation of the study findings seems well supported by the data she has presented, and she also discusses the study's limitations. While it is not the highest-quality example of a phenomenologically-based study, it does have some clinical utility.

One of the strengths of qualitative research is its reporting of raw data in the form of direct quotes from interviews. In this case, it may appear to some readers that there is a disparity between Jane's comments about her emotional response and the author's remarks about whether she may have been harmed. While the caution regarding the potential for massage to bring up difficult emotions prematurely is well taken, in Jane's case this seems a bit patronizing, based both on Jane's choice to continue the treatments even though she could have stopped, and on her comment that, "I think it was important to do it really. I've certainly felt better since."

- *Are the results applicable to other settings?*

The author states clearly that the results are not intended to be generalized. However, one can argue that this is a rich and useful study with a detailed description of clients' experience, both of having had a mastectomy and of receiving subsequent massage. The study provides a conceptual generalization that opens a window to different perspectives, and is grounded in patients' own words.

- *Are the results clinically meaningful?*

The practitioner working with women who have had mastectomies would find valuable information in the study, both in understanding possible issues such clients may face, and in inferring ways that massage therapists may choose to interact with and work with them. It is a clinically meaningful study in terms of showing how massage therapy can affect recipients who are struggling with difficult physiological and psychosocial issues on multiple levels.

Study Example #2: Massage During Chemotherapy

The Experience of Massage During Chemotherapy Treatment in Breast Cancer Patients

Annika Billhult, Elisabet Stener-Victorin, Ingegerd Bergbom The Sahlgrenska Academy at Göteborg University, Göteborg, Sweden

Clinical Nursing Research, Vol. 16, No. 2, 85-99 (2007)
DOI: 10.1177/1054773806298488 © 2007 SAGE Publications

This study aimed to describe the experience of massage for breast cancer patients during chemotherapy treatment. Ten patients received massage at five occasions. They were interviewed and analysis was conducted using Giorgi's ideas of phenomenological research. The essential meaning of getting massage during chemotherapy was described as a retreat from the feeling of uneasiness toward chemotherapy. Results revealed five themes: the patients experienced distraction from the frightening experience, a turn from negative to positive, a sense of relaxation, a confirmation of caring, and finally they just felt good. In conclusion, the findings of this study show that massage offered a retreat from uneasy, unwanted, negative feelings connected with chemotherapy treatment. It is a treatment that can be added to the arsenal of treatment choices available to the oncological staff.

Keywords: *breast carcinoma; chemotherapy; experience; massage therapy*

Breast cancer is the most common cancer form in females, affecting about 6,500 women yearly in Sweden (Socialstyrelsen, 2006). Not only do women need to face the worries of a serious illness but also they must go through tough treatment. Treatment options available for breast cancer are surgery, chemotherapy, radiation, and hormonal therapy. These treatments often entail numerous troublesome side effects, such as pain, nausea, weakness, and fatigue (Foltz, Gaines, & Gullatte, 1996; Hickok et al., 1999). Patients continue to experience discomfort despite pharmacological treatment.

Many patients, therefore, seek nonpharmacological treatments to complement mainstream care (Henderson & Donatelle, 2004; Lengacher, Bennett, Kipp, Berarducci, & Cox, 2003). Massage is a form of complementary therapy that has existed for 3,000 years. Historically, massage has been used worldwide in many cultures with their unique forms for various types of medical applications, health and fitness, as well as for spiritual development (Tappan, 1998). Traditionally, massage has not been widespread in the field of oncology. Therefore, in the current study, patient experience of massage during chemotherapy was of interest.

There are many massage techniques, such as petrissage, effleurage, hacking, friction, and kneading (Vickers & Zollman, 1999). Before the current study started, various massage techniques were voluntarily tested on patients with cancer. Techniques, such as effleurage and petrissage, and combinations of these techniques were tested; however, according to patients' experience and opinions, they preferred effleurage. Effleurage was therefore the technique used in the current study.

Problem

The Effect of Massage

Gate control theory (GCT) is often used to explain the pain relief of massage (Melzack & Wall, 1965). It is based on the theory that activation of large diameter afferents, A beta fibres, activate interneuron that via the release of gamma-amino butyric acid (GABA) inhibits pain transmission via small diameter, A delta and C fibres, in the spinal cord. Based on this theory, the central nervous system is not a passive receiver of pain stimuli but can modulate incoming information. Tactile stimuli can, according to this theory, be pain reducing by inhibiting nociception and, therefore, pain. Furthermore, massage has been shown to boost serotonin concentrations associated with mood enhancement (Hernandez-Reif et al., 2004).

Earlier Research

Massage has previously been shown to relieve pain; reduce depression, suffering, anxiety; and lower blood pressure in patients with cancer (Ferrell-Torry & Glick, 1993; Grealish, Lomasney, & Whiteman, 2000; Hernandez-Reif et al., 2000; Smith, Kemp, Hemphill, & Vojir, 2002; Soden, Vincent, Craske, Lucas, & Ashley, 2004; Weinrich & Weinrich, 1990; Wilkie et al., 2000; Wilkinson, Aldridge, Salmon, Cain, & Wilson, 1999). Furthermore, massage relieves nausea in patients with cancer (Grealish et al., 2000). In addition, one study examined the effect of massage on immune function in breast cancer patients. Hernandez-Reif et al. (2004) tested immune function in a randomized controlled study where 27 women were allocated either to massage (n = 15) or a control consisting solely of standard medical care. Results revealed an increase in natural killer (NK) cell number and lymphocytes. Hernandez-Reif et al. also investigated the effect of massage therapy compared to progressive muscle relaxation. The massage therapy group showed increased levels of dopamine, NK cells, and lymphocytes (Hernandez-Reif et al., 2005).

Qualitative Studies

The effects of massage are usually studied through blood pressure, pain, and nausea (Grealish et al., 2000; Hernandez-Reif et al., 2000; Weinrich & Weinrich, 1990). Only a few studies of cancer patients' experience of massage were found. One study (Billhult & Dahlberg, 2001) described patient experience of massage integrated into daily care at an oncology unit. The results revealed the essential meaning of receiving massage as getting meaningful relief from suffering. Five themes were identified: an experience of being special, a positive development with the personnel, a sense of feeling strong, a balance between autonomy and dependence, and just feeling good. Corner, Cawley, and Hildebrand (1995) reported positive effects of massage such as relaxation, release of tension and stiffness, and pain relief in a quasi-experimental study of 52 patients with cancer.

As to our knowledge no qualitative studies have been published concerning massage during chemotherapy treatment for patients with breast cancer. With the current study, we wanted to discover additional dimensions of experiences of massage during a treatment that is often experienced as uncomfortable. In this way the current study complements earlier studies of massage.

Purpose

The objective of the current study was to describe the experience of massage in patients with breast cancer during chemotherapy treatment.

Design

Phenomena and human experience are central to phenomenological research. The current study focused on the meaning of massage for patients with breast cancer during chemotherapy, therefore phenomenology was chosen as the methodological and epistemological framework.

Phenomenology

Qualitative research is the most appropriate method to study experience. Phenomenology is the bedrock of most qualitative research (Porter, 1996). The aim of phenomenology is to understand the essential structure of a phenomenon under investigation. It is a method where human experience as it is lived is in focus, along with meaning and intersubjectivity (Merleau-Ponty, 1964).

Phenomenology is grounded on Husserl's philosophical ideas. Husserl meant that the way to access the material world was through consciousness. His method entails intentionality, phenomenological reduction, description, and essence (Baker, Wuest, & Stern, 1992). Intentionality means that the mind consciously directs its attention toward a phenomenon (Holloway & Wheeler, 1996). To focus on the phenomena under investigation, one needs to put aside prejudices of the world, or preunderstanding. This is also called bracketing or phenomenological reduction *and is central to phenomenological work (Giorgi, 2005). One also needs to be open, near but also distant, aware of the unique, and open to meaning to retrieve rich interviews suitable for phenomenological analysis.In this way, the phenomena can be described and their essential structure or essence can be revealed. Researchers have taken Husserl's ideas forming research methods inspired by phenomenological philosophy. Colaizzi (1978), Van Kaam (1969), and Giorgi (1985), for example, developed methods suitable for caring science research.*

Sample

Ten patients were recruited from an oncology clinic in a county hospital in southwestern Sweden. They were scheduled for chemotherapy every third week for a total of seven sessions. Inclusion criteria for the study were (a) diagnosed breast cancer, (b) female gender, (c) scheduled for chemotherapy treatment, and (d) available to participate in the study with their physician's approval. Mean age was 50 years, ranging from 34 to 63 years. Average time from diagnosis to interview was 5 months ranging from 4 to 6 months. All had nonrecurrent breast cancer at the time of the interviews. Furthermore, one patient was diagnosed with Stage 1, five patients with Stage 2A, three patients with Stage 2B, and one patient with Stage 3A according to the tumour, nodes, metastasis (TNM)-classification (Sobin & Wittekind, 2002). The patients' occupations varied and were, for example, accountant, nurse, and information technology technician. Nine of the patients had a lumpectomy and one had a mastectomy in combination with axillary node dissection.

Method

The patients received a letter of information on the current study at the second chemotherapy session. A week later, they received a phone call concerning participation in the current study. After accepting the current study conditions, patients received massage during five of the seven chemotherapy sessions. A total of 10 patients were asked to participate; all 10 accepted.

The massage technique, that is, effleurage, was given by five hospital staffers. The staffers received one day of instruction in the effleurage technique by the first author, and in addition, they had vast previous experience and competence in massaging cancer patients. The massage took place at the chemotherapy ward during chemotherapy infusion. The massage consisted of soft strokes, so-called effleurage, and lasted 20 to 30 minutes. The patients were able to choose between foot and/or lower leg or hand and/or lower arm massage. There was no difference in duration between the two. A cold-pressed vegetable oil was used to reduce friction. The limb was then wrapped in a towel immediately following massage.

Patients were given five massage treatments based on the estimate that five treatments would be sufficient to tell about the experience of the massage. Patients were interviewed by the researcher (AB) after the last massage session so that they could tell about their experience of all five treatments together, as opposed to the experience of single massage treatments. Therefore, one interview was chosen and assessed to provide information rich enough for analysis. Interviews took place in the chemotherapy ward during ongoing infusion lasting about 1 hr. The researcher (AB) began by asking patients: "Please tell me about your experience of the massage." Follow-up questions such as "Could you tell me more about that?" were asked to gain understanding of the patient's experience of the massage. To better focus on the phenomena, the researcher strived to maintain an open mind, thereby setting all prior understanding of the phenomena aside during data collection (bracketing). To achieve openness, the researcher strived to maintain intimacy but also to keep a distance to establish a comfortable level of involvement. The idea of openness requires immediacy to prevent missing important information from informants. With this in mind, the researcher could better illuminate the target phenomenon which, in this case, was the experience of massage for breast cancer patients during chemotherapy. The interviews were carried out, audiotaped, and transcribed by the first author. The study was reviewed and approved by The Research Ethics Committee of the University (no. Ö 666-01).

Data Analysis

The analysis was conducted using the ideas of Giorgi (2000), meaning that the researcher was descriptive, worked within the phenomenological reduction, and, using free imaginative variation, searched for individuated meanings and then the most invariant or essential meaning (Giorgi, 1997). The naïve description of the interviews was analyzed in three steps: whole-parts-whole. The text was first read several times in its entirety to become acquainted with the narratives and the data as a whole. It was then broken down into units, revealing similarities and differences, thus forming a pattern of categories. These categories or units were scrutinized for meaning and transformed into scientific language. As patterns emerged, Phase 3 began. The researcher then returned to the whole and synthesized the insights into an essence. The essence is thus the unvarying core of the phenomenon, forming the general structure.

Findings

The essence of receiving massage during chemotherapy can be described as a retreat from the feeling of uneasiness toward chemotherapy. Chemotherapy treatment is often connected with hair loss, nausea, fatigue, and general ill being. This creates a feeling of uneasiness despite modern side effect treatments. The patients in the current study have to face not only troublesome side effects but also troublesome thoughts of having a life-threatening disease. Because chemotherapy was not optional to the patients, the retreat from the feeling of uneasiness became very valuable. Patients were offered a means to ease their feelings about the treatment, that is, the massage could balance that with something optional and good. The patients' experiences of receiving massage is described as a distraction from the frightening experience, a turn from negative to positive, a sense of relaxation, a confirmation of caring, and finally to just feel good.

A Distraction from the Frightening Experience

Massage during chemotherapy was a retreat because the patients perceived the experience of chemotherapy as frightening. It was an experience that brought about a feeling of something that was new and unknown and something that was good to get away from for a while. In addition to the treatment being unknown, the patients connected chemotherapy with something unpleasant and repulsive. The massage offered a distraction from the worries and the frightening experience. Thoughts were expressed as follows:

> *[Can you describe what it feels like?] Yes, otherwise I have my focus on these medicines that must go inside my body, I think that it is unpleasant. During the massage though I don't think about that...It [the treatment] becomes less repulsive.*

> *I think about the future, how I am going to feel after the treatment, but then I think, oh, I am going to get massage. Then I get calm and relaxed going up the stairs.*

> *[What were your thoughts when you were given (the massage) for the first time?] I thought it felt good to be distracted from the other stuff that was going on [chemotherapy].*

> *I think it feels very good when she comes to give massage because I get away from this a little bit. I would rather not look at these bottles [the bottles with chemotherapy].*

> *Before she [the massage person] came, and the infusion started I felt sick. I don't know if it was the infusion or if I just knew I was going to get sick but it disappeared when she started the massage...it [the sick feeling] sort of fades away during the massage.*

> *It [the massage] is a little luxury in the middle of disaster...it makes you relax and it is not only frightening to come here and that has been important to me.*

> *The surroundings at the chemotherapy ward were not perceived as soothing. The massage created an opportunity to escape from the surroundings...it feels good to get away from this environment a while.*

> *I think that it [the massage] is calming...it feels safe and I think it is good to get away from this environment.*

A Turn From Negative to Positive

Despite the fact that modern anti-emetics have been taken into use, patients still experience discomfort during chemotherapy. Patients felt that this negative association of treatment could be counteracted with massage. Massage during chemotherapy was a retreat because the patients perceived the massage as something to look forward to, and that balanced negative feelings of chemotherapy with positive feelings of massage. They expressed this as follows:

> *It has had a positive effect on me because I knew that I was going to get massage as opposed to when I didn't get it...I have looked forward to this [the massage]. [What does it mean to get this positive effect?] Well chemotherapy is connected with misery, but now I can get something positive too.*

> *[Is there anything else you feel in your body?] I feel calm and it is important...I come here thinking that I am going to be sick...but the massage makes it positive, so I can come here and get massage and then it [the chemotherapy] is not so scary.*

> *[Is there anything that has been particularly important to you?] I have said that when I am coming here, I am going to get massage with chemotherapy. I have said it in that way, because I have a positive experience and then I mention it [the massage] first.*

A Sense of Relaxation

Furthermore, the massage was a retreat because the patients experienced relaxation as a contrast to the inner tense feeling associated with chemotherapy treatment. The serious situation of the patients in the current study meant that they were under a great deal of stress and tension. A chance to get relaxation meant a chance to get a retreat from the uneasiness of treatment. Some examples are as follows:

> *[Please tell me how you have experienced the massage.] Well in the beginning I was tense. I didn't know what to expect, I have been very tense every time and I have been afraid of the chemotherapy. She [the massage person] felt that. But I have relaxed and feel calmer.*

> *I feel like I really relax when she starts to massage.*

> *I know that she is coming and I feel that I can relax, that I don't get so tense.*

> *When you feel the massage you start to relax and concentrate on relaxing, it feels good.*

A Confirmation of Caring

To be a patient means that you become dependent on the care of the hospital staff. In addition, the body has changed depending on the operation and treatment given. Hair loss, weight gain or loss, in combination with fatigue and nausea, can alter body image. The massage was experienced as a retreat because it counteracted the feeling of being "sick and ugly." To be confirmed and feel important was experienced very strongly because patients felt unworthy of being touched because of appearance and illness.

> *Sometimes I feel lonely with this disease and when I get massage it feels like my well-being is very important. [How does that feel?] Nice...I feel mutilated and you know, no hair. I feel like here, you dare to touch me, but the others [family members] are afraid to touch and be near me.*

> *I think it is that the person massaging does not reflect upon it as being weird. She gives me massage regardless if I am as I was before or as I am now.*

> *Well, it feels like caring, you get cared for a little more [when being massaged], which feels positive.*

> *A feeling of well-being...the massage makes you feel like someone cares.*

> *What I feel is that I really get confirmed when someone touches me...I really get taken seriously because they even want to touch me, you know. I feel ugly with no eyebrows or eyelashes. Someone wants to touch me, even though right now, I feel really ugly...touching me, with no conditions.*

To Just Feel Good

Finally, the massage was a retreat from the feeling of uneasiness because it just felt good. Getting massage during chemotherapy meant that patients were able to enjoy something they perceived as a luxury, something that was normal in their serious situation.

> *[How does feel in the body?] It is a feeling of well-being; it is a feeling that you feel good...*

> *[How does it feel?] It feels good; I think it just feels good to be massaged.*

> *Nice, it feels good because I am, I am kind of tense before treatment...I don't really know how to explain it, it just feels good when she starts. Well-being.*

Discussion

The current study was carried out using a phenomenological method. As researcher and patients are subjective beings, one needs to proceed with caution, adhering to the intention of phenomenology as far as possible. It must be the researcher's full intention to give an accurate description of the phenomenon. As bracketing is central to this method, it is a target for critique. By being aware of one's past knowledge, it is necessary to adopt as open a mind as possible to avoid missing aspects of the phenomenon. The researcher can also utilize Husserl's idea of free imaginative variation. By doing this, the researcher seeks the most invariant structure of the phenomenon by envisioning variation of the characteristics of the phenomenon, thereby confirming the general structure or essence (Beck, 1994).

Furthermore, the analysis of the current study was not confirmed with participants. However, Giorgi (1989) does not encourage validation of findings using participants as evaluators. The participants have described experiences of everyday life, whereas the researcher seeks the meaning of everyday experience.

Furthermore, all the patients in the current study expressed positive feelings about the massage. They had the opportunity to express negative thoughts but did not. One explanation for this may be that all patients in the current study accepted to participate and had not done so if they did not like being massaged, or were hesitant due to, for example, concern about stimulating recurrence.

It is important to emphasize that it was not intended to investigate the effect of massage on specific symptoms or side effects of chemotherapy. The focus was primarily on the experience of massage during a treatment situation such as chemotherapy.

The current study showed that massage during chemotherapy could give the patient a retreat from the feeling of uneasiness toward chemotherapy. Chemotherapy is often not optional to the patient, and although it has been used for a long time, the numerous side effects have not always been successfully treated. Not knowing how treatment affects the body can make the experience frightening and threatening. The patients thought that the massage gave a moment of relief from this new and unknown experience.

The patients experienced a distraction from the frightening experience, a turn from negative to positive, a sense of relaxation, a confirmation of caring, and finally they just felt good.

Distraction From the Frightening Experience

Massage provided distraction from chemotherapy not only because it was perceived as safe and calm but also because attention was taken away from the very visible physical attributes of chemotherapy bottles. Chemotherapy treatment and the effects were for many of the patients unknown, generating a frightening feeling. The massage could then distract the patients with something known and familiar. Massage offered patients an opportunity to retreat within themselves.

This finding is supported by another study (Vasterling, Jenkins, Tope, & Burish, 1993) where the effect of distraction was investigated on anticipatory nausea due to chemotherapy treatment.

A Turn From Negative to Positive

With the help of massage, a thought process different from that of just receiving chemotherapy was initiated. This meant that at the following chemotherapy treatment, negative feelings of chemotherapy were replaced by positive ones, through thoughts of massage. A positive feeling took over, thus easing treatment.

To Be Relaxed

Chemotherapy made patients tense whereas massage relaxed them. This may seem unimportant; however, given the high tension level of the patient, relaxation became even more important. This is consistent with a randomized controlled trial by Wilkie et al. (2000). In this study conducted in a hospice setting, massage gave patients immediate relaxation when measured by pulse and respiratory rate. Another study confirmed the same results investigating the effect of foot massage on relaxation in patients with cancer (Grealish et al., 2000).

A Confirmation of Caring

Treatment for breast cancer transforms the body. Surgery leaves the body permanently changed, and chemotherapy drastically alters appearance with considerable hair loss. This leaves patients with a feeling of despair, a feeling of being "ugly." They felt that unconditional caring and touching made them feel important and "deserving," despite their altered body image. This is consistent with a pilot study investigating breast cancer patients' experience of massage in relation to body image (Bredin, 1999). One woman in the current study reported that massage helped her when her body felt repulsive. Another study by Corner et al. (1995) confirmed these findings. Cancer patients received massage and reported feelings of security and acceptance.

To Just Feel Good

Nausea is the most common side effect of chemotherapy (Foltz et al.,1996). Despite this, nausea was not a main issue for patients in the current study. One explanation is that massage decreased nausea by providing positive feelings overpowering nausea. Another explanation is that patients were adequately treated pharmacologically for nausea. This enabled patients to just feel good. This finding was also evident in another study by Billhult and Dahlberg (2001), where patients in an oncology unit received massage in their daily care.

Retreat and Well-Being

The essence of massage during chemotherapy could be described as a retreat from feeling uneasiness toward chemotherapy. This meant experiencing a sense of well-being despite a troublesome situation. Perhaps massage contributed to making the chemotherapy experience more tolerable by balancing the feeling of uneasiness with something positive.

Application

It is clear that chemotherapy is distressful for patients. They experience fear and tension, in addition to the physical side effects of breast cancer treatment, which is necessary for their survival. We wanted to illuminate the experience of massage when given at the same time as a troublesome treatment such as chemotherapy. The current study showed that massage offered a retreat from these uneasy, unwanted, negative feelings. It is a treatment that can be added to the arsenal of treatment choices available to the oncological staff.

It is important to note that massage can be offered to those patients benefiting from it, within a short time. Based on the descriptions of the patients, their experience of massage could balance the uneasy feeling study could be generalized to similar situations concerning unwanted treatment other than chemotherapy treatment. However, we cannot be certain that the results can be applied to all caring situations.

Meta-analyses and further research are needed to explore the effects of massage and cultural differences in relation to massage for patients with cancer. As the patient with cancer encounters new care situations, the need for complementary treatments may be altered. Research is therefore needed in other contexts of care to broaden the knowledge of the utility of massage for patients with cancer.

References

1. Baker, C., Wuest, J., & Stern, P. N. (1992). Method slurring: The grounded theory /phenomenology example. *Journal of Advanced Nursing, 17, 1355-1360.*

2. Beck, C. T. (1994). Reliability and validity issues in phenomenological research. *Western Journal of Nursing Research, 16, 254-262.*

3. Billhult, A., & Dahlberg, K. (2001). A meaningful relief from suffering experiences of massage in cancer care. *Cancer Nursing, 24, 180-184.*

4. Bredin, M. (1999). Mastectomy, body image and therapeutic massage: A qualitative study of women's experience. *Journal of Advanced Nursing, 29, 1113-1120.*

5. Colaizzi, P. (1978). Psychological research as the phenomenologist views it. In R. Valle & M. King (Eds.), *Existential-phenomenological alternatives for psychology* (pp. 48-71). New York: Oxford University Press.

6. Corner, J., Cawley, N., & Hildebrand, S. (1995). An evaluation of the use of massage and essential oils on the wellbeing of cancer patients. *International Journal of Palliative Nursing, 1, 67-73.*

7. Ferrell-Torry, A. T., & Glick, O. J. (1993). The use of therapeutic massage as a nursing intervention to modify anxiety and the perception of cancer pain. *Cancer Nursing, 16, 93-101.*

8. Foltz, A. T., Gaines, G., & Gullatte, M. (1996). Recalled side effects and self-care actions of patients receiving inpatient chemotherapy. Oncology Nursing Forum, 23, 679-683.

9. Giorgi, A. (1985). Phenomenology and psychological research. Pittsburgh, PA: Duquesne University Press.

10. Giorgi, A. (1989). Some theoretical and practical issues regarding the psychological and phenomenological method. Saybrook Review, 7, 71-85.

11. Giorgi, A. (1997). The theory, practise, and evaluation of the phenomenological method as a qualitative research procedure. Journal of Phenomenological Psychology, 28, 235-260.

12. Giorgi, A. (2000). The status of Husserlian phenomenology in caring research. Scandinavian Journal of Caring Sciences, 14, 3-10.

13. Giorgi, A. (2005). The phenomenological movement and research in the human sciences. Nursing Science Quarterly, 18, 75-82.

14. Grealish, L., Lomasney, A., & Whiteman, B. (2000). Foot massage. A nursing intervention to modify the distressing symptoms of pain and nausea in patients hospitalized with cancer. Cancer Nursing, 23, 237-243.

15 Henderson, J. W., & Donatelle, R. J. (2004). Complementary and alternative medicine use by women after completion of allopathic treatment for breast cancer. Alternative Therapies in Health and Medicine, 10, 52-57.

16. Hernandez-Reif, M., Field, T., Ironson, G., Beutler, J., Vera, Y., Hurley, J., et al. (2005). Natural killer cells and lymphocytes increase in women with breast cancer following massage therapy. International Journal of Neuroscience, 115, 495-510.

17. Hernandez-Reif, M., Field, T., Krasnegor, J., Theakston, H., Hossain, Z., & Burman, I. (2000). High blood pressure and associated symptoms were reduced by massage therapy. Journal of Bodywork and Movement Therapies, 4, 31-38.

18. Hernandez-Reif, M., Ironson, G., Field, T., Hurley, J., Katz, G., Diego, M., et al. (2004). Breast cancer patients have improved immune and neuroendocrine functions following massage therapy. Journal of Psychosomatic Research, 57, 45-52.

19. Hickok, J. T., Roscoe, J. A., Morrow, G. R., Stern, R. M., Yang, B., Flynn, P. I., et al. (1999). Use of 5-HT3 receptor antagonists to prevent nausea and emesis caused by chemotherapy for patients with breast carcinoma in community practice settings. Cancer, 86, 64-71.

20. Holloway, I., & Wheeler, S. (1996). Qualitative research for nurses. Oxford, UK: Blackwell Science.

21. Lengacher, C. A., Bennett, M. P., Kipp, K. E., Berarducci, A., & Cox, C. E. (2003). Design and testing of the use of a complementary and alternative therapies survey in women with breast cancer. Oncology Nursing Forum, 30, 811-821.

22. Melzack, R., & Wall, P. D. (1965). Pain mechanisms: A new theory. Science, 150, 971-979.

23. Merleau-Ponty, M. (1964). The primacy of perception. Evanston, IL: Northwestern University Press.

24. Porter, S. (1996). Qualitative research. In D. F. S. Cormack (Ed.), The research process in nursing (pp. 113-122). Oxford, UK: Blackwell Science.

25. Smith, M. C., Kemp, J., Hemphill, L., & Vojir, C. P. (2002). Outcomes of therapeutic massage for hospitalized cancer patients. Journal of Nursing Scholarship, 34, 257-262.

26. Sobin, C. W., & Wittekind, C. (2002). Breast cancer. In TNM classification of malignant tumours – International Union Against Cancer (UICC) (6th ed., pp. 131-141). New York: Wiley-Liss.

27. Socialstyrelsen [National Board of Health and Welfare]. (2006). Cancer incidence in Sweden, 2004. Stockholm: Statistics – Health and Diseases. Retrieved May 12, 2006, from www.socialstyrelsen.se/Statistik/statistik_amne/Cancer

28. Soden, K., Vincent, K., Craske, S., Lucas, C., & Ashley, S. (2004). A randomized controlled trial of aromatherapy massage in a hospice setting. Palliative Medicine, 18, 87-92.

29. Tappan, F. (1998). Healing massage techniques. Norwalk, CT: Appleton and Lange.

30. Van Kaam, A. (1969). Existential foundations of psychology. New York: Doubleday.

31. Vasterling, J., Jenkins, R. A., Tope, D. M., & Burish, T. G. (1993). Cognitive distraction and relaxation training for the control of side effects due to cancer chemotherapy. Journal of Behavioral Medicine, 16, 65-80.

32. Vickers, A., & Zollman, C. (1999). ABC of complementary medicine. Massage therapies. British Medical Journal / British Medical Association, 319, 1254-1257.

33. Weinrich, S. P., & Weinrich, M. C. (1990). The effect of massage on pain in cancer patients.Applied Nursing Research, 3, 140-145.

34. Wilkie, D. J., Kampbell, J., Cutshall, S., Halabisky, H., Harmon, H., Johnson, L. P., et al. (2000). Effects of massage on pain intensity, analgesics and quality of life in patients with cancer pain: A pilot study of a randomized clinical trial conducted within hospice care delivery. Hospice Journal, 15, 31-53.

35. Wilkinson, S., Aldridge, J., Salmon, I., Cain, E., & Wilson, B. (1999). An evaluation of aromatherapy massage in palliative care. Palliative Medicine, 13, 409-417.

Annika Billhult is a physical therapist and doctoral student at the Department of Physiotherapy, Institute of Neuroscience and Physiology, Sahlgrenska Academy, Göteborg University, Sweden.

Elisabet Stener-Victorin is an associate professor in neuroendocrinology at Sahlgrenska Academy, Göteborg University in Sweden, and is appointed as full-time researcher and assistant head of the

Department of Physiology at the Institute of Neuroscience and Physiology, Department of Physiology, Sahlgrenska Academy, Göteborg University, Sweden. Her research involves both clinical and experimental studies evaluating the effect of sensory stimulation in pain and disease. Ingegerd Bergbom is a professor at the Institute of Health and Caring Sciences at Sahlgrenska Academy, Göteborg University, Sweden. She is a registered nurse, nurse teacher, and holds a PhD in nursing. Her research is mainly within intensive care and focuses on patients' experiences and memories, and the impact of high tech environment on nursing care from patients', relatives', and nurses' perspectives.

Critical Evaluation

- *Is the research question clearly articulated?*

Yes. The authors state the research question quite clearly in both the study abstract and in the section labeled "Purpose" in the body of the article.

- *What assumptions underlie the study; what qualitative approach forms its theoretical basis?*

Certainly this is a qualitative study, although some quantitative information is contained in the description of the study participants. It is clear from both the title and the abstract that phenomenology is the qualitative approach employed by the authors.

- *What are the qualifications, experience, and perspective of the researcher(s)?*

From looking at the institutional affiliations of all the authors, we can tell that the study was conducted in Sweden. From the author information listed at the end of the paper, and from research cited in the review of the literature contained in the section labeled "Earlier Research," we know that the lead author is a physical therapist and doctoral student who has been involved in at least one other prior study employing qualitative methods in a similar population. The second author is a neuroendocrinologist with prior research experience in sensory stimulation that probably involved both animal and human studies. The third author appears to be a PhD-prepared professor of nursing with previous experience in qualitative research. Taken altogether, this team appears well-qualified and experienced regarding the qualitative approach. From the authors' statements in the text discussing the use of "bracketing" to put aside preconceived ideas, and what it means for the researcher to be "open" and "near but also distant," we can also infer that they intend to take a balanced and unprejudiced perspective.

- *What techniques and methods were used to ensure the integrity of the results as well as their accuracy and verifiability?*

Participants with varying stages of breast cancer were identified and recruited based on stated inclusion criteria. During their chemotherapy sessions in the hospital infusion center they received five massages from different providers with experience in oncology massage, after which they were interviewed by the lead author using open-ended questions and follow-up prompts. These were included in the description of the study methods. All 10 hour-long interviews were audiotaped and transcribed by the same author.

- *Are the methods used in data collection and analysis described in sufficient detail?*

Yes. There is a helpful description of the phenomenological approach for readers who may be unfamiliar with qualitative research methods. Contrast this description with that provided in the methods section of the previous study. The participants and setting for the interviews are described with some degree of detail. The intervention is described in sufficient detail for replication.

The method of data analysis is also described, although whether the analysis was performed with the aid of computer software is not stated. Given the sample size of 10, it is quite feasible that the lead author who performed the analysis used the traditional method of reading and marking text by hand.

- *Given the theoretical approach and the purpose of the study, are the methods used appropriate?*

It appears so. Phenomenology is certainly the most appropriate qualitative approach to meet the study's stated objective, and the authors have taken some pains to explain their rationale for the choices they made in employing the methods used, which are described in some detail.

- *Are the results credible?*

The quotations from the participants certainly support the authors' interpretation of the themes synthesized from the responses to the open-ended interview questions. It is easy to see the repetition of key words and concepts in the participants' own statements.

- *Do the results justify the conclusions?*

Yes, the results certainly support the authors' conclusions. However, the authors do not address any limitations in the study design or improvements that could be made for future studies. A potential limitation of many qualitative studies that should be considered in relation to the research question is that they require participants who are knowledgeable and articulate in order for the researcher to collect useful data. Based on the description of the study participants, they appear to be quite well-educated, which is common in phenomenological studies. On the other hand, the phenomenological approach does attempt to distill universal attributes of a particular experience. Sampling to redundancy and seeking out additional participants with more varied backgrounds would certainly increase the rigor of the study, as would the use of triangulation in the data analysis.

- *Are the results applicable to other settings?*

This question is addressed directly by the authors, who suggest that the results are applicable to other patients who are receiving chemotherapy, and that the potential of massage therapy to provide a positive contrasting experience during negatively perceived medical treatments needs to be explored. This exploration in turn may offer new contexts in which massage can be effectively used in oncology care.

- *Are the results clinically meaningful?*

Most definitely. The authors make a compelling case through describing in the patients' own words the distress they experience as they undergo chemotherapy, and the benefits that massage offers in ameliorating that distress. In addition, they note that massage therapy is a relatively simple intervention that can be easily and quickly implemented. Overall, the study is a good example of a credible phenomenological study, and it stands in some contrast in terms of its methods and procedures to the previous example in this chapter.

Mixed Methods: Combining Quantitative and Qualitative Methods

As we have noted previously, qualitative and quantitative research methods have different viewpoints and assumptions, approaches to data collection and analysis, and perspectives on the nature of reality. Yet they can be complementary in that the strengths of each methodology generally compensate for the weaknesses of the other. It would seem like common sense to combine both within a single study to gain a more complete picture of the research question under investigation and increase its rigor. It is surprising that the use of mixed methods is such a relatively recent development in health care research, and that guidelines for researchers employing this approach are still evolving. A PubMed search conducted on May 24, 2008 using the search term "mixed quantitative and qualitative methods" with the exclusion "not biological not chemical" yielded only 311 articles. Of those, 181, or slightly more than half (58%), were published since 2005, with the earliest study published in 1991.[5]

In the next example we examine a study using a mixed methods approach. No specific protocol is presented; however, concepts used in evaluating both kinds of research methodologies are considered in the critique that follows, so keep in mind what you have learned thus far about weighing the evidence presented in both quantitative and qualitative journal articles. Remember that no matter what methodological approach is used, the key issue is whether the study design, methods, and procedures suggest a plausible alternate explanation for the results, and whether the author's conclusions are supported by the results presented.

Study Example #3: Body-Oriented Therapy and Child Sexual Abuse

Body-Oriented Therapy in Recovery from Child Sexual Abuse: An Efficacy Study

Cynthia Price, PhD
Alternative Therapies in Health and Medicine. 2005;11(5):46–57.

Context: There has been little research on body therapy for women in sexual abuse recovery. This study examines body-oriented therapy—an approach focused on body awareness and involving the combination of bodywork and the emotional processing of psychotherapy.

Objective: To examine the efficacy and the perceived influence on abuse recovery of body-oriented therapy. Massage therapy served as a relative control condition to address the lack of touch based-comparisons in bodywork research.

Design: *A 2-group, repeated measures design was employed, involving randomization to either body-oriented therapy or massage group, conducted in 8, hour-long sessions by 1 of 4 research clinicians. Statistical and qualitative analysis was employed to provide both empirical and experiential perspectives on the study process.*

Setting: *Participants were seen in treatment rooms of a university in the northwestern United States and in clinician's private offices.*

Participants: *Twenty-four adult females in psychotherapy for child sexual abuse.*

Interventions: *Body-oriented therapy protocol was delivered in three stages, involving massage, body awareness exercises, and inner-body focusing process. Massage therapy protocol was standardized. Both protocols were delivered over clothes.*

Main Outcome Measures: *The outcomes reflected 3 key constructs—psychological well being, physical well-being, and body connection. Repeated measures included: Brief Symptom Inventory, Dissociative Experiences Scale, Crime-Related Post Traumatic Stress Disorder Scale, Medical Symptoms Checklist, Scale of Body Connection and Scale of Body Investment. Results were gathered at 6 time points: baseline, 2 times during intervention, post-intervention, and at 1 month and 3 months follow-up. To examine the experiential perspective of the study process, written questionnaires were administered before and after intervention and at 1 month and 3 months follow-up.*

Results: *Repeated measures analysis of variance (ANOVA) indicated significant improvement on all outcome measures for both intervention groups, providing support for the efficacy of body therapy in recovery from childhood sexual abuse. There were no statistically significant differences between groups; however, qualitative analysis of open-ended questions about participant intervention experience revealed that the groups differed on perceived experience of the intervention and its influence on therapeutic recovery.*

For women in therapeutic recovery from childhood sexual abuse, recovery is intimately related to integration of the self — involving on the one hand reassociation with the self, and on the other hand, reduction of dissociation.[1,2] Integration of the self is addressed in experiential psychology, which holds the premise that healthy functioning results when as many parts of the self as possible are integrated in awareness.[3] The dissociative strategies that are protective in dealing with childhood abuse involve fragmentation of self and separation from sensory and emotional experience and can inhibit healing from trauma.[1,4] Dissociation involves psychological and physical distress and is associated with post-traumatic stress disorder (PTSD),[5] affect dysregulation and somatization,[6] and problems with gastrointestinal health.[7] Sexual symptoms and dysfunction, also frequent consequences of sexual abuse,[8,9] are closely related to dissociation from the body.[10,11] Women with a history of childhood sexual abuse have higher levels of psychological and physical distress than non-abused women,[12] which likely contribute to the common lack of emotional and sensory awareness—or body connection—seen clinically in this population.[13,14] Problems with affect regulation and physiological regulation are also common among female survivors of childhood trauma,[6,15] which indicates the importance of self-regulation as a primary goal in therapeutic recovery with this population.

In recent years, there has been increased attention to the clinical importance of addressing the body to facilitate integration of sensory and emotional awareness in sexual abuse recovery.[2,16-19] Body psychotherapy approaches for trauma recovery include teaching patients and facilitating their ability to incrementally access and sustain inner body awareness, which increases the capacity for body connection and thus facilitates dissociation reduction and reassociation or integration with the self.[19-21] Body psychotherapy is psychotherapy focused on the interactions between the patient's mental representations and their bodily phenomena.[22] To date, there has been little clinical research in body psychotherapy approaches in sexual abuse recovery. This is a study of body-oriented psychotherapy, an approach well-suited to the process of integration. Body-oriented therapy falls under the auspices of body psychotherapy and involves the combination of bodywork an—umbrella term for touch therapy modalities (e.g., massage, polarity, acupressure) and the emotional processing of psychotherapy.

The therapeutic goal of body-oriented therapy is to promote integration of psyche and soma, a shared and stated purpose within body psychotherapy.[22] Body psychotherapy approaches often use proprioceptive sensing to enhance somatic awareness.[23-25]

Making Sense of Research

Examples of proprioceptive sensing include the internal awareness of physiological release in tight muscle tissue during a massage and the internal awareness of the underlying emotion associated with stomach "knots." Touch therapy, when combined with proprioceptive sensing, provides a focal point for inner awareness, serving to facilitate access and sustained presence in bodily attention.[26,27] Engaging in proprioceptive sensing is not a passive process; as in biofeedback, there is a reciprocal "feedback loop" that increases self-regulation.[28]

There is both anecdotal and experimental evidence that body-oriented therapy is beneficial for therapeutic recovery from sexual abuse.[2,29] A pilot-test comparison of body-oriented therapy found a decrease in psychological symptoms, physical symptoms, and PTSD for the body-oriented therapy group compared to a wait-list control among women in psychotherapeutic recovery from childhood sexual abuse.[29] The body-oriented therapy approach used in this study was designed to teach proprioceptive sensing to access inner-body sensory awareness and to facilitate integration of psyche and soma using a combination of verbal and touch therapies. This study, which follows up on the pilot, compares the body-oriented therapy process to a standardized massage.

Whereas many studies have examined the benefits of massage,[30] a search of such literature databases as the Cumulative Index to Nursing and Allied Health Literature (CINAHL), PubMed, PsycINFO revealed little research focused on the potential benefits of body-oriented therapy. Consequently, we know little about the relative efficacy of body-oriented therapy interventions or the mechanisms by which they are purported to work. As a relatively new area of study within mind-body research, there are many elements that need to be systematically developed and examined to build a strong basis of research in body-oriented therapy. These include comparing body-oriented therapy to other bodywork approaches to address the lack of touch-based comparison groups in bodywork research; testing the feasibility of developing and implementing a body-oriented therapy protocol; developing measures that are specific to the bodywork process; and addressing ethical issues as they pertain to human subjects concerns and high-risk populations.

This study tested the efficacy of body-oriented therapy as an adjunct to psychotherapy and the hypothesis that body-oriented therapy compared to massage would result in increased psychological well-being (decreased PTSD, dissociation, and psychological distress); increased physical well-being (decreased physical symptoms); and increased body connection (increased body awareness, body association, and body investment) among women in psychotherapeutic recovery from childhood sexual abuse. In addition, this study examined the experience and impact of the interventions through qualitative analysis of open-ended questions on written questionnaires.

Methods

Design

A two-group repeated measures design was used to test the efficacy of body-oriented therapy as an adjunct to psychotherapy in comparison to a standardized massage and to explore the perceived influence of these interventions on abuse recovery using a follow-up written questionnaire. Participants were randomly assigned to receive 8, hour-long sessions of either body-oriented or massage therapy. Measures were administered at 6 time points: at baseline, after 2 weeks of sessions, after 4 weeks of sessions, one week after the intervention, and at 1 month and 3 months follow-up. Four research clinicians, 2 massage therapists and 2 body-oriented therapists, provided the study interventions.

Subjects and Procedures

· Recruitment and Selection

Women currently in psychotherapy for recovery from childhood sexual abuse were recruited for study participation via flyers posted at a university in the northwest and in mental health clinics, as well as from psychotherapy referrals and referrals from friends. Prospective participants were screened during the initial phone contact. Study inclusion required that participants be female, over the age of 25, engaged in an established psychotherapeutic relationship of at least 2 months, have a minimum of 2 years of psychotherapy, and agree to not seek bodywork treatment during study involvement.

Study exclusion included a change in psychotropic medication during the past 8 weeks, addiction to alcohol or drugs, current abusive relationship, hospitalization for psychological care within the past 12 months, diagnosis or medication for psychosis, pregnant by more than three months, and prior body-oriented therapy (more than 20 sessions). Participants were told that at the initial appointment there would be additional screening for severe dissociation and that severe dissociation would not be an appropriate fit for the study. This screening involved the use of the Dissociative Experiences Scale Taxon (DES-T), which has a cut-off indication for probable dissociation disorder.

· *Enrollment and Background Characteristics*

During the enrollment period, 50 women expressed interest in study participation. Twenty-four individuals were not eligible based on screening criteria. Of the 26 women who were eligible for study participation, 1 never enrolled in the study, and 1 withdrew from the study after 2 sessions (massage group) because she felt the experience was too stimulating at this point in her recovery. The final number of participants was 24.

The study participants ranged in age from 26 to 56 years, with a median age of 41. Of the participants, 1 was Native American, 1 was Hispanic, 2 were black, and 20 were white. Overall, they were highly educated, the household incomes varied widely, and the majority had endured extensive childhood abuse (Table I).

· *Data Collection*

Measures were administered at 6 time points: at baseline, after 2 weeks of sessions, after 4 weeks of sessions, one week after the intervention, and at 1 month and 3 months follow-up. The investigator administered baseline measures and the initial questionnaire at the first appointment. Within a week of the initial appointment, participants were randomly assigned to intervention groups and informed of the assignment. The randomization process involved paired blocking so that for every 2 study participants who completed the initial appointment, 1 was assigned to the body-oriented therapy group and 1 was assigned to the massage group. The interventions were both delivered as 8,

TABLE I – Demographics and Baseline Characteristics (N = 24)

Characteristics	
Age, median (range)	41 (26-56)
Racial/ethnic identity	
White	20
Black	2
Hispanic	1
Native American	1
Income (range)	$4,000-$200,000
< $30,000	8
$30,000 to $50,000	11
> $50,000	5
Education	
Completed high school	24
Completed college	18
Graduate student	5
Completed graduate program	6
Massage history	
None	3
Minimal (1-10 sessions)	15
Moderate (10-30 sessions)	6
Regularly scheduled (< 30 sessions)	3
Body-oriented therapy	
None	20
Minimal (1-10 sessions)	4
Abuse history	
Childhood sexual abuse over multiple years	18
Childhood sexual abuse over multiple years, from multiple perpetrators	9
Physically abused by parent(s)	11
Subsequent date rape in early adulthood	8
Psychotherapy in years, mean (range)	5 (2.5-15)

hour-long sessions within a 10-week period. The mid-intervention measures were completed by the participants prior to the third and fifth intervention sessions. At 1 week after completion of the intervention, the investigator contacted the participants to schedule a final appointment for administration of measures and the final questionnaire. One month and 3 months after the final appointment, a follow-up set of measures and the follow-up questionnaire was sent by mail to participants.

· *Training and Fidelity*

The research clinicians were licensed to practice massage in the state of Washington; the body-oriented therapists had, in addition, graduate-level education in psychology. They all had a minimum of 5 years in practice, plus experience working with women with a childhood sexual abuse history. The investigator provided the training and supervision. She was a bodywork practitioner for 17 years and has a master's degree in counseling and psychology. She developed the body-oriented therapy protocol based on her extensive therapeutic work with women in sexual abuse recovery as a body-oriented therapist. The training included instruction in the study procedures and study protocols and was provided using verbal and hands-on instruction with the investigator, as well as a training manual provided to each interventionist. Compliance with and quality of the intervention were evaluated by the investigator by (a) listening to sessions, which were audiotaped, and (b) reviewing process evaluation forms completed by the research clinicians immediately after each session. The investigator provided weekly individual feedback and separate supervision meetings with the massage therapists and the body-oriented therapists to review research protocol and to discuss clinical or research-related issues.

· *Intervention Procedures*

The body-oriented therapy and massage therapy interventions were similar in that both involved the therapeutic use of touch. However, the therapeutic goals and strategies of each approach differ. The therapeutic goal of body-oriented therapy is focus on sensory and emotional awareness, using a combination of hands-on and verbal therapy to promote integration of psyche and soma. The therapeutic goal of massage is to apply massage techniques with the intention of improving the client's health and well-being.[31] The massage group received a standardized massage, similar to that one might receive at a spa; the protocol contained no verbal therapeutic elements or educational components.

· Massage Group

The massage group received a standardized protocol similar to that used in research at the Touch Therapy Institute in Miami, Fla,[32,33] The protocol was modified to: a) cover a longer period of time (60 versus 30 minutes) and b) be carried out with the recipient clothed. Massage therapists often work over clothes to minimize anxiety and discomfort related to nudity and touch, particularly with abuse survivors during the initial weeks of building the relationship and familiarizing the client with touch.[34] The massage protocol had two primary elements: sense of safety and massage. Sense of safety refers to the participant's physical and emotional comfort. It was attended to throughout the sessions with use of frequent check-ins (i.e., asking client about the acceptability of touch) to assess comfort level and, if necessary, modification of the protocol to ensure participant comfort. Check-ins provided the massage therapist with feedback regarding her level of tactile pressure, the acceptability of touch in a particular area of the body, the participant's general physical comfort, and room temperature. The check-in was also used to access information that might indicate participant emotional discomfort (ie, dissociation, fear, aversion to touch). Massage techniques were used throughout the session to facilitate relaxation (Table II).

· Body-oriented Group

The body-oriented therapy protocol was separated into 3 stages to facilitate study of the different components of the intervention (Table III). Stage 1 included sessions 1 and 2 and involved massage with body literacy. Stage 2 included sessions 3 and 4 and involved massage with body literacy and body awareness exercises. Stage 3 included sessions 5 to 8 and involved massage with body literacy and delving practice. Each session began seated, with 10 minutes of intake. The next 40 minutes of each session involved the therapeutic elements particular to Stage 1, 2 or 3; all sessions were conducted with the participants

TABLE II – Overview of Massage Protocol

Face Up	Face Down
1) Head and Neck	5) Legs
• Traction to neck	• Calf stretch
• Stroke on both sides of neck	• Knead calf muscle
• Forehead stroke	• Strokes up and down full leg
• Circular stroke on jaw	6) Back
• Shoulder pressure	• Low back stretch
2) Arms	• Thumb pressure along vertebrae
• Arm traction	• Knead tops of shoulders
• Hand massage	• Circles around shoulder blades
• Strokes up and down arms	• Strokes down both sides of spine
• Shoulder circles	• Sacrum press
• Hand trigger point	• Thumb circles in gluteus muscles
3) Torso	• Connecting stroke from shoulders to feet
• Rocking at ribcage	• Gentle rocking with hands on back
• Deep breaths into belly	
4) Legs	
• Leg traction	
• Foot massage	
• Strokes up and down legs	

clothed. The last 10 minutes of each session was seated, and involved 10 minutes of session review. Session review included identification of body awareness homework for the interim week. Key elements of the intervention are detailed below.

1. Sense of safety was verified throughout the sessions. Check-ins specific to the intervention allowed research clinicians to assess participant engagement in the process, and to determine if increased skill training or change in pace was necessary.

2. Intake involved asking participants questions about their emotional and physical well-being to guide the therapeutic focus of the session.

3. *Massage with body literacy involved massage, using the standardized protocol to facilitate relaxation. It was accompanied by body literacy, the practice of identifying and articulating what is noticed in the body and the best words to describe the sensations. The therapists asked questions such as, "What are you noticing in your body right now?" and, "How would you describe how it feels in this area?"*

4. *Inner body awareness exercises involved 4 approaches to accessing somatic experience. Participants were taught how to (a) direct exhalation to facilitate movement of breath through the body; (b) use the power of mental intention to release tension; (c) deepen inner awareness, particularly in areas associated with physical and emotional difficulty; and (d) access the inner body through bringing conscious attention, or presence, to specific areas of the body.*

5. *Delving is derived from focusing, which involves "tuning in," or listening to the inner bodily self to identify and attend to an overall sense of oneself (the "felt sense") in relation to an identified problem area.[23] Delving is similar to mindfulness meditation in that it involves maintaining a compassionate, accompanying presence within the self while observing internal processes. However, delving is designed specifically for bodywork therapy and thus is distinct from both processes in the following ways: (a) the focal point is a specific area within the body rather than the general sensing orientation of focusing or the mental processes of mindfulness; (b) it involves the use of nonanalytic, sustained presence in internal awareness, whereas focusing involves switching back and forth between inner sensing and cognitive processing; (c) it involves scanning different aspects of awareness such as image, emotion, form, and sensation as a way to increase bodily self-awareness, a process guided by the therapist; and (d) it is carried out in conjunction with touch.*

6. *Session review involved therapist facilitation of participants' verbal review of session highlights to promote integration of the therapeutic elements in the session.*

7. *Homework consisted of a take-home practice in body awareness. It was developed through collaboration between the participant and the therapist and was based on the*

participant's experience in the session. For example, during an exercise in Stage 2, a participant focused on softening her jaw. She experienced a lessening of muscle tension in this area and wanted this exercise to be her daily take-home practice. The therapist suggested that she gently hold her jaw with both hands to increase the focus of her softening intention and to compare the tension in her jaw before and after the exercise.

TABLE III – Body-Oriented Therapy Intervention

Key Elements	Stage 1	Stage 2	Stage 3
Sense of safety	X	X	X
Intake	X (10)	X (10)	X (10)
Massage with body literacy	X (40)	X (10)	X (10)
Inner body awareness exercises		X (30)	
Delving			X (30)
Session review	X(10)	X (10)	X (10)
Homework	X	X	X

Minutes spent on each element are specified in parentheses.

Elements of Research Design

The study was designed to address important elements for building a strong basis of research in body-oriented therapy. Standardized massage was used as the comparison group to address the lack of touch-based comparison groups in body therapy research. The study tested the feasibility of developing and implementing a body-oriented therapy protocol through training and supervising research clinicians in the body-oriented therapy process. Last, to address ethical issues as they pertain to human subjects concerns and high-risk populations, the intervention protocols were designed to be flexible and sensitive to the emotional comfort of participants; the design of the study involved body therapy as an adjunct to psychotherapy to ensure adequate psychological support for study participants.

Measurement

The outcome measures reflected 3 key constructs—psychological well-being, physical well-being, and body connection—to serve the aims of this study. Psychological well-being was an assessment of intrapersonal and interpersonal health, both in relation to general measures of psychological health (Brief Symptom Inventory), and in relation to trauma history (Crime-Related Post-Traumatic Stress Disorder Scale; Dissociative Experiences Scale). Sense of safety was included within this construct (Bowerman Touch Empathy Scale). Physical well-being was an assessment of physical symptoms of discomfort (Medical Symptom Checklist). Body connection was an assessment of body awareness, body association, and body investment (Scale of Body Connection; Body Investment Scale). Measures were scored such that high values reflected higher levels of the construct. Validity and reliability coefficients reported below were derived from other, larger samples.

Measures

· *Psychological Well-being*

The Brief Symptom Inventory (BSI) has 53 items for 9 subscales (a = .71-.85); distress is rated on a 5-point scale (0-4). This study reported the "global severity index (GSI)," the mean of all endorsed items, and was used to indicate overall level of psychological distress. Test-retest reliability is .68-.91 with a 2-week interval; the reliability and validity of the scale are well documented.[35]

The Crime-Related Post-Traumatic Stress Disorder Scale (CR-PTSD) is based on 28 selected items from the BSI[35] and the Symptoms Checklist-90 Revised (SCL-90)[36] that indicate post-traumatic stress disorder. Crime-related victimization includes sexual assault from any time in life, including childhood. With excellent internal consistency (a = .93), the scale effectively discriminates between individuals with and without crime-related PTSD (F = 98.2, P < .001).[37]

Dissociative Experiences Scale (DES) contains 28 items and measures the frequency of dissociative experiences, from 0% = never to 100% = always, on an 11-point scale. The coefficient alphas for internal consistency ranged from .83 to .93, and the test-retest reliability was .79 with a 6-8-week test-retest interval; reliability and validity of the scale are well-documented.[38]

The DES-T consists of 8 items taken from the DES that represent severe dissociation and may indicate a dissociative disorder; the scale effectively discriminates between individuals with and without a dissociative disorder.[39]

The Bowerman Touch Empathy Scale is a 26-item, Likert-type scale (a = .93) that assesses empathy and quality of touch administered by a practitioner. Item responses range from "extremely" to "not at all" for questions about the quality of the therapist-client interaction. Construct validity was achieved through factor analysis.[40]

· Physical Well-being

The Medical Symptoms Checklist measures the number and frequency of 26 common physical symptoms and associated discomfort. The number and frequency of symptoms is rated 0 (never) to 8 (constant) on a 2-point scale. The degree of discomfort of each symptom is rated on an 11-point scale (0 = none to 10 = extreme). The scale has been used in other mind-body studies.[41,42]

· Body Connection

The Scale of Body Connection (SBC) has 2 distinct, uncorrelated dimensions measuring body awareness and body association. A 5-point scale, 12 items measure body awareness (a = .85) and 8 items measure body association (a = .79). Body awareness measures conscious attention to sensory cues indicating bodily state (e.g., tension, nervousness, peacefulness). Body association measures connection to or separation from body, including emotional connection (e.g., ease or difficulty attending to emotion). The scale, which was developed for this study, has demonstrated construct validity through exploratory and confirmatory factor analysis.[43]

The Body Investment Scale (BIS) is a 24-item, 5-point scale assessing attitudinal relationship to the body. It consists of 4 factors: (a) attitude and feeling (a = .75), (b) body care (a = .86), (c) body protection (a = .92), and (d) comfort in touch (a = .85).[44]

· *Demographic and Intervention Experience Questionnaires*

The initial questionnaire gathered demographic information (i.e., age, education, occupation, income); psychological history (i.e., number of years in psychotherapy, mental health concerns and symptoms); general abuse history information (i.e., age of abuse, identity of abuser, duration of abuse); and responses to questions about motivation (i.e., reasons for seeking body therapy).

The final questionnaire asked questions about experience of bodywork and perceived impact of study participation on therapeutic recovery. Key questions included: "What was the most important experience(s) that came from receiving massage?", "Did you learn something new during the intervention? If yes, what are the most important things that you learned?", "Were you 'ready' for bodywork at this point in your recovery (i.e., did you feel that massage was appropriate and therapeutic for you at this time)?", and "Do you think that the massage intervention influenced your psychotherapy? If yes, please comment on how."

The follow-up questionnaire asked about bodywork received subsequent to the intervention. Additional questions for the body-oriented group addressed the use and experience of body-oriented therapy techniques after the intervention; for example, "Have you done anything that you learned or practiced from the study during your daily life since your last bodywork session? If yes, please describe."

Analysis

Statistical and qualitative analyses were used to provide both empirical and experiential perspectives on the study process, which are particularly appropriate in such a new field of study. These analytical methodologies represent different epistemological perspectives. The triangulation of findings supports the primary goals of this study: to test the efficacy of body-oriented therapy and to advance understanding of the intervention process.

Statistical Analysis

Preliminary analysis included sample statistics, evaluation of baseline equivalence of the study groups, evaluation of outcome equivalence by a research clinician within study *groups, and regression analysis to determine if variables predicted intervention response. Repeated measure analysis of variance (ANOVA) was used to compare the effects of the interventions across 6 time points. Trend analysis was used to test the effectiveness of the massage and body-oriented therapy interventions and to describe the pattern of change for both interventions across time. The analysis was conducted using the Statistical Package for the Social Sciences, version 11.5 (SPSS, Chicago, Ill). Follow-up comparisons between groups and across time periods were conducted using t-tests and percent reduction equations. Because of the small sample size and the exploratory nature of this study, P value was set at <.10.*

Qualitative Analysis

Content analysis, along with analytic tools from discourse analysis, was used to describe the qualitative responses of the massage and body-oriented therapy intervention. The investigator conducted the analysis, using the final questionnaire and the follow-up questionnaire. The first step of the qualitative analysis involved categorizing types of general response to the questions across intervention groups. The second step involved evaluating the use of specific words and meaning in the narrative response. If distinctions between groups appeared in either step of the process, responses were separated by group (massage versus body-oriented) to enhance clarity of the similarities and differences in word use, phrasing, and meaning. To verify interpretation of meaning, word use and phrasing in responses to other questions were examined to support or refute the interpretation.

Results

Sample Characteristics

The psychological and physical symptom profile at baseline indicated generally high levels of psychological and physical symptoms among participants in both groups. With one exception, all participants scored above the 50% percentile rank on the global severity index (GSI) for psychological distress compared to the normed mean (50%) for nonpatient females; 15 were at or above the 90% percentile rank. PTSD scores at baseline were similarly high; 15 of the 24 participants were at, or above, the cut-off for active PTSD.[37]

Dissociation was elevated, with a mean score of 12.4 compared to the average range of 4.4-7.8 for the general public. To indicate physical symptom distress, the scores ranged from 3 to 21 symptoms endorsed out of a possible 26. Nineteen out of 24 participants endorsed between 10-21 physical symptoms. Frequency of symptoms occurred, on average, once a week for each symptom for 13 of the 24 participants. Although the endorsed items varied among individuals, common symptoms included back pain, headache, gastrointestinal discomfort, nausea, and insomnia.

Quantitative Findings

Preliminary Analysis

The demographic and sample characteristic data were examined for equivalence between groups and to determine whether or not they predicted outcomes after the intervention or at 3-month follow-up. The groups were equivalent, and none of the characteristics were associated with intervention outcomes.

The intervention groups were examined for equivalence at baseline and for equivalence on outcomes by the research clinicians (2 for each intervention) using repeated measures ANOVA. The t-tests and nonparametric tests revealed no significant baseline group differences or therapist effect.

There was baseline equivalence between the intervention groups on demographics, sample characteristics, sense of safety with research clinician, and on all baseline outcome measures. Likewise, there were no therapist effects in the massage or body-oriented therapy groups.

Sense of safety is considered fundamental for therapeutic activity among sexual abuse survivors receiving touch therapy.[34] Both intervention groups had a mean score of 4.3 (out of 5.0) on the Bowerman Empathy Scale, which indicated a high sense of safety among study participants. Using independent samples t-tests, there was equivalence in sense of safety by research clinician both within study groups and between study groups.

Change Across Time Comparing Intervention Groups

Repeated measures were administered at 6 points across time. The results indicate little difference between groups (massage versus body-oriented) on outcomes (Table IV). The results showed no significant group-by-time linear trends. The hypothesis that the

TABLE IV – Means and Standard Deviations (SD) for Massage and Body-Oriented Therapy

	Baseline		At 2 weeks		At 4 weeks		Post-Intervention		1-Month Follow-Up		3-Month Follow-Up	
	Mean	(SD)	Mean	(SD)	Mean	(SD)	Mean	(SD)	Mean	(SD)	Mean	(SD)
Psychological symptoms												
massage (n = 11)	.92	(.47)	.72	(.42)	.70	(.59)	.48	(.37)	.65	(.43)	.51	(.42)
body-oriented (n = 12)	1.2	(.61)	.95	(.55)	.86	(.38)	.66	(.45)	.59	(.33)	.56	(.37)
Crime-related PTSD												
massage (n = 11)	1.0	(.40)	.81	(.45)	.79	(.61)	.51	(.35)	.66	(.43)	.53	(.42)
body-oriented (n = 11)	1.2	(.61)	.98	(.52)	.90	(.40)	.65	(.35)	.62	(.40)	.56	(.34)
Dissociation experiences												
massage (n = 11)	12.1	(7.5)	9.6	(5.7)	8.3	(6.9)	5.5	(4.6)	4.6	(3.9)	3.7	(3.4)
body-oriented (n = 12)	12.4	(6.8)	11.3	(9.1)	8.5	(6.8)	7.8	(5.8)	6.5	(6.4)	5.4	(5.4)
Body awareness												
massage (n = 11)	2.7	(.88)	3.1	(.80)	3.2	(.66)	3.5	(.43)	3.3	(.59)	3.2	(.45)
body-oriented (n = 11)	2.7	(.65)	2.9	(.58)	3.0	(.61)	3.4	(.68)	3.4	(.60)	3.4	(.62)
Body association												
massage (n = 11)	3.3	(.73)	3.5	(.38)	3.6	(.50)	4.0	(.35)	3.5	(.55)	3.6	(.41)
body-oriented (n = 12)	3.1	(.81)	3.2	(.64)	3.3	(.50)	3.7	(.58)	3.7	(.35)	3.6	(.55)
Body investment												
massage (n = 11)	3.4	(.61)	3.4	(.55)	3.6	(.54)	3.7	(.53)	3.7	(.41)	3.8	(.46)
body-oriented (n = 12)	3.4	(.55)	3.5	(.60)	3.6	(.46)	3.9	(.49)	3.9	(.46)	3.8	(.60)
Number of physical symptoms												
massage (n = 11)	14	(5.3)	14	(6.1)	12	(4.9)	12	(5.4)	12	(7.1)	10	(7.1)
body-oriented (n = 12)	12	(5.2)	13	(5.3)	13	(5.4)	12	(5.1)	11	(4.6)	6.8	(4.5)
Physical symptom discomfort												
massage (n = 10)	54	(23)	48	(32)	47	(30)	42	(28)	37	(28)	35	(32)
body-oriented (n = 10)	48	(24)	49	(29)	42	(20)	40	(25)	30	(25)	26	(20)

body-oriented therapy group would demonstrate greater improvements in outcomes across time than the massage group was not supported. Rather, the groups showed equally significant improvements as demonstrated by the statistically significant changes across time for psychological well-being (psychological symptoms, PTSD, dissociation experiences) physical well-being (medical symptoms), and body connection (body awareness, body association, and body investment) (Table IV).

Change Across Time for Both Intervention Groups

The repeated measures ANOVA revealed significant linear changes in psychological well-being, body connection, and physical well-being experienced by participants in both interventions (massage and body-oriented therapy), as displayed in Table V.

TABLE V – Repeated Measures Analysis: Linear Trends Across Intervention Groups

Outcome Measure	df	MS	F	P
Psychological symptoms	1	3.8	27.0	.00
Post-traumatic stress disorder	1	4.5	34.0	.00
Dissociation experiences	1	98	33.0	.00
Body awareness	1	6.9	15.0	.00
Body association	1	3.2	8.0	.01
Body investment	1	3.3	20.0	.00
Number of physical symptoms	1	287	20.0	.00
Physical symptom discomfort	1	6,428	20.0	.00

df=degrees of freedom; MS=mean squares; F=F-ratio

The significant increase in psychological well-being can be interpreted by comparisons with normative data from the Brief Symptom Inventory (BSI) and Crime-Related PTSD scale. The percentile rank in psychological symptoms (based on normed mean GSI) dropped from 93% to 80% from baseline to 3-month follow-up. For dissociation, 10 of the 24 participants had scores within the normal range for the general public; at post-intervention 18 of the participants were within normal range. This reduction in *scores was maintained through 3-month follow-up. The reductions in PTSD scores were also indicative of the increase in psychological well-being. At post-intervention, only 4 participants (2 from each intervention group) had scores reflecting active PTSD compared to the 15 participants (7 in massage group and 8 in body-oriented therapy group) with active PTSD at baseline. These overall PTSD reductions were maintained into follow-up; only 5 participants had scores reflecting active PTSD (3 in massage group and 2 in body-oriented therapy group). These overall findings demonstrate the significant clinical effectiveness of both interventions in sexual abuse recovery.*

Qualitative Findings

Qualitative study looks at the subjective experience of the participant, which is important for understanding the experience and impact of an intervention. The triangulation of empirical and interpretive methodologies can bring insight to quantitative data.

Reasons for Seeking Bodywork

Analysis of the initial questionnaire responses indicated that the primary reason participants sought study participation was to increase body connection. On the final questionnaire, participants who had received pre-study bodywork were asked to comment on similarities or differences compared to past bodywork in: a) their bodywork experience, b) reasons for seeking bodywork, and c) the role that bodywork played in their health and healing. Their responses to these questions were analyzed to determine whether participants distinguished between motivation for study participation compared to motivation to seek bodywork before the study. More than half of the participants (11 of 18 who had more than one previous bodywork session) described different reasons for seeking bodywork before the study than for study participation. Before the study, they sought bodywork primarily for relaxation and relief from muscle tension. In contrast, with respect to this study, they sought bodywork primarily to increase body connection and enhance their abuse recovery. The similarity in responses to the initial and final questionnaires indicates the participants' sincerity and motivation for study involvement. The responses highlight the perceived importance of body connection in abuse recovery.

Experiential Perspective of the Intervention

Written responses to questions from the final questionnaire about the experience of receiving the massage or body-oriented therapy interventions and the perceived influence on abuse recovery were examined. Distinct differences emerged between the massage and body-oriented therapy group responses. The experiential distinction between interventions is best explained as 2 perspectives in relationship to the bodily self: a behavioral perspective and a somatic perspective. The behavioral perspective is akin to a psychological framework of self-perception. It is characterized by the ability to gain an observational and objective (from outside the body) perspective that involves recognizing the body as part of the self and provide insight into behavior.[25] The somatic perspective is akin to the concept of "embodiment" in anthropology,[45] in which the bodily self is the foundation of self-knowledge. It is characterized by access to proprioceptive sensing, or inner body awareness.[25]

Intervention Experience

Written responses to questions on the final questionnaire about the experience of receiving the massage or body-oriented therapy intervention were examined. All participants responded to these questions. The massage group responses reflected a shift toward increased awareness of self, specifically, awareness of behaviors that were linked to childhood abuse history. These responses generally fell into 2 primary categories: recognizing the impact of dissociation and increased self-care. As an example of recognizing the impact of dissociation, one participant wrote that the most important thing she learned from the massage was, "Owning just how disconnected I realize I am at this point with my body." Increased self-care was commonly expressed as, "I'm trying to learn to connect, accept, nurture, and take care of my body."

In contrast, the body-oriented group responses highlighted learning specific tools for body-focused attention, which indicated their use of proprioceptive sensing. These responses fell into two primary categories: experiencing emotional self and learning to access inner bodily self. As an example of experiencing emotional self, one participant

Making Sense of Research

wrote, "[I] feel body and emotion connection was solidified." "I relaxed those deep abdominal muscles and I just started to weep. I was shocked that this 'weeping and sadness' was in me." A common example of inner body awareness was, "I learned to relax my muscles from the inside. I was able to stay inside parts of my body rather than just looking at myself from the outside."

Intervention Influence on Recovery

Written responses to questions from the final questionnaire about the perceived impact or lack of impact of the intervention on abuse recovery were examined. All participants responded to these questions. Distinct differences in response to these questions emerged between massage and body-oriented therapy groups. In the massage group, 3 of the 12 participants did not think that receiving the massage intervention influenced their recovery from childhood sexual abuse. For the 9 who did, the influence of massage on recovery was expressed as a combination of newfound volition (self-efficacy) and budding self-care. A common response reflecting self-efficacy was, "I find myself planning to learn and do things I've wanted to for a long time. I seem to have a slightly to greatly improved belief in my ability to make positive lifestyle change." In an example of budding self-care, one participant said, "The massage was a contradiction to having been abused and a contradiction to helplessness. By committing to these sessions, I was demonstrating to myself that I was taking care of my body, and myself, in a way I could not do as a child." The influence of massage on psychotherapy was overwhelmingly expressed as jump-starting psychotherapy, particularly around healing from the vestiges of childhood abuse. A common response was, "I've been avoiding talking about [abuse] stuff with [a] therapist because [it is] so painful, but now I want to. It's a relief to get it out. I think about this [abuse] while on the massage table. I can accept that this [abuse] really contributed to some life problems; I was in such denial for such a long time."

All participants in the body-oriented therapy group thought that receiving the intervention influenced their recovery. The influence of body-oriented therapy on recovery was expressed as increased understanding and insight emerging from somatic experience. For example, one participant wrote, "This strategy has really opened me up to ways that I can *stay in my body more often without fearing for my life. I am learning that being inside my body can be empowering and enjoyable." The influence of body-oriented therapy on psychotherapy was expressed as the inclusion of somatic experience in psychotherapy sessions, enhancing psychotherapeutic work. For example, one participant described this process as, "After delving, I found that my emotions were more reachable, which assisted in psychotherapy." "...an increase in internal cues allowed me to focus or telegraph my recovery work in psychotherapy. This telegraphing had a profound effect on me in that it propelled and intensified my recovery work."*

In sum, the findings suggest that the massage group acquired a behavioral perspective, increasing self-care behavior and relationship to bodily self. These, in turn, influenced abuse recovery by stimulating self-efficacy and jump-starting psychotherapy. For the massage group, the behavioral perspective was familiar, demonstrated by the ease with which they pursued self-motivated therapeutic activity during massage sessions; reflecting the behavioral orientation of our culture and their psychotherapeutic experience.

In contrast, the body-oriented group acquired a somatic perspective, learning specific tools to access somatic experience and increased sensory and emotional awareness. These, in turn, facilitated somatically-based insight and understanding. All body-oriented group participants perceived that body-oriented therapy influenced abuse recovery by providing new ground for self-knowledge and information, enhancing psychotherapy through the inclusion of somatically-based process and information. For the body-oriented therapy group, the somatic perspective was new, demonstrated by their descriptions of learning new tools that facilitated somatic experience, indicating the typical lack of sensory and emotional awareness among this population.

Motivation for Increased Body-Mind Connection

Participant responses to the final questionnaire administered post-intervention were examined to explore the role of motivation in the study process. All participants indicated that they felt "ready" for body therapy in their abuse recovery. The indication of readiness for bodywork and the strong desire for increased body connection among all study

Making Sense of Research

participants may have contributed to the retention (100%) of participants throughout the study. The motivation to increase body connection in recovery appears to have played a role in the positive outcomes. The role that motivation played was expressed differently in the massage and body-oriented therapy groups.

Motivation in Massage Group

The motivation to address recovery through attention to the body became apparent in process evaluation of the intervention and in the participants' responses to the final questionnaire. The massage group, despite receiving a nonverbal, standardized massage, used the massage experience as a catalyst for therapeutic activity. Notably, they did this privately. The session audiotapes did not reveal their inward processes. Rather, as appropriate to the protocol, the taped sessions reflected the nonverbal emphasis of the intervention; conversations that did occur were fairly mundane. On the final questionnaire, however, the massage group participants repeatedly described self-motivated therapeutic activity during the massage session. A common example involved the purposeful attention to dissociation during the massage. For some participants, this involved general awareness of dissociative response to massage; for others, it involved practicing various behavioral strategies to increase capacity for presence while receiving massage. Ten of the 12 massage group participants described some degree of self-motivated therapeutic activity during massage sessions.

The engagement in self-motivated therapeutic activity during massage was perceived as the stimulus for the increased self-care behavior and psychotherapeutic engagement; 9 of the 12 massage group participants described increased engagement in psychotherapy. For example, one participant described how the therapist check-ins facilitated her ability to attend to her comfort needs by asking for less tactile pressure, an extra blanket, etc. The positive and supportive response by the therapist further enabled her to attend to her comfort needs both during subsequent massage sessions and in her daily life. She described these positive changes in interpersonal behavior as indications of massage influence on therapeutic recovery. Another participant described privately reflecting on her dysfunctional childhood home environment during the massage sessions, making important and new *connections regarding her own problematic patterns of behavior. She attributed this process to staying present rather than dissociating during the massage. She described the process as painful but exceedingly helpful for recovery and for stimulating psychotherapy.*

The high level of self-motivated therapeutic activity during the massage intervention was remarkable given that (a) the non-verbal protocol provided no facilitation of sensory or emotional processing, (b) the majority of participants were naïve to bodywork therapy, and (c) with one exception, the participants had no experience with using bodywork to address recovery. The engagement in self-motivated therapeutic activity reflects the great sense of safety participants felt with their practitioners; many commented on the safety inherent in the predictability of the massage and the clinician responsiveness to feedback, both fundamental elements of the protocol. The participants' descriptions of their massage experience suggest that they responded differently to the study massage compared to previous massage experiences, most likely due to the safety inherent in participating in a study specific to abuse recovery that involved experienced and carefully supervised bodywork clinicians.

Motivation in the Body-Oriented Therapy Group

The body-oriented therapy group's motivation for change was equally apparent but expressed differently. In contrast to the massage intervention, the body-oriented protocol was designed to teach participants to access inner somatic experience and to facilitate the incorporation of these skills into daily life.

All body-oriented therapy group participants demonstrated consistent and profound engagement in the intervention, apparent in the audiotaped sessions and reflected in the weekly process evaluations by the research clinicians. Each participant kept a daily log documenting frequency and duration of homework practice during the 8 weeks of the intervention. All body-oriented therapy group participants engaged in regular and frequent body awareness homework each week. At the 3-month follow-up, 11 of the 12 participants reported that they regularly incorporated at least one of the somatic experiencing techniques from the body-oriented intervention into daily life (approximately 2-5 times per week). They described their motivation for continued use of body awareness practice during follow-up as facilitating emotional connection, increasing sense of well-being, and reducing tension and anxiety. The motivation for, and continued practice of, body awareness techniques during follow-up reflected the perceived therapeutic usefulness of learning techniques to access somatic experience.

Discussion

The results demonstrate improvement for both the massage and body-oriented therapy groups, which provides preliminary support for the efficacy and effectiveness of body therapy in recovery from childhood sexual abuse. The improvements in psychological well-being and physical well-being were similar to the pre-intervention to post-intervention findings in a pilot-test comparison of body-oriented therapy as an adjunct to psychotherapy with this population[21] and to the pre-intervention to post-intervention improvements in anxiety and depressed mood in a randomized control trial of massage therapy for female sexual abuse survivors.[33] Particularly remarkable were the maintained improvements on all outcomes from post-intervention through 3-month follow-up for both groups. Few body therapy studies have gathered longitudinal data, and no body therapy studies have measured these particular markers of psychological and physical well-being and body connection into a follow-up period. The similar benefits for both groups despite the differences in intervention were not expected and did not support the study hypothesis. The standardized massage was expected to evoke less therapeutic response and consequently less improvement in outcomes compared to the more individualized and skill-building orientation of the body-oriented therapy intervention. Although concurrent psychotherapy likely contributed to the improved and maintained health outcomes, qualitative findings and process evaluation provide insight into the massage and body-oriented therapy contribution to health outcomes.

The motivation to address recovery through attention to the body appears to have played a role in the positive outcomes and likely contributed to the similarity in outcomes between groups. This was most clearly demonstrated by the massage group. Dissociation reduction was the primary focus of self-motivated therapeutic activity by the massage group, and likely facilitated the decrease in dissociation evident in the outcomes. Given the role that massage played in providing the opportunity for body-focused, self-directed therapeutic activity, it is unlikely that the positive outcomes among the massage group resulted from psychotherapy alone. It is likely that significant improvements in outcomes were a result of increased psychotherapeutic engagement facilitated by activation of a behavioral perspective on bodily self. This does not diminish the role of massage therapy, but rather supports the importance of bodywork as an adjunct to psychotherapy in recovery from sexual abuse. The impact of motivation in the body-oriented therapy group is more clearly tied to engagement in the specific therapeutic process of the intervention. Although concurrent psychotherapy likely contributed to the improved and maintained health outcomes, it is unlikely that the improvement in outcomes in the body-oriented therapy group resulted from psychotherapy alone; this is further supported by the pilot study findings of body-oriented therapy as an adjunct to psychotherapy with this population that found little change from pre-intervention to post-intervention among the wait-list control group compared to the experimental group.[21]

The intervention approaches stimulated different types of therapeutic activity, due in large part to the difference in behavioral-versus-somatic perspective in relationship to bodily self. The intervention group differences were not apparent on "body connection" outcomes, possibly because of the measures' inability to capture the subtle differences in body awareness, association, and investment that contribute to these distinct perspectives on self. Though distinct, these body awareness perspectives are considered equally important modes in relation to bodily self.[25] The similar statistical change on outcomes between groups supports the clinical perspective that behavioral and somatic perspectives are both therapeutically important. In particular, both groups experienced shifts in perspective that likely contributed to the reduction in dissociation, a result of increased body awareness that facilitated change in perception from disembodied to embodied self.

Clinical Implications

These findings contribute to the scientific basis for the practice of massage and body-oriented therapy. First, this is the second study indicating that women in psychotherapy for childhood sexual abuse recovery who seek out bodywork tend to be extremely committed to their healing.[46] For many, the opportunities to address the body in recovery have been limited by the lack of attention to the body in psychotherapy, the expense of bodywork therapy, and the relative lack of bodyworkers skilled in trauma recovery. This study provided such an opportunity and tapped a needed resource, evidenced by the completion of study enrollment only weeks after recruitment, and points to the need for therapeutic attention to body-mind connection in therapeutic recovery among abuse survivors.

Second, abuse history is generally severe among women who seek body therapy as an adjunct to psychotherapy for abuse recovery, and the women have a concomitant level of psychological and physical distress.[46] It is important the sexual abuse survivors are psychologically ready for the integrative work of body therapy. Given the prevalence of abuse trauma in the general population, basic bodywork education must address the therapeutic needs of sexual abuse survivors. More advanced training and graduate programs that address trauma recovery using bodywork and body-oriented therapy also are needed.

Third, the similar effectiveness of both massage and body-oriented therapy approaches, combined with the qualitative findings suggesting distinctly different experiential and therapeutic processes, raises questions about who would be best served by each approach. The clinical emphasis on inner body awareness for integration in sexual abuse recovery points to the need to clarify the construct of body awareness to more accurately interpret the clinical relevance of experiential differences in body awareness among women in sexual abuse recovery. It is possible that one approach is more appropriate than another at any given stage of abuse recovery. Likewise, it is possible that there would be differences in the long-term impact of any one body therapy approach on therapeutic recovery from childhood sexual abuse.

Study Limitations and Future Research

The study limitations highlight the need for future research in this area. First, the study sample is small, limiting interpretation of comparative results and generalization of study findings. Also, this study compared 2 treatment approaches but lacked an absolute control condition, a limitation of study design that also restricts result interpretation. Future research calls for a larger sample, randomly assigned to multiple treatment arms (including an absolute control condition). Second, the measures of body awareness did not distinguish between bodily self perspective (behavioral versus somatic), which indicates the need for increased specificity and sensitivity to the body-oriented therapy intervention. This study also points to the need for additional measures that address skill-acquisition in body-oriented therapy. There is a positive association between somatic perspective and self-regulation in biofeedback[47] that is particularly relevant because it presents the possibility that access to somatic experience in body-oriented therapy may facilitate self-regulation. Because lack of self-regulation is a common and primary issue among adult sexual abuse survivors in psychotherapeutic recovery, it is important to measure loci of control and self-regulation in future body therapy research with this population. Third, the design did not account for the impact of sense of safety or the use of self-directed therapeutic activity, both of which appear to have influenced the character of the comparison intervention (i.e., it did not simulate a spa massage). Consequently, future study design will need to address the impact of sense of safety and the use of self-directed therapeutic activity on therapeutic outcomes in comparative intervention studies. Fourth, the investigator collected and analyzed the data, so the investigator was not masked to study condition during the phases of data collection and analysis, a limitation of the study design. Great care was taken toward equanimity in these aspects of the research process, but it is possible that the role of the investigator in data collection may have influenced participant responses on questionnaires or the interpretation of findings.

Last, high educational background, a prominent demographic feature, may be typical of women in psychotherapy for childhood sexual abuse who seek adjunctive body therapy. It may also reflect the exclusion criteria, which excluded women not currently in psychotherapy and women with more severe mental health concerns. These exclusions were chosen to increase homogeneity among such a small sample. Ideally, future study will allow for a more inclusive sample. This will require greater education among and greater supervision of research clinicians and will increase generalization of study results.

Conclusion

This is an important study of massage and body-oriented therapy approaches for women recovering from childhood sexual abuse. This study demonstrated the feasibility of body-oriented therapy intervention training and implementation and the development of ethical protocols and study design for a vulnerable population. The significant benefit of both intervention approaches supports the use of body therapy in sexual abuse recovery. The triangulation of methodologies facilitated understanding of study findings and addressed the intricacies of clinical experience and research, raising important clinical and research questions about the role of body therapy in abuse recovery. Likewise, the similar positive outcomes between groups, the role of motivation among both groups, and the positive experience of the intervention suggest that the expectations and interpersonal element of the therapist-client relationship were significant factors underlying the combined and comparative intervention effects. The qualitative results indicate that both massage and body-oriented interventions influence abuse recovery in important but distinct ways, involving different perspectives in relationship to self. This distinction is important for future studies examining the role of body therapy as an adjunct to psychotherapy in recovery from childhood sexual abuse. The findings also raise more general questions about the role of somatic integration in health and healing.

Acknowledgements

Thanks to Elaine Thompson, PhD, who mentored me through this project, the women who participated in this study, and the practitioners who provided the study interventions—Hilary Bolles, Kay Monahan, Laurie Purpuri, and Sari Spieler. Funding support from the National Center for Complementary and Alternative Medicine at National Institutes of Health (F31 AT01053), the McLaws Nursing Research Fund from the University of Washington School of Nursing, UW School of Nursing Curriculum Training Grant in Complementary Therapies (I R25 AT01240), and the UW School of Nursing Department of Psychosocial and Community Health.

Footnote

Cynthia Price, PhD, is a postdoctoral fellow in the School of Nursing, University of Washington, Seattle.

References

1. Herman, J. *Trauma and Recovery.* New York, NY: HarperCollins Publishers; 1992.

2. Timms, R.; Connors, P. *Embodying Healing: Integrating Bodywork and Psychotherapy in Recovery from Childhood Sexual Abuse.* Orwell, Vermont; The Safer Society Press: 1992.

3. Greenberg, L.; Van Balen, R. The theory of experience-centered therapies. In: Greenberg L, Watson J, Lietaer G. , editors. *Handbook of Experiential Psychotherapy.* New York NY: Guildford; 1998.

4. van der Kolk, B.;van der Hart, O.; Marmar, C. Dissociation and Information Processing in Posttraumtatic Stress Disorder. In: van der Kolk B, McFarlane C, Weisaeth L. , editors. *Traumatic Stress: the effects of overwhelming experience on mind, body and society.* New York NY: Guilford Press; 1996. pp. 303–327.

5. Feeny NC, Zoellner LA, Fitzgibbons LA, Foa EB. Exploring the roles of emotional numbing, depression, and dissociation in PTSD. *J Trauma Stress.* 2000;13:489–498.

6. van der Kolk BA, Pelcovitz D, Roth S, Mandel FS, McFarlane A, Herman JL. Dissociation, somatization, and affect dysregulation: the complexity of adaptation of trauma. *Am J Psychiatry.* 1996;153:83–93.

7   Salmon P, Skaife K, Rhodes J. Abuse, dissociation, and somatization in irritable bowel syndrome: towards an explanatory model. *J Behav Med.* 2003;26:1–18.

8. Beitchman JH, Zucker KJ, Hood JE, daCosta GA, Akman D, Cassavia E. A review of the long-term effects of child sexual abuse. *Child Abuse Negl.* 1992;16:101–118.

9. Briere J, Elliott DM. Prevalence and symptomatic sequelae of self-reported childhood physical and sexual abuse in a general population sample of men and women. *Child Abuse Neglect: Intern J.* 2003;27:1205–1222.

10. Maltz W. Identifying and treating the sexual repercussions of incest: a couples therapy approach. *J Sex Marital Ther.* 1988;14:142–170.

11. Maltz, W. *The Sexual Healing Journey: A Guide for Survivors of Sexual Abuse.* New York NY: Quill; 2001.

12. McCauley J, Kern DE, Kolodner K, et al. Clinical characteristics of women with a history of childhood abuse: unhealed wounds. *JAMA.* 1997;277:1362–1368.

13. Courtois, C. *Healing the Incest Wound: Adult Survivors in Therapy.* New York NY: WW Norton; 1996.

14. Kepner, J. *Healing Tasks: Psychotherapy with Adult Survivors of Childhood Abuse.* San Francisco Calif: Jossey-Bass; 1995.

15. Kendall-Tackett K. Physiological correlates of childhood abuse: chronic hyperarousal in PTSD, depression, and irritable bowel syndrome. *Child Abuse Negl.* 2000;24:799–810.

16. Fitch P, Dryden P. Recovering body and soul from Post-Traumatic Stress Disorder. *Mass Ther J.* 2000;39:41–62.

17. Levine, P. *Waking the Tiger: Healing Trauma.* Berkeley Calif: North Atlantic Books; 1997.

18. Van der Kolk, B. *Beyond the Talking Cure: Somatic Experience, Subcortical Imprints, and the Treatment of Trauma.* Proceedings of The United States Association For Body Psychotherapy "Emergence & Convergence: The Body in Psychotherapy". Baltimore, Md: 2002.

19. Aposhyan, S. *Body-Mind Psychotherapy: Principles, Techniques, and Practical Applications.* New York NY: Norton; 2004.

20. Ogden P, Minton K. Sensorimotor Psychotherapy: One method for processing traumatic memory. *Traumatology.* 2000;7:1–20.

21. Price C. Body-oriented therapy as an adjunct to psychotherapy in recovery from childhood abuse: a case study. *J Bodywork Move Ther.* 2002;6:228–236.

22. European Association of Body-Centered Psychology. *What is body-psychotherapy?* Available at: http://www.eabp.org. Accessed July 2005.

23. Gendlin, E. *Focusing.* New York NY: Bantam; 1981.

24. Gendlin, E. *Focusing-Oriented Psychotherapy: A Manual of the Experiential Method.* New York NY: Guilford; 1996.

25. Hanna, T. *What is Somatics?* In: Johnson D. , editor. *Bone, Breath and Gesture: Practices of Embodiment.* Berkeley Calif: North Atlantic Books; 1995. pp. 341–352.

26. Ogden, P. *Hakomi integrated somatics: hands-on psychotherapy.* In: Caldwell C., editor. *Getting in Touch: The Guide to New Body-Centered Therapies.* Wheaton Ill: Quest; 1997.

27. Price C. Fantastic voyage/fantastic voyagers: connecting and imagery in bodywork. *Somatics.* 1999;12:32–34.

28. Hanna, T. *The body of life: Creating new pathways for sensory awareness and fluid movement.* Rochester, Vt: Healing Arts; 1993.

29. Price C. Body-oriented therapy in sexual abuse recovery: a pilot-test comparison. *J Bodywork Move Ther.* 2005. (In press).

30. Moyer C, Rounds J, Hannum J. A meta-analysis of massage therapy research. *Psychol Bull.* 2004;130:3–18.

31. American Massage Therapy Association. *Enhancing your health with therapeutic massage.* Available at: http://www.amtamassage.org. Accessed July 2005.

32. Field T, Grizzle N, Scafidi F, Schanberg S. Massage and Relaxation Therapies' Effects on Depressed Adolescent Mothers. *Adolescence.* 1996;31:904–911.

33. Field T, Hernandez-Reif M, Hart S, et al. Effects of sexual abuse are lessened by massage therapy. J Bodywork Move Ther. 1997;1:65–69.

34. Benjamin B. Massage and bodywork with survivors of abuse, Part V. Massage Ther J. 1996:1–18.

35. Derogatis, L. The Brief Symptoms Inventory. Minneapolis MN: National Computer Systems Inc: 1993.

36. Derogatis, L. The SCL-90-R: Administration, scoring, and procedures manual. Baltimore Md: Clinical Psychometric Research; 1977.

37. Saunders B, Arata C, Killpatrick D. Development of a crime-related post-traumatic stress disorder scale for women within the symptom checklist-90-revised. J Trauma Stress. 1990;3:439–448.

38. Carlson E, Putnam F. An update on the dissociative experiences scale. Dissociation. 1993;6:16–27.

39. Waller N, Putnam F, Carlson E. Types of dissociation and dissociative types: A taxometric analysis of dissociative experiences. Psycholog Meth. 1996;1:300–321.

40. Bowerman, S. The effect of empathic touch and expectations on mood change during a therapeutic massage treatment. Unpublished Doctoral Dissertation. California School of Professional Psychology. 1989.

41. Kroenke K, Spitzer RL. Gender differences in the reporting of physical and somatoform symptoms. Psychosom Med. 1998;60:150–155.

42. Nakao M, Fricchione G, Myers P, et al. Anxiety is a good indicator for somatic symptom reduction through behavioral medicine intervention in a mind/body medicine clinic. Psychother Psychosom. 2001;70:50–57.

43. Price C. Measuring Dimensions of Body Connection: Body Awareness and Body Dissociation. Manuscript in preparation, 2004.

44. Orbach I, Mikulincer M. The Body Investment Scale: Construction and Validation of a Body Experience Scale. Psychological Assessment. 1998;10:415–425.

45. Csordas T. Embodiment as a paradigm for anthropology. Ethos. 1990;18:5–47.

46. Price C. Characteristics of women seeking bodywork as an adjunct to psychotherapy during recovery from childhood sexual abuse. J Bodywork Move Ther. 2004;8:35–42

47. Criswell, E. Biofeedback and Somatics: Toward a Personal Revolution. Novato Calif: Freeperson; 1995.

Critical Evaluation

First, notice that this mixed methods study was originally published in a peer-reviewed journal. When we examine the sources of financial support for the study, we see that it was funded in part by a grant from the National Center for Complementary and Alternative Medicine, part of the National Institutes of Health. Because it was funded through NIH, a copy of the author's manuscript is available through PubMed Central as required by federal regulations, so that the full text is available free of charge.

From a qualitative evaluative perspective, the author appears to be well-qualified academically, with a background in both body-oriented therapy and bodywork, and previous experience in both quantitative and qualitative research. From a quantitative evaluative perspective, we see that the article uses a standardized abstract. Based on the information contained there, we will want to look more closely at the details regarding participant selection, the descriptions of the protocols for the two interventions being compared, and the methods used in the analysis of both the quantitative and qualitative data.

As we consider the introduction to the study, the research objective and specific hypotheses to be tested are stated clearly. The context for the study and significance of the research question are well established. Childhood sexual abuse has lasting physiological and psychological effects on female survivors, recovery is challenging, and body therapy appears to offer benefits, yet little research on its use for this population has been conducted.

In the methods sections, the description of the study's approach and procedures is weighted more toward the quantitative side, with some consideration of qualitative methods used in the analysis of the interview data. Inclusion and exclusion criteria necessary in high-quality quantitative research are stated and seem appropriate to the study's research question. Given the sensitive nature of the study question, the method of recruitment and selection of study participants appears reasonable. Random assignment to either the body-oriented therapy or the comparison massage group is stated to have been used, but the exact method of randomization is not described. Blinding as to group assignment was not used, but would likely not have been possible given the study design. The massage and body-oriented therapy protocols are both described in detail sufficient for replication of the study.

Most of the quantitative outcome measures are well-described, with good reliability and validity reported. One measure, the Scale of Body Connection, was developed for this study, but the actual validity data for this measure are not reported. A manuscript in preparation containing this information is cited in the references. The demographic questionnaire and the intervention experience questionnaire used to collect the qualitative data in written form are also described in some detail. The sample size of 24 is small in relation to the number of outcomes measured (8), and no power analysis is reported. Plans for both the quantitative and qualitative analysis are described in advance. Given the exploratory nature of the study, setting the level of statistical significance at 0.10 rather than the customary 0.05 seems reasonable. The use of repeated measures ANOVA, and measuring participants across six time points helps to increase the statistical validity of the study.

No particular theoretical approach is mentioned in the plans for the qualitative data analysis; however, content analysis of the open-ended written questionnaire data is specified, and was performed by the author. In addition, all intervention sessions were audiotaped.

In the results section, the methods of both quantitative and qualitative analysis are described. Based on the demographic and baseline data, randomization appears to have been successful, with no significant preexisting difference between the two groups. The tables are clearly labeled, and means and standard deviations are provided. All outcomes measured are reported. There appears to have been some attrition during the course of the study; in Table 4, the *n* reported for each outcome does not add up to 24, and this discrepancy is not addressed. The repeated measures ANOVA used did not show a statistically significant difference between the two groups on any of the outcomes measured; however, the linear trend for both groups over the study time period is significant. Note the scores for each group at the different time points – they are quite close to each other, but both are different from beginning to end. If we were to graph the scores of the two groups for any of the outcome measures over the study time period, we would have a graph that looks like the one following, with the lines for each group parallel and both lines starting higher and ending relatively lower. Also pay attention to the use of scaling on the right hand side of the graph. By marking symptom scores in increments of 0.5, the data points for the time intervals are father apart than if increments of 1.0 had been used.

Basically, from the quantitative results it appears that both interventions reduced the self-reported physical and psychological symptoms for study participants, and these

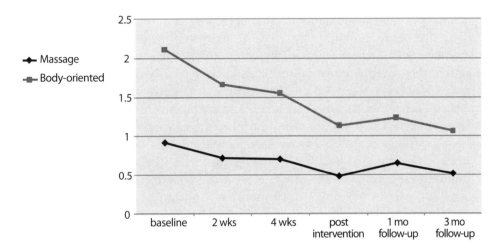

Figure 8.1 Psychological Symptoms

improvements in well-being were maintained over the three-month follow-up period. A frequent criticism of before-and-after treatment studies is that only the immediate effects of the treatment are measured. In this study, the addition of follow-up data increases the credibility and clinical utility of the findings. The qualitative data showed a difference between groups in their perceived experience of the intervention and its role in recovery, which was supported by the statements of the participants. Analysis and incorporation of the qualitative data helped to explain the quantitative results, which is one of the strengths of using a mixed methods approach in health care research.

In the discussion section, the author clearly states that no statistically significant differences were found between groups, that the study hypothesis was not supported, and that this finding was unexpected. Generalizability of the quantitative findings is limited, and is included in a thorough discussion of the inherent limitations of the study, along with suggestions for future research in this area. The clinical significance of the results is discussed. References appear to be pertinent and succinct.

This is a rich and layered study, and at the time it was conducted and published, unusual in its integration of quantitative and qualitative methods. Inclusion of both methodologies increases the validity of the study and its findings, especially when considering that the study explored a topic about which little research had previously been conducted. The study also piloted two different body-centered interventions for a vulnerable population and demonstrated both their feasibility and safety. The use of the repeated measures design helps to compensate for the small sample size relative to the number of outcome variables measured. Although the study findings were unexpected, they are internally consistent, and consistent with the study objective. The comparison between the two groups over time also illustrates the efficacy paradox described by Walach – because both treatments show a positive result, comparing means showed no difference between the two, which could be misinterpreted as evidence of no effect. The results of the qualitative data analysis inform the quantitative analysis and provide important information for designing future studies. Overall, the study conclusions are supported by the results presented – body therapy, whether massage alone or body-oriented therapy – does appear to be helpful in recovery for women who are survivors of childhood abuse. While there are some limitations in the study, chance, bias, or confounding do not provide sufficiently plausible alternate explanations for the study findings.

Summary

Qualitative research approaches have evolved from a variety of social science fields, including sociology, anthropology, psychology, education, and philosophy. Its units of data collection and analysis are words rather than numbers. These approaches, such as grounded theory, ethnography, and phenomenology, are employed to answer research questions related to describing, observing, and understanding complex situations and experiences, rather than determining whether a cause-and-effect relationship exists between treatment and outcome. Credible qualitative research adds a human dimension to health care research that is well-reasoned and verifiable, and often engaging to read.

Although the perspectives, approaches, and methods in qualitative health care research are different from those in quantitative research, the logic and common sense approach that underlie its evaluation are similar. Qualitative research requires equal rigor in its design, conduct, and analysis. Methodological flaws in any type of research are often related to practical and logistical issues, and the reader must judge these realistically. No study is perfect, whether qualitative or quantitative, and the informed reader should assess both the merits and flaws of any given study to determine its credibility. Ideally, a mixed methods approach can increase the overall validity of a study because of the triangulation created through using complementary research approaches.

References

1. Patton MQ. *Qualitative evaluation and research methods*. Newbury Park, CA: Sage Publications, Inc.; 1990.

2. Glaser BG & Strauss AL. *The discovery of grounded theory: Strategies for qualitative research*. Hawthorne, NY: Aldine; 1967.

3. Lincoln YS & Guba EG. *Naturalistic inquiry*. Newbury Park, CA: Sage Publications, Inc.; 1985.

4. Greenhalgh T. *How to read a paper: The basics of evidence-based medicine*. London: BMJ Publishing Group; 2001.

5. Parkhurst PE, Lovell KL, Sprafka SA, Hodgins M. Evaluation of videodisc modules: a mixed method approach. *Proc Annu Symp Comput Appl Med Care* 1991:747–51.

Exercises

1. *If you were going to replicate the first study example given in this chapter, what changes to the research design would you make to improve the credibility of the study?*

2. *For any of the quantitative study examples given in previous chapters, describe a qualitative component that could be added to the design to strengthen it and provide additional information.*

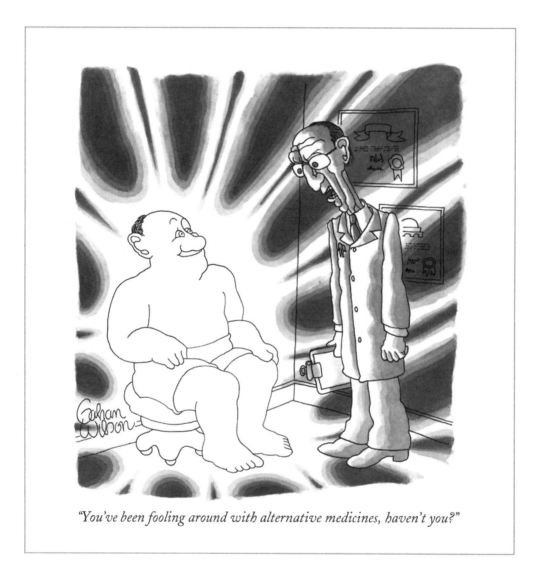

"You've been fooling around with alternative medicines, haven't you?"

Chapter 9:

Writing a
Case Report

*No number of lectures, seminars, or other verbal
communications can take the place of a contribution to
a learned journal.*

P. B. Medawar

Learning Objectives

After completing this chapter,
the reader should be able to:

· *Define a case report.*

· *Give three reasons for publishing a case report.*

· *List the first four steps involved in planning a case report.*

Chapter 9: Writing A Case Report

At this point, the reader has become more knowledgeable regarding the research process, understands basic concepts involved in scientific research, and can locate health care research articles of interest and critically evaluate them. In this chapter, we move from evaluating the work of others to considering the creation of our own, focusing on how to design and conduct case reports. Some general suggestions about writing for publication are also included.

As we discussed in Chapter 4, a case report is a detailed account of the history, presenting symptoms, observations, assessment, treatment, and follow-up of an individual client or patient. A case series is the report of a series of patients or clients presenting with the same symptom or who have other features in common. Many people use the term "case study" synonymously with case report; technically speaking, "case report" is used more often in health care research, while "case study" is used more often in the social sciences. The case report or study is the simplest form of practice-based research, and one that is within the grasp of any interested practitioner. It also allows for the use of a mixed methods approach to research design through the incorporation of both quantitative and qualitative data.

Review the criteria for evaluation of case reports in Chapter 4. Remember that case reports are based on the observation and description of an individual case, and are not intended to provide strong evidence of cause and effect – by their very nature they cannot. Instead, a good case report emphasizes the clinical usefulness of the information presented, and places a single instance into a larger context.

The Uses of Case Reports

Let us first consider some of the reasons why practitioners read and write case reports. Of primary importance is the fact that a case report is an original contribution to the research literature. What separates the case report from a clinical anecdote is its level of organization, clear focus, and pertinent detail. Case reports in the health care literature most often describe an unusual event, such as the uncommon presentation of a condition, a rare condition, or an adverse response to a treatment. Case reports are also employed to describe a useful approach to the treatment or management of a common condition, or to demonstrate the feasibility of a new therapeutic application.

A case report may also be the first step in developing a hypothesis. Ideally, the case report provides an opportunity for inductive reasoning through moving from the specific instance to a more general statement that could be tested in a larger study. A good case report advances our understanding, and is rewarding for the author to write and for practitioners to read. Through reading case reports, the practitioner has access to the clinical experience of others.

Before we discuss the construction of our own case reports and studies, it will be helpful to look at a few examples and to note their similarities and differences.

Some writers have dismissed the case report as "merely anecdotal" in that its descriptive nature makes its capacity to link cause and effect weaker compared with that of an experimental RCT with an n in the thousands. Remember, however, that all good science begins with observation and description. For this reason alone, the case report is valuable in its own right. It is particularly valuable in the field of epidemiology for its ability to notify the health care community that something out of the ordinary is happening. Consider the following report of a series of five cases, first published in the Centers for Disease Control publication *Morbidity and Mortality Weekly Report* on June 4, 1981:

Pneumocystis Pneumonia -- Los Angeles

As part of its commemoration of CDC's 50th anniversary, MMWR is reprinting selected MMWR articles of historical interest to public health, accompanied by a current editorial note. On June 4, 1981, MMWR published a report about Pneumocystis carinii pneumonia in homosexual men in Los Angeles. This was the first published report of what, a year later, became known as acquired immunodeficiency syndrome (AIDS). This report and current editorial note appear below.

Gottlieb, M. "Pneumocystis pneumonia -- Los Angeles." MMWR Weekly August 30, 1996 45(34);729-733. © 1996 Centers for Disease Control and Prevention

In the period October 1980 - May 1981, 5 young men, all active homosexuals, were treated for biopsy-confirmed Pneumocystis carinii pneumonia at 3 different hospitals in Los Angeles, California. Two of the patients died. All 5 patients had laboratory-confirmed previous or current cytomegalovirus (CMV) infection and candidal mucosal infection. Case reports of these patients follow.

Patient 1: A previously healthy 33-year-old man developed P. carinii pneumonia and oral mucosal candidiasis in March 1981 after a 2-month history of fever associated with elevated liver enzymes, leukopenia, and CMV viruria. The serum complement-fixation CMV titer in October 1980 was 256; in May 1981 it was 32.* The patient's condition deteriorated despite courses of treatment with trimethoprim-sulfamethoxazole (TMP/SMX), pentamidine, and acyclovir. He died May 3, and postmortem examination showed residual P. carinii and CMV pneumonia, but no evidence of neoplasia.

Patient 2: A previously healthy 30-year-old man developed P. carinii pneumonia in April 1981 after a 5-month history of fever each day and of elevated liver-function tests, CMV viruria, and documented seroconversion to CMV, i.e., an acute-phase titer of 16 and a convalescent-phase titer of 28* in anticomplement immunofluorescence tests. Other features of his illness included leukopenia and mucosal candidiasis. His pneumonia responded to a course of intravenous TMP/SMX, but, as of the latest reports, he continues to have a fever each day.

Patient 3: A 30-year-old man was well until January 1981 when he developed esophageal and oral candidiasis that responded to Amphotericin B treatment. He was hospitalized in February 1981 for P. carinii pneumonia that responded to oral TMP/SMX. His esophageal candidiasis recurred after the pneumonia was diagnosed, and he was again given Amphotericin B. The CMV complement-fixation titer in March 1981 was 8. Material from an esophageal biopsy was positive for CMV.

Patient 4: A 29-year-old man developed P. carinii pneumonia in February 1981. He had had Hodgkins disease 3 years earlier, but had been successfully treated with radiation therapy alone. He did not improve after being given intravenous TMP/SMX and corticosteroids and died in March. Postmortem examination showed no evidence of Hodgkins disease, but P. carinii and CMV were found in lung tissue.

Patient 5: A previously healthy 36-year-old man with a clinically diagnosed CMV infection in September 1980 was seen in April 1981 because of a 4-month history of fever, dyspnea, and cough. On admission he was found to have P. carinii pneumonia, oral candidiasis, and CMV retinitis. A complement-fixation CMV titer in April 1981 was 128. The patient has been treated with 2 short courses of TMP/SMX that have been limited because of a sulfa-induced neutropenia. He is being treated for candidiasis with topical nystatin.

The diagnosis of Pneumocystis pneumonia was confirmed for all 5 patients ante-mortem by closed or open lung biopsy. The patients did not know each other and had no known common contacts or knowledge of sexual partners who had had similar illnesses. The 5 did not have comparable histories of sexually transmitted disease. Four had serologic evidence of past hepatitis B infection but had no evidence of current hepatitis B surface antigen. Two of the 5 reported having frequent homosexual contacts with various partners. All 5 reported using inhalant drugs, and 1 reported parenteral drug abuse. Three patients had profoundly depressed in vitro proliferative responses to mitogens and antigens. Lymphocyte studies were not performed on the other 2 patients.

* Paired specimens not run in parallel.

Reported by MS Gottlieb, MD, HM Schanker, MD, PT Fan, MD, A Saxon, MD, JD Weisman, DO, Div of Clinical Immunology-Allergy, Dept of Medicine, UCLA School of Medicine; I Pozalski, MD, Cedars-Mt. Sinai Hospital, Los Angeles; Field Services Div, Epidemiology Program Office, CDC.

Editorial Note

Pneumocystis pneumonia in the United States is almost exclusively limited to severely immunosuppressed patients.[1] The occurrence of pneumocystosis in these 5 previously healthy individuals without a clinically apparent underlying immunodeficiency is unusual. The fact that these patients were all homosexuals suggests an association between some aspect of a homosexual lifestyle or disease acquired through sexual contact and Pneumocystis pneumonia in this population. All 5 patients described in this report had laboratory-confirmed CMV disease or virus shedding within 5 months of the diagnosis of Pneumocystis pneumonia. CMV infection has been shown to induce transient abnormalities of in vitro cellular-immune function in otherwise healthy human hosts.[2,3] Although all 3 patients tested had abnormal cellular-immune function, no definitive conclusion regarding the role of CMV infection in these 5 cases can be reached because of the lack of published data on cellular-immune function in healthy homosexual males with and without CMV antibody. In 1 report, 7 (3.6%) of 194 patients with pneumocystosis also had CMV infection; 40 (21%) of the same group had at least 1 other major concurrent infection.[1] A high prevalence of CMV infections among homosexual males was recently reported: 179 (94%) of 190 males reported to be exclusively homosexual had serum antibody to CMV, and 14 (7.4%) had CMV viruria; rates for 101 controls of similar age who were reported to be exclusively heterosexual were 54% for seropositivity and zero for viruria.[4] In another study of 64 males, 4 (6.3%) had positive tests for CMV in semen, but none had CMV recovered from urine. Two of the 4 reported recent homosexual contacts. These findings suggest not only that virus shedding may be more readily detected in seminal fluid than in urine, but also that seminal fluid may be an important vehicle of CMV transmission.[5]

All the above observations suggest the possibility of a cellular-immune dysfunction related to a common exposure that predisposes individuals to opportunistic infections such as pneumocystosis and candidiasis. Although the role of CMV infection in the pathogenesis of pneumocystosis remains unknown, the possibility of P. carinii infection must be carefully considered in a differential diagnosis for previously healthy homosexual males with dyspnea and pneumonia.

References

1. Walzer PD, Perl DP, Krogstad DJ, Rawson PG, Schultz MG. Pneumocystis carinii pneumonia in the United States. Epidemiologic, diagnostic, and clinical features. Ann Intern Med 1974;80:83-93.

2. Rinaldo CR, Jr, Black PH, Hirsch MS. Interaction of cytomegalovirus with leukocytes from patients with mononucleosis due to cytomegalovirus. J Infect Dis 1977;136:667-78.

3. Rinaldo CR, Jr, Carney WP, Richter BS, Black PH, Hirsch MS. Mechanisms of immunosuppression in cytomegaloviral mononucleosis. J Infect Dis 1980;141:488-95.

4. Drew WL, Mintz L, Miner RC, Sands M, Ketterer B. Prevalence of cytomegalovirus infection in homosexual men. J Infect Dis 1981;143:188-92.

5. Lang DJ, Kummer JF. Cytomegalovirus in semen: observations in selected populations. J Infect Dis 1975;132:472-3.

Editorial Note -- 1996

The June 4, 1981, report of five cases of Pneumocystis carinii pneumonia (PCP) in homosexual men in Los Angeles was the first published report about acquired immunodeficiency syndrome (AIDS). This report in MMWR alerted the medical and public health communities 4 months before the first peer-reviewed article was published.[1]

The timeliness of this report can be credited to the public health sensitivity of the astute reporting physicians and the diligence of CDC staff. Dr. Gottlieb and his colleagues at the University of California at Los Angeles School of Medicine and Cedars-Mt. Sinai Hospital worked closely with the CDC Epidemic Intelligence Service Officer assigned to the Los Angeles Department of Health Services to summarize the data and draft this brief report. When news of these cases reached CDC, scientists in the Parasitic Diseases Division of CDC's Center for Infectious Diseases already were concerned about other unusual cases of PCP. That division housed the Parasitic Diseases Drug Service and requests for pentamidine isethionate to treat PCP in other similar patients in New York had been called to the attention of these scientists by the CDC employee who administered the distribution of this drug (which was not yet licensed and was available in the United States only from CDC).

In July 1981, following the report of these cases of PCP and cases of other rare life-threatening opportunistic infections and cancers,[2] CDC formed a Task Force on Kaposi's Sarcoma and Opportunistic Infections. A key first task facing CDC was to develop a case definition for this condition and to conduct surveillance. The CDC case definition was adopted quickly worldwide. Results from active surveillance conducted in the United States rapidly established that the syndrome was new, and the number of cases was increasing rapidly.[3] By the end of 1982, the distribution pattern of cases strongly suggested that AIDS was caused by an agent transmitted through sexual contact between men[4,5] and between men and women[6,7] and transmitted through blood among injecting-drug users and among recipients of blood or blood products.[8-10] Cases also were identified among infants born to women with AIDS or at risk for AIDS,[11] and the epidemic extended beyond the life-threatening reported cases to include persistent unexplained lymphadenopathy.[12]

To prevent transmission of AIDS, in 1983 the Public Health Service used epidemiologic information about the condition to recommend that sexual contact be avoided with persons known or suspected to have AIDS and that persons at increased risk for AIDS refrain from donating plasma or blood.[10,13] In addition, work was intensified toward developing safer blood products for persons with hemophilia. These recommendations were developed and published only 21 months after the first cases were reported and well before the first published reports identifying what is now termed HIV as the etiologic agent of AIDS.[14,15] Isolation of HIV enabled development of assays to diagnose infections; characterization of the natural history of HIV; further protection of the blood supply; development of specific antiviral therapies; and expansion of surveillance criteria to include other conditions indicative of severe HIV disease. Research and prevention programs for HIV have contributed greatly to scientific and programmatic approaches to other public health problems.

During 1981-1996, approximately 350 reports related to AIDS were published in MMWR, an average of two per month since June 1981. Throughout the HIV epidemic, timely publication of reports about AIDS and related topics in MMWR have continued to play a crucial role in alerting health professionals and the public.

In 1996, HIV transmission occurs worldwide and has an impact in all countries.[16] In the United States, prevention efforts have been successful at reducing HIV transmission. For example, blood-donor deferral and blood screening have virtually eliminated HIV transmission through blood and blood products, and adoption of less risky behaviors has greatly reduced sexual transmission between men; most recently, therapeutic advances have reduced transmission from mother to newborn.[17] However, in the United States, AIDS has been diagnosed in 548,000 persons, and 343,000 have died. HIV infection has become the leading cause of death for persons aged 25-44 years, and an estimated 650,000-950,000 persons are living with HIV infection. Throughout the world, HIV continues to spread rapidly, especially in impoverished populations in Africa, Asia, and South and Central America. The emergence of the HIV pandemic demonstrates the vulnerability of the world's populations to previously unknown infectious diseases.

The first 15 years in the recorded history of AIDS have included remarkable scientific successes and countless examples of individual courage and accomplishment. Although these accomplishments provide hope for the future, further efforts are needed to halt the steady spread of HIV throughout the world.

Editorial Note by: James W. Curran, M.D., Dean, Rollins School of Public Health of Emory University (Atlanta); Coordinator of the 1981 Task Force on Kaposi's Sarcoma and Opportunistic Infections; and former Director of the Office of HIV/AIDS, CDC.

References

1. *Hymes KB, Cheung T, Greene JB, et al. Kaposi's sarcoma in homosexual men: a report of eight cases. Lancet 1981;2:598-600.*

2. *CDC. Kaposi's sarcoma and Pneumocystis pneumonia among homosexual men -- New York City and California. MMWR 1981;30:305-8.*

3. *CDC Task Force on Kaposi's Sarcoma and Opportunistic Infections. Epidemiologic aspects of the current outbreak of Kaposi's sarcoma and opportunistic infections. N Engl J Med 1982;306:248-52.*

4. *CDC. A cluster of Kaposi's sarcoma and Pneumocystis carinii pneumonia among homosexual male residents of Los Angeles and Orange counties, California. MMWR 1982;31:305-7.*

5. *Jaffe HW, Choi K, Thomas PA, et al. National case-control study of Kaposi's sarcoma and Pneumocystis carinii pneumonia in homosexual men: part 1, epidemiologic results. Ann Intern Med 1983;99:145-51.*

6. *CDC. Immunodeficiency among female sexual partners of males with acquired immune deficiency syndrome (AIDS) -- New York. MMWR 1983;31:697-8.*

7. *Harris C, Small CB, Klein RS, et al. Immunodeficiency in female sexual partners of men with the acquired immunodeficiency syndrome. N Engl J Med 1983;308:1181-4.*

8. *CDC. Pneumocystis carinii pneumonia among persons with hemophilia A. MMWR 1982;31:365-7.*

9. *CDC. Possible transfusion-associated acquired immune deficiency syndrome (AIDS) -- California. MMWR 1982;31:652-54.*

10. *CDC. Acquired immune deficiency syndrome (AIDS): precautions for clinical and laboratory staffs. MMWR 1982;31:577-80.*

11. *CDC. Unexplained immunodeficiency and opportunistic infections in infants -- New York, New Jersey, and California. MMWR 1982;31:665-7.*

12. CDC. Persistent, generalized lymphadenopathy among homosexual males. MMWR 1982;31: 249-51.

13. CDC. Prevention of acquired immune deficiency syndrome (AIDS): report of inter-agency recommendations. MMWR 1983;32:101-3.

14. Barre-Sinoussi F, Chermann JC, Rey F, et al. Isolation of a T-lymphotropic retrovirus from a patient at risk for acquired immune deficiency syndrome (AIDS). Science 1983;220:868-71.

15. Gallo RC, Salahuddin SZ, Popovic M, et al. Frequent detection and isolation of cytopathic retroviruses (HTLV-III) from patients with AIDS and at risk for AIDS. Science 1984;224:500-3.

16. Mann J, Tarantela D, eds. AIDS in the world II. New York: Oxford University Press, 1996.

17. CDC. Recommendations of the U.S. Public Health Service Task Force on the Use of Zidovudine to Reduce Perinatal Transmission of Human Immunodeficiency Virus. MMWR 1994;43(no. RR-11).

This brief and informative article was the first published report describing acquired immunodeficiency syndrome, and it appeared four full months before the first large-scale observational study. It alerted the public health and medical communities about this unusual cluster of opportunistic infections in previously healthy young men, and played a crucial role in mounting the health care community's response to the crisis posed by the disease. It has since become a classic in the medical literature. Even though its ability to demonstrate a link between cause and effect is relatively weaker, we can see in this example how case reports can suggest future hypotheses to be tested and directions to be explored in subsequent studies.

The next example is a case report from Japan, which details an adverse event following a shiatsu massage:

Internal Jugular Vein Thrombosis Associated with Shiatsu Massage of the Neck

Y Wada, C Yanagihara, Y Nishimura Department of Neurology, Nishi-Kobe Medical Center, Hyogo, Japan

Journal of Neurology Neurosurgery and Psychiatry 2005;76:142-143
© 2005 BMJ Publishing Group Ltd

Keywords: internal jugular vein thrombosis; shiatsu massage

Thrombosis of the internal jugular vein is a relatively rare condition that can be induced by a variety of mechanical injuries.[1,2] Acupressure, or "shiatsu", is an oriental massage technique and many acupoints on the body surface, known as "tsubos", are used for shiatsu. Shiatsu of tsubos in the nape of the neck is known to improve tension headache due to neck and shoulder aches. However, we recently came across a case of internal jugular vein (IJV) and cerebral sinus thrombosis after shiatsu massage of the neck.

Case Report

A 35 year old man, a non-smoker, was suffering from a stiff neck. He consulted a shiatsu masseur, who performed shiatsu massage on the right side of his neck and right shoulder for 30 minutes. Immediately after the shiatsu massage, the patient noticed pain and swelling of the right side of the neck, both of which subsided within seven days. Two days after the shiatsu massage, he developed a severe, constant right occipital headache and consulted his attending physician. His cervical radiograph was normal. The patient continued to have severe headache, however, and on the seventh day after the massage, he developed blurred vision. On the twentieth day, he developed weakness and paraesthesia of his right arm and leg, and mild agraphia for kanji characters. When he also developed focal motor seizure, he was admitted to our hospital. He underwent a neurological examination on the twenty-third day after the shiatsu massage.

The patient did not have any history of recent trauma, dental procedures, or upper respiratory infection. There was no history of any other relevant medication including homoeopathic or herbal medicines, or pathologic conditions. There was no family history of premature stroke or thrombotic events.

Physical examination was normal and no neck mass was detected. On neurological examination, he showed normal consciousness and orientation. Funduscopic examination revealed bilateral papilloedema without haemorrhage, but the remaining cranial nerves were intact. He had mild muscle weakness and sensory deficit in the right arm and leg. Ataxia was not detected in any of the limbs and trunk. Mild agraphia for kanji characters was observed.

Laboratory analysis showed prothrombin time, partial thromboplastin time, antithrombin III, protein C, and protein S were normal, but values for anticardiolipin antibody IgG and lupus anticoagulant were negative. Plasma homocysteine was within normal limits. Autoantibodies and cryoglobulins were absent. No evidence of any systemic disease was found on investigation. Cerebrospinal fluid was clear without pleocytosis, but the cerebrospinal fluid pressure was 350 mm H_2O.

Magnetic resonance imaging (MRI) scan of the brain showed infarction with haemorrhage in the left parietal lobe and an area of increased signal intensity in the area of the right transverse and superior sagittal sinuses (Figure 1). In addition, MRI of the neck with and without enhancement revealed thrombosis of the right IJV, starting from the junction with the right subclavian vein (see Figure 1). However, there were no structural abnormalities adjacent to the right IJV, and the carotid arteries were normal. Digital subtraction venous angiography confirmed extensive thrombosis in the right IJV, the right sigmoid sinus, the right transverse sinus, and the superior sagittal sinus (see Figure 1). The rest of the intracranial dural sinuses were patent, and no vascular malformation was detected.

Phenytoin and valproic acid were promptly administered resulting in improvement in the patient's focal motor seizures. He was also given heparin and warfarin and the intracranial hypertension was treated with a lumboperitoneal shunt. The headache and papilloedema slowly improved over the next three weeks, after which the patient was discharged. Neurological examinations over the past several months have revealed only mild clumsiness and paraesthesia of his right hand and leg.

Discussion

Our patient started complaining of a swelling and pain in the right side of the neck immediately after the shiatsu massage of the neck. Subsequently, over a period of about a month, he developed progressive headache, right extremity paralysis, papilloedema, and partial seizures. Although it may be coincidental, the possibility of a causal link between the shiatsu massage and IJV thrombosis is supported by the patient's claim of a massage induced swelling and pain in his neck, and by the temporal relation between the massage and the onset of symptoms that progressed to IJV and cerebral venous sinus thrombosis.

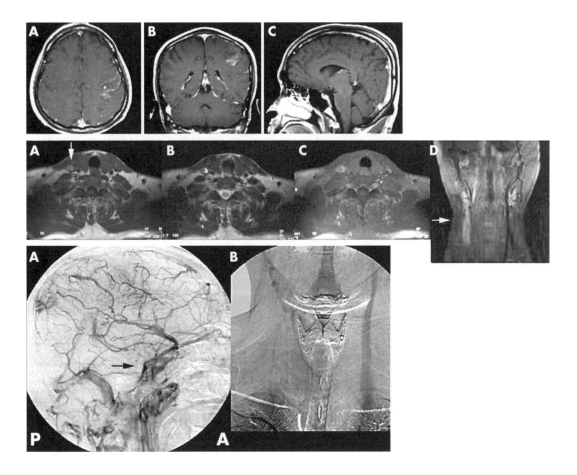

Figure 1 *Top panel: post enhancement T1-weighted magnetic resonance (MR) image of the head (A) axial, (B) coronal, and (C) sagittal. (A) and (B) show the left parietal haemorrhagic infarct. The superior sagittal sinus and right transverse sinus show high intensity signal within the lumen instead of the normal "flow void", indicating thrombosis. Middle panel: MR image of the neck (A) T1-weighted, (B) T2-weighted, (C) post enhancement T1-weighted, and (D) coronal T2-weighted showing right internal jugular vein thrombosis without other structural abnormalities (arrows). Bottom panel: digital subtraction angiogram (A) lateral view of the head during the early venous phase of right carotid digital subtraction angiography confirms the non-opacification of the superior sagittal sinus, the deep cerebral venous system and the transverse sinuses. The predominant venous drainage is via the sphenoparietal sinus (arrow). (B) Anteroposterior view of the neck—the right jugular vein had an area of obstruction at its junction with the right subclavian vein.*

It is difficult to determine the exact mechanism of the IJV thrombosis in our patient. One possibility is that direct trauma or pressure may have induced both venous stasis and vascular injury during the shiatsu massage. The other possibility is that extrinsic compression of the IJV by tissue swelling subsequent to trauma during the shiatsu massage may have induced venous stasis, resulting in thrombosis at this unusual site.

Various forms of trauma have been reported in association with IJV thrombosis, such as jugular thrombosis after catheterisation[1] and Glisson traction for the neck.[2] To the best of our knowledge, IJV and cerebral venous sinus thrombosis possibly caused by shiatsu massage has not been previously reported. Our case may thus represent a newly identified traumatic aetiology.

Chiropractice is a popular alternative therapy in Western countries, and there are several reports of a relation between chiropractic manipulation and stroke.[3] Shiatsu massage, an oriental technique of massage, is a popular alternative therapy in Japan and other Asian countries. Recently this therapy, including the use of a mechanical shiatsu-type massager, is becoming increasingly popular in Western countries. In addition, it is generally accepted that this technique is risk free. However, there are two other reports of vascular complications following shiatsu massage in the literature.[4,5] Tsuboi[4] reported a case of retinal and cerebral artery embolism directly caused by shiatsu massage of the neck. Elliott and Taylor[5] also reported two cases of carotid dissection that occurred after use of a shiatsu-type massaging machine. We would therefore like to draw attention to the possibility that shiatsu massage of the neck may cause serious neurological complications.

References

1. *Larkey D, Williams CR, Fanning J, et al. Fatal superior sagittal sinus thrombosis associated with internal jugular vein catheterization. Am J Obstet Gynecol 1993;169:1612–14.*

2. *Simmers TA, Bekkenk MW, Vidakovic-Vukic M. Internal jugular vein thrombosis after cervical traction. J Intern Med 1997;241:333–5.*

3. *Peters M, Bohl J, Thomke F, et al. Dissection of the internal carotid artery after chiropractic manipulation of the neck. Neurology 1995;45:2284–6.*

4. *Tsuboi K. Retinal and cerebral artery embolism after "shiatsu" on the neck. Stroke 2001;32:2441.*

5. *Elliott MA, Taylor LP. "Shiatsu" sympathectomy ICA dissection associated with a shiatsu massager. Neurology 2002;58:1302–4.*

Notice that only relevant details are included in the description of the case, and that the discussion contains both a review of the literature and a suggestion that the events described represent a potentially new source of trauma. This case report also illustrates the need for informed consent of the patient or client whose case is being reported upon, and the value of supporting documentation such as photographs, imaging, or results of other clinical tests as part of the data presented. Note that although the temporal proximity of symptom onset relative to exposure is suggestive, it is not conclusive and would need more data to determine whether a cause-and-effect relationship does in fact exist between the shiatsu treatment and the client's vascular and neurological problems.

Case Report and Case Study Design

There are two basic ways to approach the design of case reports and studies:

1. the **retrospective case report**, which makes use of existing data that has already been observed and recorded

2. the **prospective case report**, in which data is collected in order to meet a research objective or answer a specific research question

An example of a retrospective case report follows. In it, the author reports an unusual event, reviews the related literature in some detail, and discusses the implications of this individual case.

Long-term Survival of a Patient With Widespread Metastases
From Epithelial Ovarian Carcinoma Receiving Mind-Body
Therapies: Case Report and Review of the Literature

Shahar Lev-ari, MSc, LLb, Yair Maimon, OMD, and Neora Yaal-Hahoshen, MD

SL-a and YM are in the Unit of Complementary Medicine and NY-H is in the Department of Oncology, Tel Aviv Sourasky Medical Center, affiliated with the Sackler Faculty of Medicine, Tel Aviv University, Tel Aviv, Israel.

Integrative Cancer Therapies, Vol. 5, No. 4, 395-399 (2006)
DOI: 10.1177/1534735406294221 © 2006 SAGE Publications

Five-year survival of patients with stage IV epithelial ovarian carcinoma not treated after recurrence is almost nonexistent in oncological literature. The authors report a patient almost 30 years after surgery of the primary epithelial ovarian carcinoma lesion and 15 years after recurrent disease and incomplete chemotherapy who is alive without evidence of disease. She received no conventional oncological therapy during the past 15 years but rather used many types of alternative medicine, predominantly mind-body therapies. The authors review the relevant literature on this subject and describe what they believe to be the first report of long-term survival of such a patient.

Keywords: *epithelial ovarian carcinoma; metastases; long-term survival; complementary and alternative medicine (CAM); mind-body therapy*

Epithelial ovarian carcinoma (EOC) represents a clinically significant health problem in Western countries, ranking fifth highest in cancer incidence and fourth highest in site-specific causes of cancer deaths in women. In the United States, approximately 25,000 new ovarian cancer cases and 16,000 ovarian cancer deaths were expected in 2004.[1] Although ovarian cancer is potentially curable by surgery and chemotherapy, most cases are still diagnosed at advanced stages, and the 5-year overall survival of stage IV patients with recurrent disease not treated by chemotherapy is almost nonexistent.

Case Report

A 20-year-old woman presented with vomiting and fullness in the abdomen after slight fever several days before presentation in March 1975. An abdominal puncture yielded almost 6 L of hemorrhagical fluid. Physical examination revealed enlarged lymph nodes on the left supraclavicular area and in both axillae.

At that time, a biopsy from the left supraclavicular area revealed a mucoid adenocarcinoma. Chest x-ray showed a small amount of fluid in the left pleura. X-rays of the upper gastrointestinal (GI) tract were normal. She underwent laparotomy, during which a mass was found adjacent to the uterus, and a primary ovarian tumor was suspected. After reviewing the pathological slides, it was decided that the primary lesion was probably in the GI tract. Chemotherapy with 5-FU was started and continued for 5 months, and a clinical complete response was achieved. In September 1975, an enlarged lymph node in the left axilla reappeared while the patient was still on chemotherapy. Cyclophosphamide was added to the 5-FU, and there was a second complete clinical remission after 4 months of this treatment. She continued to receive the combined chemotherapy for an additional month. The ascites reappeared in June 1977, and she received for 6 months a course of adriamycin, but only a partial response was achieved. The abdominal disease progressed, and in May 1978, she was given a combination of methotrexate, cyclophosphamide, vincristine, and prednisone, which led to a partial remission. In August 1978, 2 masses were palpated in the pelvis, and the patient underwent a total abdominal hysterectomy (TAH) and bilateral salpingooophorectomy (BSO). Pathology revealed a well-differentiated adenocarcinoma in both ovaries with cytological positive ascites. At that time, chemotherapy with cisplatinum was offered to the patient, but she refused it and any other conventional treatment after having been told by her oncologist that her life expectancy was estimated as being about 3 months.

The patient was essentially asymptomatic until the end of 1991, when a subcutaneous mass, about 2 cm in diameter, was detected in the lower right abdomen. The fine-needle aspiration biopsy results were compatible with ovarian carcinoma. Other tests including blood biochemistry, tumor markers, and chest and abdomen computerized tomographic scans were normal. In December 1991, the patient underwent a wide resection of this abdominal mass. Laparoscopy revealed 3 small (<5 mm each) peritoneal nodules, and pathological examination showed malignant cells in 2 of them. She refused to undergo the recommended platinum-based chemotherapy and embarked on intensive use of many types of mind-body therapies, predominantly the Reich technique and dance therapy.

Currently, almost 27 years later, the patient is well and free of symptoms and any clinical sign of cancer.

Discussion

We describe a very young patient who essentially failed several lines of chemotherapy for an apparent primary ovarian malignancy and who, 27 years after abdominal surgery *without any adjuvant chemotherapy, is alive and clinically free of disease. She had undergone TAH + BSO, which would be considered as being inadequate surgery according to current standard guidelines of treatment. In addition, she did not receive any oncological therapy despite having laparotomy-positive ascites.*

This case represents a very rare outcome in the oncological literature. In a review of 192 patients[2] with stage IV EOC as defined in 1985 by the International Federation of Gynecology and Obstetrics, the 5-year survival rate was 7.6%, with only 6 patients surviving more than 5 years. In that report, 25 patients (14.8%) were left with only microscopic residual disease or less than 2 cm of macroscopic residual disease, 13 were disease free after surgery (2 became long-term survivors), 13 had residual disease less than 2 cm (1 survived long term), and 12 had residual disease greater than 2 cm after interval debulking surgery. The median progression-free survival was 7.1 months, and the median overall survival was 13.4 months. Univariate and multivariate analysis showed that the parameters associated with a shorter survival time were visceral involvement (lung or liver) and diagnosis before 1984. Six patients (age range, 41-54 years) survived more than 5 years: all of them received platinum-containing regimens.

In another recent published analysis,[3] the authors described long-term survival in patients with stage III to IV ovarian cancer treated about the same time as our patient but with very good conventional therapy (platinum-including chemotherapy or whole abdominal radiation). Overall survival of their patients was 21% at 5 years, 13.5% at 10 years, and 12% at 15 years. The important prognostic factors for long-term survival were disease-free or minimal residual disease (a single remaining deposit < 2 cm) at initial surgery with tumor grade 1 and good performance status. Compared with the normal population (1995 data), the ratio of observed to expected deaths after the start of chemotherapy at 5 years was 14.1 (P < .001), 4.9 at 9 to 10 years (P = .0033), dropping to 2.75 at 11 to 15 years (P = .090). In this study, patients with advanced cancer of the ovary who survive 11 years or longer have a life expectancy that is very similar to that of the normal population of women of the same age.

In another recent large population-based study,[4] survival following ovarian cancer was poor, with only 33% of women surviving 5 years. Stage was the strongest predictor of survival, and women diagnosed with stage III or IV disease had 5-year survival estimates of 28% and 10%, respectively, similar to figures in other reports.[5,6] Having either poorly differentiated tumors or unknown grade tumors was associated with decreased survival, and this effect held after controlling for multiple factors including stage. The impact of grade on survival remains inconsistent, however, with several studies having reported that the influence of grade on survival disappears in multivariate analysis.[7-9]

Kosary examined more than 21,000 cases reported to Surveillance, Epidemiology, and End Results between 1973 and 1987 and found that after adjusting for multiple factors, the relative risk of death increased significantly by 24% for moderately differentiated cases and by 104% for poorly differentiated cases, compared to well-differentiated cases.[9] It may be that the smaller studies lacked the statistical power to identify any significant effect of grade. As with grade, the impact of histology on survival is inconclusive in the published literature. In Kosary's study, only clear cell histology differed significantly from the reference group of endometrioid histology. Adjusting for stage, chemotherapy, and comorbidity considerably decreased the risk of death associated with being 75 years or older, but elderly women still had twice the risk of dying from ovarian cancer compared to young women. Similar to stage, the prognostic importance of age is well known, with the risk of death from ovarian carcinoma highest in elderly patients. The distribution of chemotherapy by grade mirrored that of stage: 74% of women with well-differentiated disease were treated compared to 80% to 89% of women with other grades. Chemotherapy was associated with improved survival in women with advanced-stage disease but not for those with early stage disease. According to Kosary's findings, advanced age continues to be associated with decreased survival even with consideration of treatment and comorbid illness. Moreover, women with comorbid conditions were at 1.4 times the risk of death compared with women with no other health conditions. The results of that study also suggest that there may be major regional differences in cancer survival. American and European studies of survival trends have shown an increase in survival for younger but not older women, from the 1970s to the 1990s. Regional variation has been previously reported in a study of US mortality trends, different health services, or Northern European ancestry.[6] Regional differences were also reported in a EUROCARE study of 17 European countries, with women in Eastern European countries having markedly decreased rates of survival.

Complementary and alternative medicine (CAM) is becoming increasingly popular, particularly among patients with cancer. Ernst and Cassileth systematically reviewed the use of CAM among cancer patients as reported in 26 studies from 13 countries.[10] The average rate of CAM use was 31.4%, with rates ranging from 7% to 64%. Higher rates of CAM use were reported by women with gynecological and/or breast malignancies.[11,12]

CAM encompasses a wide range of treatment modalities, which the National Center for Complementary and Alternative Medicine (NCCAM)[13] classifies into 5 categories:

1. alternative medical systems, which are whole medical systems that are built on complete systems of theory and practice (e.g., homeopathic, naturopathic, and traditional Chinese medicine);

2. mind-body interventions, which include a variety of techniques designed to enhance the mind's capacity to affect bodily function and symptoms (e.g., meditation, prayer, mental healing, and art therapy);

3. biologically based therapies, which include biological substances found in nature (such as herbs, foods, and vitamins);

4. manipulative and body-based methods, including manipulation and/or movement techniques of 1 or more parts of the body (e.g., chiropractic, osteopathic manipulation, and massage); and

5. energy therapies, intended to affect energy fields that allegedly surround and penetrate the human body by applying pressure and/or manipulating the body through these fields (examples include qi gong, Reiki, and Therapeutic Touch).

The objectives of CAM treatments are diverse and include reduction of radiochemotherapy associated toxicity, improvement of cancer-related symptoms, enhancing of the immune system, and even direct antineoplastic effects.[14] Recent clinical trials have generated data on the efficacy of CAM mainly in improvement of chemotherapy-associated toxicity and cancer-related symptoms, but evidence-based data on the effect of most CAM modalities on disease recurrence and survival are lacking.[15,16] Application of CAM-based approaches was reported as being beneficial in cancer patients in chemotherapy-associated nausea and vomiting,[17] pain,[18] fatigue,[19] relaxation,[20,21] and anxiety and mood disturbances (for a review, see Deng and Cassileth[22]). Furthermore, prominent cancer centers, such as M.D. Anderson (Houston, Tex), Dana-Farber (Boston, Mass), and Memorial Sloan Kettering (New York, NY), currently employ protocols that integrate conventional and complementary medicine for oncological patients.

The patient reported in this article made intensive use of mind-body modalities, predominantly the Reich technique and dance therapy.

According to the NCCAM, mind-body medicine focuses "on the interactions among the brain, mind, body, and behavior, and the powerful ways in which emotional, mental, social, spiritual, and behavioral factors can directly affect health."[13] Mind-body interventions constitute more than 30% of the adult US population's use of CAM.[23] Evidence from multiple studies with various types of cancer patients suggests that mind-body interventions can reduce pain and improve quality of life.[24-26] Several mind-body therapies were also reported to enhance the immune system.[27-29]

Reichian therapy[30] is an original body-oriented psychotherapy, developed by the Austrian psychoanalyst Dr Wilhelm Reich, who worked closely with Sigmund Freud. He employed many Freudian concepts in his work, but unlike Freud, he applied mainly body work and breathing techniques in his therapies. Reich described the tendency of the body to hold on to emotional and psychological stress as "armoring." Reich believed that physical armor develops from the chronic tightening of the muscles of the body to prevent the expression of the emotion that is being suppressed and prohibited. For example, a stiff neck can be due to the tightening of the neck muscles that prevents the patient from freely expressing the words or emotions (such as crying) that he or she does not allow himself or herself to express. Breathing work, deep tissue massage, and communication can be used for an emotional release.

The use of dance in the context of healing has been reported in ancient societies in which dance was used in spiritual growth and healing rituals.[31] Dance therapy is described by the American Cancer Society[32] as "therapeutic use of movement to improve the mental and physical well being of a person which focuses on the connection between the mind and body to promote health and healing." It was proposed by several authors that dance therapy may enhance the healing process by helping to (1) develop positive body image and self-esteem; (2) decrease stress, anxiety, and depression; (3) reduce chronic pain and body tension; (4) decrease isolation, increase communication skills, and enhance interpersonal interaction; and (5) encourage a sense of well-being and completeness.[33,34] Several nonrandomized small trials have shown a benefit for dance therapy in psychological and spiritual adaptation[35,36] to breast cancer. Sandel et al[37] recently assessed the efficacy effect of a dance and movement program on quality of life and shoulder function in breast cancer survivors treated within the preceding 5 years. Thirty-five women completed a 12-week intervention, using the Lebed method, which focuses on healing through movement and dance. The study design was a randomized controlled crossover trial, and the analysis of the results showed that breast cancer quality of life was significantly improved in the intervention group compared to the control group.

We are not aware of any published report on long-term, disease-free survival of a patient with stage IV ovarian cancer and recurrent disease not treated by aggressive chemotherapy after surgery. The patient we describe is now 27 years after first diagnosis and recurrences and remains clinically free of disease. Based on this report and the data in the literature, we recommend further scientific research to assess the efficacy of CAM modalities for patients with cancer.

References

1. Jemal A, Tiwari RC, Murray T, et al. Cancer statistics, 2004. CA Cancer J Clin. 2004;54:8-29.

2. Bonnefoi H, A'Hern RP, Fisher C, et al. Natural history of stage IV epithelial ovarian cancer. J Clin Oncol. 1999;17:767-775.

3. Lambert HE, Gregory WM, Nelstrop AE, Rustin GJS. Long-term survival in 463 women treated with platinum analogs for advanced epithelial carcinoma of the ovary: life

Making Sense of Research

expectancy compared to women of an age-matched normal population. *Int J Gynecol Cancer.* 2004;14:772-778.

4. O'Malley CD, Cress RD, Campleman SL, Leiserowitz GS. Survival of Californian women with epithelial ovarian cancer, 1994-1996: a population-based study. *Gynecol Oncol.* 2003;91: 608-615.

5. Venesmaa P. Epithelial ovarian cancer: impact of surgery and chemotherapy on survival during 1977-1990. *Obstet Gynecol.* 1994;84:8-11.

6. Balli S, Fey MF, Hanggi W, et al. Ovarian cancer: an institutional review of patterns of care, health insurance and prognosis. *Eur J Cancer.* 2000;36:2061-2068.

7. Scholz HS, Benedicic C, Haas J, Tamussino K, Petru E. Stage IV ovarian cancer: prognostic factors and survival beyond 5 years. *Anticancer Res.* 2001;21:3729-3732.

8. Markman M, Lewis JL Jr, Saigo P, et al. Epithelial ovarian cancer in the elderly. The Memorial Sloan–Kettering Cancer Center experience. *Cancer.* 1993;71:634-637.

9. Kosary CL. FIGO stage, histology, histologic grade, age and race as prognostic factors in determining survival for cancers of the female gynecological system: an analysis of 1973-87 SEER cases of cancers of the endometrium, cervix, ovary, vulva, and vagina. *Semin Surg Oncol.* 1994;10:31-46.

10. Ernst E, Cassileth BR. The prevalence of complementary/alternative medicine in cancer: a systematic review. *Cancer.* 1998;83:777-782.

11. Navo MA, Phan J, Vaughan C, et al. An assessment of the utilization of complementary and alternative medication in women with gynecologic or breast malignancies. *J Clin Oncol.* 2004;22:671-677.

12. Shen J, Andersen R, Albert PS, et al. Use of complementary/alternative therapies by women with advanced-stage breast cancer. *BMC Complement Altern Med.* 2002;2:8.

13. National Center for Complementary and Alternative Medicine. Available at: http://nccam.nih.gov/.

14. Vickers AJ, Cassileth BR. Unconventional therapies for cancer and cancer-related symptoms. *Lancet Oncol.* 2001;2:226-232.

15. Deng G, Cassileth BR, Yeung KS. Complementary therapies for cancer-related symptoms. *J Support Oncol.* 2004;2:419-429.

16. Cassileth BR, Deng G. Complementary and alternative therapies for cancer. *Oncologist.* 2004;9:80-89.

17. NIH Consensus Development Panel on Acupuncture. *JAMA.* 1998;280:1518-1524.

18. Sellick SM, Zaza C. Critical review of 5 nonpharmacologic strategies for managing cancer pain. *Cancer Prev Control.* 1998;2:7-14.

19. Vickers AJ, Straus DJ, Fearon B, Cassileth BR. *Acupuncture for postchemotherapy fatigue: a phase II study. J Clin Oncol. 2004;22:1731-1735.*

20. Bindemann S, Soukop M, Kaye SB. *Randomised controlled study of relaxation training. Eur J Cancer. 1991;27:170-174.*

21. Bridge LR, Benson P, Pietroni PC, Priest RG. *Relaxation and imagery in the treatment of breast cancer. Br Med J. 1988;297: 1169-1172.*

22. Deng G, Cassileth B. *Integrative oncology: complementary therapies for pain, anxiety, and mood disturbance. CA Cancer J Clin. 2005;55:109-116.*

23. Wolsko PM, Eisenberg DM, Davis RB, Phillips RS. *Use of mind-body medical therapies. J Gen Intern Med. 2004;19:43-50.*

24. Mundy EA, DuHamel KN, Montgomery GH. *The efficacy of behavioral interventions for cancer treatment-related side effects. Semin Clin Neuropsychiatry. 2003;8:253-275.*

25. Sloman R, Brown P, Aldana E, Chee E. *The use of relaxation for the promotion of comfort and pain relief in persons with advanced cancer. Contemp Nurse. 1994;3:6-12.*

26. Syrjala KL, Donaldson GW, Davis MW, Kippes ME, Carr JE. *Relaxation and imagery and cognitive-behavioral training reduce pain during cancer treatment: a controlled clinical trial. Pain. 1995;63:189-198.*

27. Irwin MR, Pike JL, Cole JC, Oxman MN. *Effects of a behavioral intervention, Tai Chi Chih, on varicella-zoster virus specific immunity and health functioning in older adults. Psychosom Med. 2003;65:824-830.*

28. Kiecolt-Glaser JK, Marucha PT, Atkinson C, Glaser R. *Hypnosis as a modulator of cellular immune dysregulation during acute stress. J Consult Clin Psychol. 2001;69:674-682.*

29. Collins MP, Dunn LF. *The effects of meditation and visual imagery on an immune system disorder: dermatomyositis. J Altern Complement Med. 2005;11:275-284.*

30. *The Institute for Orgonomic Science. Available at: http://www.orgonomicscience.org/.*

31. Levy F. *Dance/Movement Therapy: A Healing Art. Reston, Va: American Alliance for Health, Physical Education, Recreation and Dance; 1988*

32. *American Cancer Society. Available at: http://www.cancer.org.*

33. Hanna JL. *The power of dance: health and healing. J Altern Complement Med. 1995;1:323-331.*

34. Cassileth B. *The Alternative Medicine Handbook. New York, NY: W. W. Norton & Co; 1998.*

35. Serlin I. *Arts medicine: dance movement therapy for women with breast cancer. Conscious Res Abst. 1996:153-154.*

36. Dibbel-Hope S. *The use of dance/movement therapy in psychological adaptation to breast cancer. Arts Psychother. 2000;27:51-68.*

37. Sandel SL, Judge JO, Landry N, Faria L, Ouellette R, Majczak M. *Dance and movement program improves quality-of-life measures in breast cancer survivors. Cancer Nurs.* 2005;28:301-309.

What makes this study unusual is not the patient's original diagnosis and treatment, which is described in retrospect, but the rare outcome – she has survived her original diagnosis much longer than expected and is now apparently well and free of disease. The authors believe this to be the first such example of someone living for such an extended period of time with stage IV ovarian carcinoma without receiving conventional oncology treatments. This study is an interesting example of the reporting of anomalous data. The implication for practitioners is that although quite unusual, such an apparent spontaneous recovery is indeed possible. The patient's report of the use of mind-body therapies and attribution of her remission to these is certainly out of the ordinary and does not constitute evidence of a cause-and-effect relationship between the two. It does however suggest a remarkable area for further exploration, and could be considered what Karl Popper referred to as a "black swan" in reference to his concept of falsification. He argued that if a researcher proposes that all swans are white, the observation of even a single black swan then disproves that hypothesis.

Prospective Case Report Designs

Prospective case reports or studies can employ a quantitative, qualitative, or mixed methods approach, which involves incorporating quantitative and qualitative data as discussed in the previous chapter. Many prospective case studies employ what is in essence the before-and-after treatment design with a single patient or client. In this design, a research objective or question of interest is determined and/or a suitable client or patient is located – either may occur first. After reviewing the relevant literature and refining the research question, a methodological approach is chosen, inclusion/exclusion criteria are defined, an appropriate outcome measure (or measures) is selected, and plans for data analysis are decided upon in advance. Informed consent for participation is then obtained, the data is collected pre- and post-treatment, and then it is analyzed. The same process can be used with a consecutive or sequential series of patients to create a case series. The weakness of this design from a cause-and-effect perspective is that there is no control group for comparison. Uncontrolled studies tend to overestimate treatment effect size, as has been noted in preceding chapters. The strength of the design is often in its description of the client's condition and the treatment.

The same process, with some modification, can also be used to compare a treatment under evaluation with usual care or with no treatment. First the outcome of interest is measured during a short period of usual care or no treatment. A **wash-out period** may be necessary if usual care is discontinued, so that any effects can dissipate, and then the treatment under investigation is introduced and continued for some amount of time, and the outcome is again measured at the end of the treatment or at regular intervals. The design can be abbreviated as A-B – condition A (usual care/no treatment) followed by condition B (treatment intervention).

For example, imagine that we wish to compare acupressure to an over-the-counter NSAID for arthritic knee pain, and that our research question is whether one treatment is more effective than the other. (We could also ask a slightly different question: whether acupressure in conjunction with the NSAID confers additional benefits compared to the NSAID alone; in this case, the client would continue to take the NSAID throughout.) We recruit a suitable client who has been using an NSAID for some time but reports insufficient relief and who consents to participate. The client would rate the knee pain at baseline and continue to keep regular daily ratings for a short period of time while discontinuing the OTC medication. Then acupressure treatment would be introduced, and again daily pain ratings would be kept for the duration of the treatment intervention.

A further refinement is to reintroduce the original condition, following a wash-out period, by reinstating the medication and withdrawing the treatment, in this case the acupressure. This design is abbreviated A-B-A. After the acupressure treatment was completed, the client would go back to using the NSAID alone and keep up the daily pain ratings. An observed pattern of no change or worsening of symptoms during condition A, followed by an improvement during the treatment to be evaluated (condition B), again followed by a worsening of the symptoms when it is removed (back to condition A) is suggestive of an effect.

A treatment that is highly effective or curative will not show a worsening of symptoms once it is removed, but in this example neither treatment will permanently repair the cartilage in the osteoarthritic joint, so such a results pattern would indicate that the acupressure provides more effective symptom relief for this individual. It is important to observe that in this design, however, expectation cannot be completely ruled out as an alternate explanation, because neither the client nor the practitioner is blinded. Variations on this type of single subject design using random assignment to treatment and blinding can considerably increase the capacity of a case report to link cause and effect.

The N of 1 Trial

The **N of 1 trial** is an experimental crossover design that uses a double-blind, placebo controlled trial design for a single patient or client. Simply put, it is an RCT with an *n* of 1, hence the name. This study design was originally developed as a method to test the clinical effectiveness of a pharmaceutical for an individual patient. The physician would work in conjunction with a pharmacist who made up two bottles of medication, one genuine and one a placebo. The patient would then be randomly assigned to receive one bottle first, with both physician and patient blinded as to allocation. The outcome of interest would be measured or assessed for a suitable period of time, followed by a wash-out period for any medication given to be metabolized out of the patient's system. Then the patient would cross over to the second treatment – the first bottle thrown away and the second one begun, again measuring the target outcome. After the data were analyzed, the blinding would be unmasked. Results for the two different time periods could then be compared to see whether one treatment was more effective than the other. The advantage of this design is that the patient acts as his or her own control for comparison, and through blinding both physician and patient, it additionally rules out expectation as a plausible alternate explanation.

How can this design be applied when double or even single blinding with random assignment to condition is not possible, which is often the case for many complementary therapies? There is a method that may make it possible to use double blinding for an individual patient in many such situations. The researcher/practitioner identifies an intervention for a particular condition to be tested, and develops a protocol to provide that intervention. A different protocol, which in theory should have no effect on the condition under treatment or the outcome to be measured, is also devised. Using our knee pain and acupressure example again, two treatments, one that should be effective for relieving arthritic knee pain in this particular client, and one that should have no effect on knee pain or arthritis for this client would be created by the researcher/practitioner. Each protocol is placed in an identical envelope by a neutral third party, sealed, shuffled, and marked Protocol 1 or Protocol 2. The researcher/practitioner does not perform the treatments. A second, equally capable practitioner, who is blinded to the client's history, is assigned to randomly select one of the protocols and deliver it. The client is instructed not to offer information about his or her history to the treating practitioner. The first treatment is implemented and daily pain ratings are kept for some period of time, followed by a wash-out period if necessary. Data from a self-reported outcome measure can be collected by the client, while other data can be collected by a neutral third party. Then the second protocol is introduced and performed by the same colleague. The outcome, in this case daily pain ratings, is measured again. The two sets of results are analyzed and compared, and only then is the blinding unmasked. The client and the practitioner delivering the protocols remain blinded during the data collection period for both protocols, as also does the researcher/practitioner. For obvious ethical reasons, this kind of trial design can be used only in situations where the client will not be subject to harm by stopping or altering any current treatment being received. The A-B-A design could also be employed using this strategy. When the A-B-A design is used with blinding, it is considered the strongest possible evidence of treatment effectiveness for an individual patient.

This variation of the N of 1 design could be employed for any manual therapy, or for other modalities that use multiple therapeutic approaches such as Traditional Chinese Medicine or naturopathy. Clients who are naïve to the particular complementary therapy being studied are more likely to remain blinded. Care should also be taken in devising the second protocol to avoid giving the treating practitioner clear clues that would make the "placebo" apparent. This design has the advantage of controlling for expectation, has a high degree of clinical and ecological validity, and allows for the effect of therapeutic relationship between the client and the treating practitioner. Any of the designs described can be used to develop consecutive case series as well.

Planning and Preparation

As with any form of research, the quality of a case report is proportional to the amount of planning and preparation that go into it. There are several steps involved in developing a useful and informative case report. Many of the criteria that we have learned to use in critical evaluation are also helpful in designing an original research project – consider it a type of reverse engineering. In both critical evaluation and research design, everything evolves in relation to the study question.

At each of the first four steps in the planning list, you will likely need to go back and revise your study question, based on what you have discovered during that activity. While formal IRB approval is not usually necessary for a case report, informed consent of the client or patient is a necessity. Some journals include an informed consent statement for the client or patient to sign as part of the journal's instructions to authors, so you may want to identify potential venues for publication early in the planning process. Confidentiality of patients is generally protected by withholding any identifying information.

Steps in Planning and Preparing a Case Report

1. Develop the study objective or purpose, and define a question to be answered.

2. Search and review the literature for background information that may affect your choice of approach, design, or outcome measure(s); revise step 1 as necessary.

3. Consider the most appropriate approach to use, based on the study objective – quantitative, qualitative, or both – and what design to use – retrospective or prospective, before-and-after, or N of 1 trial with or without blinding; revise step 1 again if necessary.

4. Draft the study protocol, specifying what data will be needed, how the data will be measured and collected and by whom, as well as how it will be analyzed; revise step 1 if necessary.

5. Determine what permissions will be needed, whether from the client or patient alone, or whether notes from other providers need to be requested.

6. Collect the data.

7. Analyze the data.

8. Think about the implications of the results for clinical practice and future research.

9. Identify and select a publication venue.

10. Obtain author guidelines.

11. Write the report using the specified format in the guidelines.

12. Submit for publication.

Case reports are a form of research that is within the grasp of any interested practitioner. The following example was written by a former student of the author, who submitted it to the Massage Therapy Foundation student case report competition. It is a good example of a clinical case report dealing with a condition commonly encountered in clinical practice, and it describes a treatment approach that integrates several modalities of care. It employs a prospective before-and-after treatment design, with both quantitative and qualitative data.

A Case Report of the Treatment of Piriformis Syndrome Applying Modalities of Therapeutic Bodywork

Peggi Honig, LMT, Hypnotherapist, MPNLP, Feldenkrais Guild Authorized ATM teacher

A previous version of this article first appeared in the January 2007, Vol. 07, Issue 01 issue of Massage Today (http://www.massagetoday.com)

Abstract

Objective: *This study assessed the benefits of weekly therapeutic deep tissue massage with the application of adjunct modalities, including somatic education and a stretching program, to alleviate chronic pain caused by compression of the sciatic nerve by the piriformis muscle.*

Methods: *A protocol of ten weekly 1½ hour massages applied deep tissue techniques with adjunct modalities including: Proprioceptive Neuromuscular Facilitation (PNF); Positional Release Therapy (PRT) stretches; Feldenkrais Method of Awareness Through Movement exercises (ATM); Kripalu yoga; and myofascial work. Focus of the work centered on the tissues of the lower back and the posterior and anterior legs.*

Results: *After the first session, subject was free of any sciatic pain for five days. When pain returned, client was able to recognize what triggered the flare-up and shifted her patterns of movement to abate the discomfort. There was a reoccurrence of chronic pain in the fourth and fifth weeks due to habitual patterns and work-related stress that required massage to remedy. From the fifth week on piriformis syndrome discomfort was rarely experienced. At week eleven, one week post treatment, subject was pain-free.*

Conclusion: This study demonstrates the application of therapeutic massage with a stretching program to ameliorate chronic piriformis syndrome. Rehabilitation is greatly improved with the addition of a daily stretching program and somatic education that improves the client's awareness of habitual patterns.

Keywords/Phrases: piriformis syndrome, pseudosciatica, sciatic nerve impingement, Positional Release Therapy (PRT) applications, chronic gluteal pain

Introduction

Piriformis syndrome has, since its first description in 1928, proved problematic to diagnose, due to the lack of supporting objective evidence. It is generally the client's described pain and the supporting medical process of elimination that leads to the diagnosis of this syndrome. At least 70 to 80% of the world population suffers from some form of lower back pain in their lifetimes and of that, 50% experience piriformis syndrome.[1]

Piriformis syndrome occurs from direct cause-and-effect incidents, e.g., blunt force trauma to the gluteal region and surgery, and from the more common accumulative habitual patterns that create structural misalignment and functional compensation. Of the total world population experiencing piriformis syndrome, no more than 20% are caused by anatomical nerve abnormalities.[2] *Half of piriformis syndrome cases are due to spontaneous onset of sciatica symptoms, most commonly as a result of vigorous physical activity. The remaining half are related to: contusions; concussive blow to the pelvic region; surgery; anatomical nerve abnormalities; hyperlordosis, muscle abnormalities and hypertrophy; fibrosis as a result of trauma; myositis ossificans, pseudoaneurysms of the inferior gluteal artery; cerebral palsy; and total hip arthroplasty.*[1]

Medical doctors perform digital exams to further reveal muscular tenderness and pinpoint the appropriate muscle for injection therapy application. Diagnostic imaging, also prescribed by doctors, is less effective in diagnosing this syndrome but helps to rule out other possible conditions.[7]

As of 2004, estimated costs related to piriformis syndrome were over $16 billion dollars. This was spent in both direct medical costs and indirect expenses to ameliorate pain.[1]

Piriformis syndrome has caused many sufferers to incur a loss of productivity because of pain, but due to lack of agreement as to how to diagnosis this syndrome, time away from work is not fully documented. Reports suggest that there is a 6:1 female to male ratio for piriformis syndrome.[1]

Standard allopathic protocols show less than a 50% reduction in chronic pain for up to three months, usually followed by full recurrence of symptoms, with the application of either marcaine or botulinum neurotoxin B injection therapy.[3] Botulinum toxin A proved even less effective.[4] Limited physical therapy sessions are a part of the injection protocol. One study of 239 patients who received spinal surgery showed a 58.5% excellent outcome with the remaining patient statistics as follows: 22.6% good outcome; 13.2% limited; 3.8% no benefit and 1.9% symptoms worsened.[5] Sports medicine approaches reveal a greater reduction and elimination of piriformis syndrome with the application of regular stretching and manual therapy protocols. The greatest successes occur when the client commits to a daily regimen of a home stretching routine. In an acute flare-up of symptoms, the client must stretch every two to three hours when awake. This creates the beginning of somatic education in retraining tissues to learn to relax and return to normalized tonus. After symptoms abate, it is necessary to continue the stretching exercises to reduce the likelihood of returning to habitual patterns that may have created this syndrome. Traditional Chinese acupuncture methods are another holistic approach used to ameliorate this syndrome.[6]

Therapeutic bodywork has presented promising applications for the reduction and remedy of pain associated with sciatic nerve impingement by gluteal muscles and at tenoperiostial junctions. Cataloging of therapies suggests a greater amelioration of symptoms with non-pharmacological approaches to reduce chronic pain.[1] Emphasis on awareness of habitual patterns and movement, release of myofascial adhesions,[10] deep transverse cross fiber friction and a daily stretching protocol show the greatest results in ameliorating piriformis syndrome.[1]

Profile of Client: *Subject, a 43-year-old active female, who plays softball and walks her dogs daily, works in a corporate setting as an executive in human resources. Medical history includes the removal of her thyroid gland thirteen years ago due to cancer. Client* is clear of any reoccurrence of cancer, is under medical supervision, and takes daily doses of synthroid. Client suffers from asthma and allergies. Weekly allergy shots are given in her right deltoid muscle. In addition to the allergy shots and thyroid medication, client takes 800 mg. of ibuprofen for pain management as needed.

Subject has experienced chronic pain for the past two years. Pain is experienced on a daily basis, in the right gluteal region and traveling inferiorly along the lateral side of the leg and down along the fibula. Using a verbal numerical rating scale from 0 to 10, she reports an intensity level of 10, describing a dull, throbbing ache that can travel distally to the hallux. Under stressful situations, the pain becomes contralateral. Ibuprofen for pain management is the only form of treatment used prior to this case study. Client's desired outcome is to manage the pain with the hope of being pain free.

Table I – Profile of Client at Start of Study

Outcomes Evaluated	Baseline at Initial Intake
Level of pain	10 on a scale from 0 to 10
Frequency of pain episodes	3 to 7 times a week, sometimes more than once a day
Pharmacological use	800 mg ibuprofen as needed, 1 to 2 doses a day
Work activity	Pain triggered by sitting for long periods of time
Personal activity	Pain triggered by standing for long periods of time on hard floors, standing and walking in high-heeled shoes, or driving in her SUV

The assessments applied in this case were: Pace test to check for abduction and external rotation of pelvic muscles; Freiberg test to force internal rotation with the leg extended; Beatty maneuver to selectively contract the piriformis muscle with the client in sidelying position on the unaffected side; and functional assessment techniques, similar to the above muscle tests described by Rolfing and massage therapists Art Riggs[8] and Whitney Lowe.[9]

Assessment revealed a positional pattern of lateral rotation at the feet referring into the hips. Her left anterior superior iliac spine was elevated approximately 1" higher than her *right side, and her right leg felt heavier and denser in passive movement. Both feet resisted medial rotation in passive testing. Client's range of motion was restricted at the coxofemoral joint where congested and contracted muscles were felt. In addition her left shoulder was elevated due to habitual patterns of cradling the phone to her ear at work.*

Rationale for Treatment Approach: *The symptoms of piriformis syndrome sciatic nerve impingement are treatable with massage therapy, by addressing the shortened muscles surrounding the sciatic nerve that are compressing it. Application of deep transverse friction at tenoperiostial junctions and focus on softening and relaxing the piriformis and the other deep lateral rotators, as well as the gluteal muscles, greatly reduce symptoms of nerve impingement. Focused work on the hamstring muscles and their proximal and distal bone attachments are also important, as these muscles can compress the sciatic nerve as it branches out and travels inferiorly, dividing into the peroneal and tibial nerves. In addition to the lateral rotators, the most appropriate muscles and attachments to massage include: tensor fascia latae (TFL); iliotibial band; iliac crest; quadratus lumborum; quadriceps; hamstring group; the greater trochanter; and sacroiliac joint attachments. Based on the subject's report of pain location, special attention was given to the lateral side of the leg including vastus lateralis, peroneus longus and brevis, and extensor hallucis longus muscles, as well as the psoas.*

Assessment of the symptoms indicated sciatic nerve impingement in the gluteal region. Further research with colleagues and source literature confirmed my assessment of piriformis syndrome.

Treatment Description

The subject received a series of ten consecutive massages of 1½ hour in duration. The focus of each session was to ameliorate chronic sciatic pain radiating from the gluteal region. The weekly approach incorporated deep tissue with other bodywork modalities to address the shortened muscles and fibrous adhesions at muscular and tenoperiostial junctions of the pelvic girdle, the leg and lower leg affected by sciatic pain.

Each session began with a verbal intake and visual assessment. Generally, sessions began with the client in supine position beginning with a series of range of motion (ROM) movements at the feet, assessment of where movement was impeded, and then palpation for the impingement of the sciatic nerve by the piriformis muscle.

As the session progressed the subject was moved into at least two positions (supine/prone, supine/sidelying). The protocol of each massage alternated with deep tissue massage and adjunct modalities including CranioSacral Therapy™ (CST), PNF and PRT stretches, somatic awareness, Trager™ rocking and myofascial work.

The 15-minute conclusion of each session included a review of lengthening exercises and awareness of habitual patterns and movements for at-home focus. The last portion of closure included a verbal and visual review of client's state and postural alignment.

Focused work addressed the softening of hypertonic muscles, especially of the rectus femoris, vastus lateralis, tensor fascia latae, piriformis and gluteus maximus and medius. These muscles were most benefited by applying cross-fiber friction at tenoperiostial junctions. Friction was applied for up to five minutes. No compressions or glides were used over the piriformis to reduce any further possibility of compressing the nerve. Cross-fiber glides, as well as glides along the grain of the muscle were applied to aid in the softening of the quadratus lumborum. Cross-fiber friction from the posterior superior iliac spine along the iliac crest attachment was done with considerable gentleness as client described a bruised sensation. This "bruised feeling" was most pronounced at all of the tenoperiostial junctions of the deep lateral rotator muscles and the gluteal area, as well as in the distal aspect of the iliotibial band. Intermittently, when the iliotibial band was most restricted, the patellar tendon and ligament on the lateral side of the knee would cause discomfort. Assisted PNF stretches and PRT movements enabled the contracted muscles around the hips and knees to release, allowing for an increased range of motion. As needed, compressions of the iliopsoas were applied to balance work on the quadratus lumborum.

Deep tissue compressions and cross fiber friction of the piriformis muscle and tenoperiostial attachments at the sacrum and the greater trochanter gave the greatest softening and improvement of impingement of the sciatic nerve. In addition, cross fiber friction of attachments at the iliac crest assisted in bringing slack to the gluteus maximus muscle overlaying the piriformis. Client was very sensitive in this area, so friction techniques were administered very gently. For congestion in the TFL and rectus femoris muscles, soft fist compressions and hand glides were the preferred strokes and tools to achieve reduction in tissue density. PNF resisted stretches involved the client in the process, while PRT stretches and ROM movements brought awareness of what she habitually does, and how her body functions. This was especially useful when addressing the quadriceps muscles and iliotibial band. Somatic awareness education enabled the client to find other movement options, looking for greater ease and comfort. This led her to catch herself as she moved into a habitual pattern that created pain. She was able to find options for what she could do to improve the situation and reduce the discomfort. CST holds were applied to the occipital region to identify locations along the spinal column where movement of cerebrospinal fluid (CSF) was impeded, so that compression of the thoracic and lumbar muscles could be relieved. As the client's constricted muscles began to release, the muscles of her lower trunk and gluteal area began to soften.

List of Modalities Applied

CranioSacral Therapy™ (CST)

Cross fiber friction (XFF)

Deep Tissue Massage (DT)

Swedish and ancillary strokes

Kripalu yoga poses

Myofascial release

Proprioception Neuromuscular Facilitation (PNF)

Positional Release Therapy (PRT)

Trager™ rocking

Results

Massage therapy appeared to ameliorate the symptoms of piriformis syndrome in the subject. Deep tissue techniques proved an effective means to reduce compression of the sciatic nerve by regional muscles and connective tissue. In conjunction with deep tissue techniques, adjunct bodywork modalities that proved most effective were: resisted PNF stretches of the iliotibial band; PRT movements to increase range of motion at the hip and decompress client's coxofemoral joint; and somatic education to bring awareness to patterns of movement that resulted in compression of joints and congestion in muscles. The 1" differential in the subject's anterior superior iliac spine leveled out to approximately a ¼" variable by the end of the first session. As the sessions progressed and her muscles began to relax more, the anterior hip imbalance disappeared.

Table II – Profile of Client at Completion of Study

Field	Response from Subject
Level of pain	Intensity decreased from a level 10 to 0
Frequency of pain episodes	Decreased from 7 to 0 over 10 sessions, and often there was no pain experienced in the latter half of the study
Pharmacological use	800 mg of ibuprofen taken occasionally in response to a flare-up of symptoms
Work activity	Occasional flare-up when seated at meetings for several hours
Personal activity	Occasional flare-up when standing or walking in high-heeled shoes

Although massage did not alleviate symptoms all the time, the protocol did considerably reduce the severity of pain and the frequency of episodes of discomfort. At one week post treatment, client reported no pain. Figure 1 shows the progression of symptom reduction over the course of the ten sessions of therapeutic bodywork.

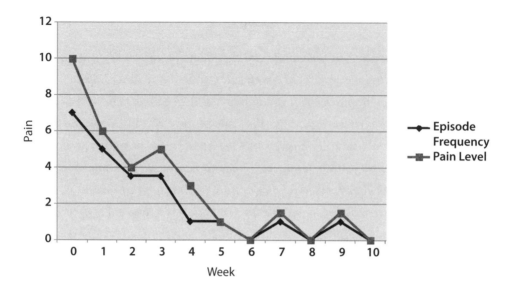

Figure 1 Pain intensity and episode frequency over the course of treatment

Somatic education appeared to enable the client to take control and recognize her movement patterns that participated in exacerbating this syndrome. Through the client's awareness of her habitual patterns and a daily stretching regimen, the compression that creates this chronic pain syndrome was greatly reduced. When the subject was not diligent in following her daily stretching exercises her symptoms were more prone to reappear. At the conclusion of the study client stated, "While the pain or discomfort may not completely go away, I can be more aware of how they get started and make adjustments early on to prevent or lessen it."

As the level of pain and frequency of discomfort diminished, the client was also able to reduce the amount of NSAID taken on a daily basis to occasional use.

Conclusion

This study demonstrates that the application of therapeutic bodywork to reduce piriformis syndrome in general, especially during a flare-up, is possible with appropriate decompression at the joints involved, relaxation of muscles that surround the sciatic nerve and a daily

Table III – Comments Made by the Client Throughout the Process

a) During or after sessions:
1st session: Feels a cool air blowing through her leg
2nd session: Bruised feeling from last session greatly reduced
3rd session: Feel compressed when pain returns
6th session: Great improvement all week with no pain
8th session: A little tweak (location is at the iliac crest)
10th session: Feeling great

b) A week after the end of the sessions:
I have become more aware of how I stand, walk and sit since all of these contribute to my discomfort.
I make adjustments more quickly to prevent or reduce the pain.
Exercises given help me stretch and release tension I build up on a daily basis.
No return of pain currently seven days after final treatment.

stretching protocol. It would be beneficial to pursue a more comprehensive study involving a larger number of subjects over a longer period of time to track the rate of improvement and the recurrence of symptoms. This could be further enhanced with observation of the duration of effects of massage therapy and stretching in addressing this condition. The inclusion of somatic awareness to learn how and what patterns of movement may contribute to piriformis syndrome were demonstrated to be of great value in reeducating the client. This practice gives individuals self-care activities that they can use themselves to alleviate discomfort. A secondary benefit of a nonpharmacological approach to this painful condition is the reduction of potential gastric upset related to the frequent use of over-the-counter NSAIDs.

Acknowledgements

I would like to thank my colleagues who influenced my thinking about treatment approaches for piriformis syndrome. Many thanks to: Bruce Hunt and Tam Gelman, Martha Menard, Ph.D, CMT; Cher Hunter, CMT; Clyde Anderson, CMT; Jonathan Foust; and Donna Blank.

References

1. *Klein, Milton J. Piriformis syndrome. eMedicine. 2004 June 14:2.*

2. *New injection technique. Anesthesiology. 2003 Jun; 98(6):1442-8.*

3. *Botulinum neurotoxin type B and physical therapy. J. Neurosurg Spine. 2005 Feb:2(2):99-115.*

4. *Botulinum toxin A. Ann Readapt Med Phys. 2003 Jul; 46(6):329-32.*

5. *J Neurosurg Spine. 2005 Feb; 2(2):99-115.*

6. *Wu, Q. Triple puncture with the bai hu yao tou maneuver. J Tradit Chin Med. 2003 Sep: 23(3):197-8.*

7. *Orthop Clin North Am. 2004 Jan; 35(1):65-71.*

8. *Riggs, Art: Deep Tissue Massage/A Visual Guide to Techniques. North Atlantic Books 2001.*

9. *Lowe, Whitney: Functional Assessment in Massage Therapy, 3rd ed. Omeri 1997.*

10. *Schultz, Louis B., Feitis, Rosemary: The Endless Web/Fascial Anatomy and Physical Reality. North Atlantic Books 1996.*

Appendix of Exercises for Piriformis Syndrome

Butterfly Pose: *Lie on your back keeping your head, neck and spine straight, bending at your knees, and bring your feet together with the heels and balls of your feet touching, then bring your feet as high up to your groin as possible and hang out – remember to breathe! When it gets too much, take another breath and hold 10 more seconds, then slowly straighten your legs and rest.*

½ Frog Pose: *Lie on your stomach and get comfortable, then as you bend your knee and lift your leg forming a 4 position, make sure that your head is turned to the same side as your raised knee. Hold this for as long as is comfortable. You may wish to slowly turn your head to the opposite side to feel what happens in your body, then rotate and address the other side. Always move very slowly.*

Feet In and Out: *Lie on your back keeping your head, neck and spine straight, then slowly while keeping your knees straight, turn your feet into the center so that your big toe touches the bed, or floor (this is medial/internal rotation), then slowly allow your feet to move straight up so that the back of your heel is resting on the bed or floor and your toes are pointing straight up, then move your feet out so that the lateral side of your foot begins to touch the bed or floor (lateral/external rotation) and then continue to rotate back to center, to medial, and repeat slowly several times. You want to pay attention to what movement is happening in your ankles, knees and hips, and breathe!*

Sitz Bones: You may do this in a chair or on the floor. Sit and with your hands pull/stretch your gluts/cheeks away from your body so that you are increasing the area touching the sitting surface. Feel your sitz bones and how you balance on them. Slowly begin to make very small movements from front to back then side-to-side, and then making a small circle all the while resting on your sitz bones, become more aware of how you are doing this and what you feel in your hips, knees and spine, and breath!

IT Band Stretch: Lie on your side on the edge of the bed so that you can let your top leg hang behind you and off of the bed. Make sure to counterbalance yourself with your top arm/hand, then slowly take a deep breath, and as you exhale, allow your top leg with straight knee to fall behind you and off the bed, hanging in the air. With each breath, become aware of how you can best allow your leg to hang, and with each exhale allow your leg to drop a little further down, feeling how the IT band slowly begins to open and lengthen. Repeat on each side.

Quad Stretch: Lie on your back on the edge of the bed and allow the leg closest to the edge to drop off the bed with your knee bent, again you will want to counterbalance yourself with your opposite hand/arm. With each exhale allow your thigh to fall down a little bit more with the feeling of it moving out and down. When you breathe have the feeling of lengthening your back onto the bed, and when you exhale allow your leg to soften and drop down allowing for a greater lengthening of the quadriceps muscles. This will also stretch the psoas muscle.

Comments

This highly descriptive case report places the client's condition into the context of previous research and discusses why it is significant. It contains a brief but relevant description of the client, and focuses on the treatment provided, including an appendix of stretches recommended for the client's use. In addition to collecting data on the frequency and severity of sciatic pain reported, the author has also incorporated qualitative data in the form of comments by the client. The conclusion notes an additional benefit to this non-pharmacological approach and makes recommendations for future research in this area.

This type of case report documents the kind of critical and clinical thinking in which health care practitioners engage every day. It authenticates the continuous and often iterative process of researching and evaluating the client's condition, determining or revising a treatment plan, and then evaluating the effectiveness of one's interventions. It can also be viewed as an example of evidence-informed practice, as described in Chapter 1.

Writing a Case Report

In the examples we have seen, the exact format of each case report or study has varied somewhat, and each journal usually has its own guidelines for authors. The general format, however, is similar to what we see in other journal articles. Author affiliation and sources of funding are standard, followed by an abstract, which may be in narrative or standardized format.

The case report should contain a review of the literature, which provides background information and a context of previous research into which this case study fits. The significance of the research question may also be addressed here. The review of the literature may also provide a rationale for any outcome measures used, along with information on their reliability and validity if these are not well known.

Usually, a pertinent description of the individual client or patient follows. It should be brief, clear, and adequate, giving relevant history and background information, describing any assessments performed and the results of any medical tests, and may include photos or other illustrations. The reference ranges or normal values for any medical tests mentioned should be included for readers who may be unfamiliar with these. A description of the treatment protocol, sufficient for general replication, should also be included.

The results section contains only the verbal and visual summary of the outcome data. It may take the form of quantitative pre- and post-treatment measures, a summary of any data analysis, and/or a qualitative analysis of the client's own words. Two BioMed Central journals, the *Journal of Medical Case Reports* and its sister publication *Cases Journal*, now include a "patient's perspective" section, authored by the patient, to add an additional layer of detail to the traditional case report format. This is a good example of the growing trend toward a mixed methods approach in health care research.

The discussion section of a case report is similar to the discussion section of other clinical journal articles. In it the author examines and discusses the evidence presented in the results in terms of the stated study question and objective. The results in relation to other relevant research may also be considered, as well as other plausible explanations for the results. Limitations of the study can be addressed here. Depending on the study objective, the author may also discuss implications for other practitioners in terms of the assessment or management of a condition. Almost always, the author makes recommendations for future research, particularly hypotheses to be explored or tested as a consequence of the information presented in the case.

The final section of a case report is the reference section. These should always be pertinent and completely accurate. Only the necessary number of relevant papers should be cited.

Preparing an Article for Submission

As part of the planning process, consider which journal is most likely to be receptive to your study. Obtain the instructions for authors from the journal's website or from a hard copy of the journal. Many journals now employ electronic submission, and will give detailed instructions for preparation and submission of the manuscript. Be sure that you follow these to the letter, especially formatting of the manuscript, organization of the sections of the article and what information should be contained in each one, and the format for the references. It can take quite some time for the article to be reviewed, and it is not unusual for an editor to request that an article be revised and resubmitted. Not every report is suitable or a good fit for every journal. If the manuscript is not accepted, choose another journal, revise the manuscript as needed, and try again. It takes time and patience. One advantage of electronic submission is that it has generally speeded up the review process, compared to even a few years ago. Do consider publishing in an open access journal – it will greatly increase the number of practitioners who can easily read and cite your work.

Venues for Publication

As this book goes to press, there are a surprisingly large number of peer-reviewed journals in which complementary therapists may publish case reports and studies. It appears that case reports, after having been considered a relatively lowly form of evidence for many years, are now making a comeback. A list of such journals is provided in alphabetical order in the box that follows, with website addresses in parentheses. By no means is this a comprehensive list, and web addresses are current as of July 2009. Most of the journals listed require electronic submission.

Acupuncture and Electro-Therapeutics Research
(http://www.cognizantcommunication.com/filecabinet/Acupuncture/acu.htm)

Acupuncture in Medicine (http://acupunctureinmedicine.org.uk/)

Advances in Mind-Body Medicine (http://www.advancesjournal.com/adv/)

Alternative Therapies in Health and Medicine (http://www.alternative-therapies.com/)

American Journal of Chinese Medicine (http://www.worldscinet.com/ajcm/ajcm.shtml)

American Journal of Homeopathic Medicine (http://www.homeopathyusa.org/journal/)

BMC Complementary and Alternative Medicine
(http://www.biomedcentral.com/bmccomplementalternmed)

Canadian Journal of Herbalism (http://www.herbalists.on.ca/journal/invite.html)

Cases Journal (http://casesjournal.com/)

Chiropractic & Osteopathy (http://www.chiroandosteo.com/home/)

Clinical Acupuncture & Oriental Medicine
(http://www.sciencedirect.com/science/journal/14611449/)

Complementary Therapies in Clinical Practice
(http://www.elsevier.com/wps/find/journaldescription.cws_home/704176/description#description/)

Complementary Therapies in Medicine
(http://www.elsevier.com/wps/find/journaldescription.cws_home/623020/authorinstructions)

European Journal of Oriental Medicine (http://www.ejom.co.uk/submissions.html)

Homeopathy
(http://www.elsevier.com/wps/find/journaldescription.cws_home/623042/description#description/)

Integrative Medicine: A Clinician's Journal (http://www.imjournal.com/)

International Journal of Clinical Aromatherapy (http://ijca.net/)

*International Journal of Therapeutic Massage & Bodywork: Research, Education, & Practice
(IJTMB)* (http://journals.sfu.ca/ijtmb/)

Journal of Alternative and Complementary Medicine
(http://www.liebertpub.com/publication.aspx?pub_id=26)

Journal of Bodywork & Movement Therapies
(http://www.elsevier.com/wps/find/journaldescription.cws_home/623047/description#description/)

Journal of Chinese Medicine (http://www.jcm.co.uk/)

Journal of Complementary and Integrative Medicine
(http://www.bepress.com/jcim/aimsandscope.html)

Journal of Midwifery & Women's Health (http://www.jmwh.com/)

Journal of Herbal Pharmacotherapy (http://www.haworthpress.com/store/product.asp?sku=J157)

Nutrition Journal (http://www.nutritionj.com/info/instructions/)

Phytotherapy Research (http://www.wiley.com/WileyCDA/WileyTitle/productCd-PTR.html)

The Massage Therapy Foundation

The Massage Therapy Foundation deserves a special mention for its efforts to advance case reporting in massage therapy research. It supports two annual competitions, one for students and one for practitioners, each with a cash prize and publication in a peer-reviewed journal for the winning study. In 2008, the Foundation also launched a peer-reviewed, open access electronic journal devoted to therapeutic massage and bodywork, the *International Journal of Therapeutic Massage & Bodywork: Research, Education, & Practice*, which is included in the preceding list. In the interest of full disclosure, the author is currently a member of the editorial board. If you are a massage or bodywork practitioner, please consider developing a case report for submission to this journal.

Summary

The case report or study tells a clinically relevant story that has unique value to the practice of health care. In a case report, the individual presentation is examined in the context of current knowledge and is shared for the purpose of educating other practitioners or stimulating further scientific inquiry and the development of new understanding or knowledge. Case reports can provide valuable "lessons learned" and enhance clinical practice. Case reports or studies are useful for communicating about a variety of clinical situations including unusual events, adverse responses, and treatment innovations. While case reports are intended to be descriptive and observational in nature, single subject designs using blinding and random assignment can also be considered strong evidence of treatment effectiveness for an individual. As well, case reports can suggest new hypotheses to be developed, and are an important original contribution to the research literature.

Conducting a case report or study requires thorough planning and preparation. An understanding of the principles of critical evaluation provides a roadmap for designing, conducting, and writing a case report for publication that will be useful to your peers. Think of the case report as a more formal documentation of the processes of evidence-informed practice and continuous clinical assessment that practitioners engage in every day.

Exercises

1. *In a small group, choose a hypothetical client you believe would make a good case report. Explain your rationale and research objective. Use the same hypothetical client for the rest of the exercises that follow.*

2. *Identify suitable search terms and perform literature searches in PubMed and BioMed Central.*

3. *Choose the most appropriate design and approaches to be used, and give a rationale for your choices. Revise your research objective if necessary.*

4. *Describe what outcomes will be assessed, and how the data will measured, collected, and analyzed.*

5. *What permissions will need to be obtained?*

6. *Identify a journal for submission of the case report; visit their website and obtain a copy of the authors' guidelines.*

Glossary

Abstract A concise summary of a research article, highlighting the objective, hypothesis, design, participants, setting, methods, results, and conclusion.

Alpha Another term for Type I error.

Alternate hypothesis Statistically, a true difference between two or more groups compared, abbreviated H_1; can also refer to plausible alternative explanations for a study's results.

Analysis of covariance (ANCOVA) A type of analysis of variance that controls for pre-existing differences between groups.

Analysis of variance (ANOVA) A commonly used test of significance for multiple groups that compares variance between groups to variance within groups.

Analytic study Another term for a quantitative, experimental study.

Audit trail In qualitative research, a written record that documents the data and the researcher's analytic process.

Before-and-after treatment design A research design comparing baseline measures taken before a treatment is given with those collected after.

Beneficence One of the three core ethical values proposed in the Belmont Report; it refers to the value of doing no harm – maximizing potential benefits and minimizing potential risks of research participation.

Best evidence synthesis A type of systematic review that combines the quantitative features of meta-analysis with a more evaluative narrative review.

Beta Another term for Type II error.

Bias Systematic error in the measurement of a variable. Problems in a study's design can also be referred to as "sources of bias."

Blinding A design strategy where knowledge of the group assignment is concealed from either participants or researchers (single blind), or both (double blind).

Boolean operators The terms "and," "not," and "or" used to limit or to expand a search for reference citations in a database such as PubMed.

Case-control design or study A type of observational study in which both the exposure(s) and outcome(s) have already occurred and are being analyzed retrospectively; often used to explore risk factors associated with chronic illness.

Case report/case study A detailed account of the history, presenting symptoms, observations, assessment, treatment and follow-up of an individual client or patient. "Case report" is used more often in the health care literature while "case study" is typically used in the social sciences.

Case series A report of a series of patients or clients presenting with the same symptom or who have other case features in common.

Ceiling or floor effect What happens when an instrument cannot measure something above or below its scale.

Chi-square test The most commonly used nonparametric test of significance; used for nominal level variables.

Citation A reference to a journal article.

Clinical trial An experimental study where the researcher randomly assigns treatment(s) to groups of participants.

Cohort A group formed at a common point in time.

Cohort study A study in which a group is defined based on the presence or absence of an exposure in common, and then the participants are followed over time to observe who develops the outcome.

Co-intervention Another procedure or treatment administered at the same time as the study intervention, occurring without the knowledge of the study investigator.

Comorbidity When a patient or research participant has multiple health conditions; usually an exclusion criterion.

Complement In probability statistics, all the other possible outcomes except those that make up an event; the odds against an event occurring.

Compliance Adherence to the study protocol.

Conceptual content analysis A method of content analysis involving identification of concepts contained in the study data and the number of times they appear.

Confidence interval An estimate of the amount of error surrounding the true score of a study as a whole, associated with a probability within which the true score lies.

Confounding variable A third, often unmeasured, variable that blurs the relationship between two other variables, making it appear that a spurious relationship or association exists. Also sometimes referred to as a "confound."

Consistency The qualitative equivalent of reliability; internal congruency of the study data.

Content analysis In qualitative research, an analysis of the content of a study's data.

Control group/Comparison group A group of study participants who do not receive the treatment being studied, or who do not have the exposure or outcome being evaluated; the group being used as a basis for comparison to the treatment group.

Correlation A statistical measure of association that indicates the strength and direction of a linear relationship between two variables.

Correlational study A study comparing an exposure and outcome using aggregated group data from a large population, such as cigarette sales by state and the number of deaths from coronary artery disease annually.

Credibility In qualitative research, a study's internal logic and cohesion that connect the study objective, methods, and results.

Cross-sectional study A study where data regarding an exposure and outcome are simultaneously collected across a population at a point in time, providing a snapshot of a situation.

Culture A particular way of defining the world, the relationship of a group to it and to each other, and accepted standards of behavior for the group. Culture is not limited to geographic location or ethnic heritage but can refer to any group of people who share a particular set of experiences, for example, in organizations, schools or workplaces.

Degrees of freedom If N is equal to the number of observations in a data set, the degrees of freedom are equal to N minus 1, or the number of deviations around the mean that are free to vary.

Demographic data Characteristics such as age, sex or gender, educational level, geographic location, ethnicity, annual income or socio-economic status, or other such that can be used to describe or classify groups.

Descriptive statistics Statistics that summarize and describe a data set, such as the range and measures of central tendency, without making any inferences that would generalize from the sample to a population.

Descriptive study A study that provides a record/description of events or activities.

Diffusion of treatment This occurs when study participants assigned to a control or comparison group seek out and obtain the active treatment.

Ecological validity The capacity of a study to accurately reflect the way a treatment is provided or implemented in clinical practice.

Effect size The magnitude of an observed effect.

Empiricism A way of acquiring knowledge by observation and verification through the physical senses.

Estimation An application of inferential statistics used to estimate some aspect of a population from a smaller representative sample.

Ethnography A qualitative research approach based on anthropology, often using participant observation and fieldwork to describe a culture.

Evidence-based medicine The conscientious, explicit and judicious use of current best research evidence in making decisions about the care of individual patients.

Experimental population The group of possible study participants, including all those who are eligible but choose not to participate for any reason.

Experimental statistics Statistical methods used in experimental designs.

Experimental study A study where the researcher manipulates events, for example, by giving a treatment and then assessing its effects.

Explanatory study A study that seeks to explain a connection between events or variables. Explanatory studies can be further divided into observational and experimental studies.

Exposure In epidemiology, the risk factor or treatment to which a study participant is subjected; analogous to independent variable in non-medical research.

External validity The capacity of a study to be generalized to other groups or clinical settings.

False negative When the negative results of a medical or statistical test are actually false; Type II error.

False positive When the positive results of a medical or statistical test are actually false; Type I error.

Falsification The idea that science progresses best through demonstrating that a hypothesis is false.

Fields Categories such as keywords, authors' names, journal titles, or textwords in an article that can be specified to limit or expand a database search.

Follow-up study Another name for a cohort study.

Generalizability Another term for external validity.

Grounded theory A qualitative approach based in sociology that attempts to generate an explanatory model that is grounded in observed data.

Grouped frequency distribution A graph of each data point in a set, which shows how often each score is repeated.

History A threat to internal validity; an event that occurs during the course of a study and influences the outcome but is unrelated to the treatment under evaluation.

Hypothesis A highly specific statement that can be demonstrated to be true or false through the methodical gathering and analysis of empirical information or data.

Hypothesis testing An application of inferential statistics used to determine whether any difference between the means of groups being compared is due to chance, or whether chance can be ruled out as an explanation for the results.

Inferential statistics Statistical tests used to draw a conclusion about a population based on a randomly selected sample of that population.

Institutional Review Board (IRB) An ethics committee at a research institution such as a university or hospital that oversees the design and conduct of research to safeguard the rights and safety of study participants.

Instrument decay A threat to internal validity when there is a change or problem with the degree of measurement possible with an instrument used in a study.

Intention to treat Statistical analysis based on the number of eligible participants originally enrolled in the study, instead of the number who completed the study.

Internal validity The capacity of a study to link cause and effect.

Interval variable A variable expressed as a number.

Intervention study Another term for an experimental or treatment study.

Iterative Describes a process of repeated development or refinement, going through several cycles.

Iterative process A process of continuous revision as new information or data becomes available.

Justice One of the three core ethical values proposed by the Belmont Report; it refers to the value of fairness in the distribution of the benefits and burdens of research participation – the researcher does not exploit vulnerable persons.

Keywords Specific words or phrases used to index an article and provide a controlled vocabulary with consistent descriptive language.

Letters to the editor A journal feature where readers write in response to previously published articles.

Literature review A critique of previous research studies on a particular topic.

Longitudinal study Another name for a cohort study.

Margin of error The estimated amount of possible statistical error in a survey's results, usually expressed as a range, such as "plus or minus 3%."

Maturation A threat to internal validity; events that occur naturally with the passage of time.

Mean The arithmetical average; the sum of a group of scores divided by the number of scores.

Measure of central tendency The middle of a data set; the mean, median, or mode.

Measures of association Statistical tests that measure the extent to which two or more variables are associated with each other.

Median A measure of central tendency where half the data set is above a certain point (the median) and half below.

Meta-analysis A summary review using a group of studies selected according to pre-established criteria, and statistically combining or "pooling" the data in those studies.

Mode A measure of central tendency describing the most frequently observed category or point in a data set.

Model fit validity When the underlying assumptions or model of the research methods used match those of the therapy being studied. Similar to ecological validity.

Mortality Another term for attrition, or when participants drop out of a study before its completion.

Multiple analysis of variance (MANOVA) Statistical test used when there are multiple outcome variables; controls for the effect of multiple comparisons.

Multiple regression A measure of association used to predict the value of a single outcome variable based upon knowledge of several exposure variables.

N of 1 trial An experimental crossover design that uses a double-blind, placebo controlled trial design for a single patient or client; an RCT with an n of 1.

Narrative review A review of the research literature examining a group of studies on a particular topic that are selected and evaluated by the author.

Negative cases Examples that are contrary to the prevailing data, deliberately sought out by the qualitative researcher to provide a more complete perspective.

Neutrality Freedom from bias in the qualitative research process and in the reporting of results.

Nocebo effect The opposite of the placebo effect – participants feel worse based on negative expectations.

Nominal variable A variable expressed as a category.

Nonparametric statistics Statistical tests that are not dependent on the data being normally distributed; used to analyze data from nominal and ordinal level variables.

Nonspecific response A more accurate term for the placebo response, which is a positive response to an inactive substance or sham treatment; sometimes used to reflect the possibility that positive clinical outcomes may be in response to factors like expectations, beliefs and attitudes.

Normal distribution The bell curve; 68% of the data points are within one standard deviation of the mean. See Figure 6.2.

Null hypothesis A hypothesis that there is no difference between the means of two or more groups being compared; abbreviated as H_0.

Observational study A study that explains a connection between naturally occurring events, such as exposure to a risk factor and subsequent development of an outcome, without manipulating those events.

Odds ratio An estimate of effect size often used in epidemiological studies; the risk of an outcome associated with a particular exposure, using dichotomous variables (yes or no).

One-tailed test A test of significance that predicts a difference in a single direction.

One-way analysis of variance A test of significance used to compare multiple groups on a single outcome measure.

Ordinal variable A variable expressed as one of a ranked order.

Outcome Any clinical endpoint of interest.

Parametric statistics Statistical tests that are based on the assumption that the data are normally distributed; used to analyze data from interval and ratio level variables.

Pearson product-moment correlation coefficient The most common correlation measure, used for two interval or ratio level variables.

Phenomenology A qualitative approach based in philosophy, used to understand the essential nature of an experience.

Post-hoc testing After reaching a statistically significant ANOVA, further comparisons between two of the multiple groups in the study.

Power analysis A calculation of the number of participants needed in a study to have an 80% probability of detecting a genuine effect if one exists.

Pragmatic trial Test of an intervention in a real-world setting under routine conditions likely to be encountered by clinicians.

Prevalence The number of cases of an existing disease or outcome per population, in other words, how common it is.

Probability The chances of a particular outcome occurring as the result of a random process.

Prospective case report A case report in which data is collected prospectively in order to meet a research objective or answer a specific research question.

Prospective study Another name for a cohort or longitudinal study.

Protocol The step-by-step description of the concrete procedures to be carried out during a research study.

Publication bias The tendency for journals to only publish articles with positive findings and reject those with negative results.

Qualitative methods/approaches Research methods that rely on the collection and analysis of word-based experiential and observational data, instead of numbers.

Quantitative methods Research methods based on the collection and analysis of numerical data.

Random assignment Assignment of study participants to group based on a random process, such as a computer-generated table of numbers.

Random sampling When every member of the total population has an equal chance of being selected, also known as "probability sampling."

Randomized controlled trial (RCT) A clinical trial whose participants have been randomly allocated to treatment and control groups; considered the "gold standard" of quantitative research.

Range The difference between the highest and lowest scores of an outcome measure.

Ratio variable A variable expressed as a numerical ratio of one thing to another.

Rationalism A way of acquiring knowledge through reason or logic.

Reactivity issues The ways in which the responses of study participants are influenced by the obtrusiveness of their being observed or measured during the course of the study.

Recall bias The tendency of study participants to distort historical information because of faulty memory or a desire to please or impress the interviewer, resulting in inaccurate data.

Reference population The larger group to which a single study's findings can be generalized.

Regression analysis A measure of association used to predict the value of one variable based upon knowledge of another.

Regression to the mean The tendency for extreme values of a baseline measure to become closer to the average upon repeated measurement.

Relational content analysis A type of content analysis that examines the relationships among concepts identified in qualitative data.

Relative risk An estimate of the size of the association between an exposure and an outcome; also an indication of the probability of developing the outcome in the exposed group compared to those not exposed.

Reliability The consistency and accuracy with which an instrument measures a tangible construct such as weight or less tangible construct such as intelligence.

Repeated measures ANOVA Statistical test used for samples that are measured at multiple points over a period of time.

Reproducibility The capacity of the study to be replicated by another investigator or in another setting.

Respect for persons One of the three core ethical values underlying research endeavors as proposed in the Belmont Report; refers to treating people as autonomous beings who can make choices based on their own interests or preferences.

Retrospective study Another name for a case-control study.

Retrospective case report A case report that makes use of existing data that have already been observed and recorded.

Review of the literature The section of a journal article that discusses pertinent prior studies that are relevant to the current research question.

Sampling The process by which participants in a study are selected to represent the experimental population. "Sample" is also used to refer to the selected subset.

Search strategy Search terms used to retrieve articles on a particular topic.

Selection bias When study participants with pre-existing and systematic differences are assigned to groups, given an intervention and then compared with each other. Any changes observed are likely attributable to the pre-existing differences and not the intervention.

Sources of bias Elements of a research design or procedures that introduce systematic error into the measurement of an outcome.

Standard deviation A measure of the variability or spread of scores around the mean.

Statistical power Based on the number of participants and outcome measures, the ability of a statistical test to detect a genuine effect if one is present.

Statistical significance Evidence that the results of a study are not due to chance or random error.

Statistical validity Whether quantitative analytic measures and procedures were properly selected and performed.

Study arm Another term for any group of participants who are all assigned to receive the same study intervention, such as a verum or a sham treatment.

Study population The specific group of participants in a given study; a subset of the total experimental population.

Systematic review A more refined version of the meta-analysis that attempts to avoid publication bias by including unpublished findings and articles from non-indexed journals, with articles weighted according to the strength and quality of evidence presented.

t-test "Student's *t*-test" is the most basic test of statistical significance, used to compare the means of two groups. The "independent *t*-test" is used to compare the means of two different, unrelated groups while the "paired" or "dependent *t*-test" is used to compare paired observations, such as subjects before and after a treatment.

Testing Learned responses to an instrument or research procedure; a threat to internal validity.

Test-retest reliability Evidence of the stability of the test or instrument used to measure an abstract concept (e.g., anxiety) over time.

Tests of statistical significance Tests that determine the statistical probability or extent to which any observed differences between two or more group means being compared are due to chance.

Textword A search field based on any word found in the text or body of an abstract.

Transferability The capacity of a qualitative study's findings to be applied to other contexts, settings, or groups.

Treatment effect The treatment group mean minus the control group mean.

Triangulation Use of more than one method or strategy of data collection or analysis in order to increase the validity/reliability of a qualitative study.

Trustworthiness Similar to credibility in qualitative research.

Two-tailed test A statistical test that predicts a difference in either a positive or negative direction.

Type I error Statistical significance mistakenly based on random error, leading to the conclusion that an effect is present when in truth it is not.

Type II error Lack of statistical significance despite the presence of a true effect; often due to lack of statistical power from too small a sample.

Validity There are many specific types of validity in research – generally, the idea that a test or instrument measures what it is supposed to measure. For example, a driving test should measure driving proficiency, not the language skills necessary to understand the directions.

Wash-out period An amount of time between ending one intervention and beginning a second, given to allow the effects of the first intervention to dissipate.

Whole systems research A research approach that studies a system of care such as naturopathy in its entirety, rather than attempting to study a system by breaking it down into its component "active" ingredients.

Index

An italic *f* following a page reference indicates the presence of a figure; an italic *t* indicates the presence of a table.

data set, 138–40, 139f, 145, 161
Declaration of Helsinki, 13
degrees of freedom (DF), 164
demographic data, 88, 96, 111, 115
    baseline, 96, 117t
descriptive statistics, 137, 138–40
    evaluation of, 161–2, 206–7
descriptive studies, 82, 83f, 84–7
    case report/study as, 305
    evaluation of, 242–5
    vs observational studies, 91
Dieppe, P., 65
diffusion of treatment, 62–3
direct observation, 17
discussion and/or conclusions (of articles), 104, 122–5
    in case reports, 314–16, 319–24
    evaluation of, 122–3, 166–7, 185–6, 209–10
    examples of, 123–5, 176–7, 199–202, 237–9, 255–8, 289–93
double blind studies, 18, 64, 159

ecological validity, 71, 160, 330
effectiveness, 97–8
effect size, 142–3, 144, 149, 153, 165, 208
efficacy, 97–8
efficacy paradox, 68, 69f
eligibility criteria, 95
EMBASE, 33
emergent theory, 216
empiricism, 9
epidemiological research methods, 80, 82, 85, 105
estimation (in inferential statistics), 140
ethical issues, 12–15
    Belmont Report, 13–14
    beneficence, 13–14
    with blinding, 64, 70
    with case reports/studies, 330
    with experimental studies, 13, 92–3
    with placebos and control groups, 62
    with sham treatments, 70
ethics review committees, 62
    IRBs, 14–15, 64, 330
ethnography, 216–17
evaluation(s) (of articles), 54–72, 156–68
    balanced perspective in, 168
    of before-and-after treatment designs, 93
    of case studies and case series, 85
    of clinical trials, 94–9
    of journals, 156–7
    of literature reviews, 81
    of methodology, 110–11
    protocol for critical evaluation, 179, 222
    of qualitative/quantitative studies, 297–300

    of qualitative studies, 219–23, 242–5, 261–3
    of quantitative studies, 156–8, 204–10
    of references lists, 125–6, 167, 187, 210, 223
    skepticism in, 156
    of study methods and procedures, 110–11, 205–7
evidence-based medicine (EBM), 3, 22–3, 27, 80, 87
evidence-based practice funnel, 26f, 27
evidence circle, 24, 99
evidence house, 24
experimental population, 94
experimental quantitative methods, 16
experimental statistics, 138
experimental studies (intervention studies), 26f, 83f, 92–3
    designs for, 21
    ethical issues, 13, 92–3
    experimental approach, 16, 24
    vs. nonexperimental, 21, 24
explanatory studies, 82, 83f, 87–94
exposure(s), 82
    binary variables, 143f
    as independent variable, 150, 161, 163
    relation with outcome, 82, 86, 87, 91, 93, 150
    and relative risk, 111
    time of measurement, 87, 88, 89
external validity, 54, 73, 98, 99
    vs. internal validity, 55, 71

false negative, 144
false positive, 144
falsification, 8, 10–11, 327
Field, Tiffany, 78
fields (in citation), 32
Finch, Paul M., 26f, 27
Fisher's exact test, 152
floor effect, 58
focus groups, 17
follow-up studies, 90
F statistic, 148, 149, 150
funding sources, 12, 98, 104, 106, 122–3, 157

Galton, Francis, 150
generalizability, 54–6, 71, 97, 182, 219, 299
Gossett, William S., 146
grounded theory, 216
grouped frequency distribution, 139–40
Guba, E.G., 219, 243
Guyatt, Gordon, 23

healing (therapeutic) relationship, 71, 87
Hill, Austin Bradford, 22
Hippocratic Oath, 13
history (event in study), 57
history (of search), 38, 39f

Hornsby, Paige, 214
Hotelling's T^2, 162
Huff, Darrell, 137
hypothesis, 9, 83f
    alternate hypothesis (H_1), 141
    in before-and-after treatment designs, 93
    case report/study as basis for, 84, 305
    and falsification, 10–11, 141
    null hypothesis(H_0), 141, 144, 152
    and statistical analysis, 60
    testing with correlational studies, 86
    testing with inferential statistics, 138
    validation of, 11
hypothesis testing, 140, 141

inconclusive results, 79
independent t-tests, 147
independent variable, 150, 161, 163
inferential statistics, 138, 140–2
    evaluation of, 161–2, 163, 206–7
    standard deviation in, 146
    testing of, 142
informed consent (of participants), 15, 64, 92, 317, 330
Institutional Review Boards (IRBs), 14–15, 62, 64, 330
instrumentation, 58, 172–3
instrument decay, 58
intention to treat, 97
internal validity, 55, 145
    in clinical trials, 97
    and instrumentation, 58
    of literature reviews, 81
    in quantitative methods, 55, 56
    and random assignment, 62
    threats to, 56–60
    vs. external validity, 55, 71
    and weighting methods, 79, 81
    See also validity
International Journal of Therapeutic Massage and Bodywork, 50, 346, 347
interval data, 152
interval variables, 137, 145–6
intervention studies. *See* experimental studies
interviews, 110–11
    open-ended, 17
    in qualitative studies, 218–19, 223
    recording of, 223
introductions (of articles), 104
    evaluation of, 108, 157–8, 180–1, 204–5, 297
    examples of, 108–9, 170–1, 189–90, 225, 246–7, 265–8, 333–4
in vitro studies, 26f
iterative process, 216

Jonas, Wayne, 24, 92, 93
journal(s)
    letters to editor, 76–7
    lists of, 48, 346
    peer-reviewed, 10, 12, 46, 106, 156, 157, 347
    quality of, 156–7
journal articles. *See* research articles
Journal of Ethnobiology and Ethnomedicine, 46
Journal of Medical Case Reports, 344
Journal of the American Medical Association, 23, 48
justice (for research participants), 14

Kaptchuk, Ted, 66, 67
Keenan, Phyllis, 78
keywords, 37, 77
    examples of, 107, 189, 246, 312, 318, 333
key words, 262
    in content analysis, 223
Kraemer, H.C., 145
Kuhn, Thomas, 12

Lancet, The, 48
learned responses, 57, 66
letters to editor, 76–7
libraries, 33, 42–4
    Library Identifier number, 44
limitations and weaknesses (of study designs), 24, 166, 185–6, 209, 244, 263
    before-and-after studies, 93
    examples of, 291–2
    of literature reviews, 77–8
Lincoln, Y.S., 219, 243
literature reviews, 77–80, 108, 223
    bibliographies of, 77
    evaluation guidelines for, 81
    in qualitative studies, 223, 225–8, 247–8, 261
    See also reference lists
Loansome Doc, 42–4, 43f
longitudinal studies, 90

Mann-Whitney-U, 152
margin of error, 141
Massage Therapy Foundation, 49, 50, 332, 347
maturation, 57
McGervey, John D., 136
mean (of variable), 138, 139f, 146, 163–4, 174t, 208
measurement
    and bias, 97
    of CAM individualized treatment, 71
    initial baseline, 59
    time of, 87, 88, 89
measurement instrumentation or tools, 58, 160–1, 172–3

measure of central tendency, 139–40, 150

measures of association, 142

median, 138–9

Medical Subject Headings (MeSH), 37

MEDLINE, 32, 33, 37, 39, 44

MEDLINE*plus*, 44

Mendel, Gregor, 152

meta-analysis studies, 21, 77, 78–9, 80, 81
    evidence in, 20*f*, 26*f*, 91*f*

methods and procedures (in articles), 104
    evaluation of, 110–11, 156–62, 181–3, 243–4, 262
    examples of, 112–15, 171–3, 191–3, 229–30, 250–1, 268–75

mixed methods (quantitative and qualitative), 18, 263, 299
    and credibility, 244, 300
    in case reports, 304, 327, 344
    in Cynthia Price study, 297
    in whole systems research, 99

mode, 138, 139

model fit validity, 70–1

Moher, David, 80

Montague, Ashley, 78

mortality (attrition), 59–60, 63, 90, 97, 204
    accounting for, 94, 162, 207, 298

multiple analysis of variance (MANOVA), 148–9, 162, 165

multiple outcomes, 60, 148, 162, 165

multiple regression, 150

multivariate analysis, 162, 165

narrative abstract, 105, 107, 188–9, 224–5, 344

narrative literature reviews, 77–8, 80

National Center for Complementary and Alternative Medicine (NCCAM), 48–9, 297, 322

National Certification Board for Therapeutic Massage and Bodywork, 71

National Commission for Protection of Human Subjects and Behavioral Research, 13

National Institutes of Health (NIH), 2, 40, 44, 45, 50, 297
    CRISP database, 50
    Office of Alternative Medicine, 2, 82

National Library of Medicine (NLM), 32, 33
    Loansome Doc, 42–4, 43*f*

negative cases, 216, 220, 243

negative results, 78, 79, 122, 144, 187

neutrality, 219

New England Journal of Medicine, The, 48

nocebo effect, 67

n-of-1 trial, 84, 329–30

"noise" vs. "signal", 66, 68

nominal variables, 137, 145, 151

nonparametric statistics, 141, 145–6, 151–2

nonresponse rate (surveys), 110

nonspecific response (nonspecific treatment effect), 65–8

normal distribution, 140*f*, 145

Norman, Geoffrey, 147, 162

null hypothesis (H_0), 141, 144, 152

Nuremberg Code, 13

Nurses Health Study, 90–1, 104, 111, 159

observational studies, 16, 25*f*, 26*f*, 82, 83*f*, 87–91
    example of, 104–30

odds ratio, 143*f*, 151

OLDMEDLINE, 33

one-tailed *t*-test. *See t*-tests

one-way analysis of variance, 148

online journals, 45–6, 48–50, 346, 347

online reference databases, 32–50, 78, 79

open access movement, 45

ordinal variables, 137, 145, 151

outcome(s), 82, 160–1, 165
    analysis of data, 115
    binary variables, 143*f*
    comprehensive reporting of, 165, 184, 208, 298
    multiple, 60, 148, 162, 165
    relation to exposure, 82, 86, 87, 91, 93, 150
    and relative risk, 88, 111
    time of measurement, 87, 88, 89

paired (or dependent) *t*-tests, 147

parametric statistics, 145–6

participants (in studies)
    accounted for in results, 163, 207–8
    allocation of, 95
    attrition of (mortality), 59–60, 90, 94, 97, 207, 298
    blinding issues with, 64
    children as, 13
    compliance of, 96
    disadvantaged persons as, 13, 14
    eligibility criteria for, 95, 158
    ethical issues concerning, 13–15, 62, 70, 92
    ID numbers for, 96
    informed consent, 15, 64, 92, 317, 330
    justice for, 14
    number needed, 143–5
    random assignment of, 61–3, 96, 159, 191
    reactivity issues, 62–3
    recall bias, 89
    selection of, 59, 158, 171–2, 181–2, 191–3
    single patient as, 329
    single patient client (example), 334–45, 339
    small sample size, 164–5, 298
    and testing, 57–8
    willingness to participate, 94
    See also control group